High Risk Diabetic Foot

High Risk Diabetic Foot
Treatment and Prevention

Edited by

Lawrence A. Lavery
University of Texas
Southwestern Medical Center
Dallas, Texas, U.S.A.

Edgar J. G. Peters
University Medical Center Utrecht
Utrecht, The Netherlands

Ruth L. Bush
Texas A&M College of Medicine
Scott & White Memorial Hospital
Temple, Texas, U.S.A.

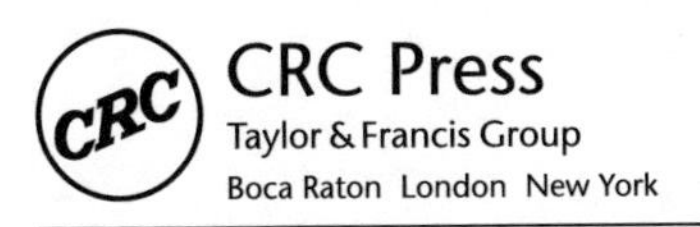

CRC Press is an imprint of the
Taylor & Francis Group, an **informa** business

CRC Press
Taylor & Francis Group
6000 Broken Sound Parkway NW, Suite 300
Boca Raton, FL 33487-2742

First issued in paperback 2017

ISBN-13: 978-1-4200-8301-9 (hbk)
ISBN-13: 978-1-138-11415-9 (pbk)

A CIP record for this book is available from the British Library.

Library of Congress Cataloging-in-Publication Data available on application.

Typeset by Aptara, Delhi, India.

Visit the Taylor & Francis Web site at
http://www.taylorandfrancis.com

and the CRC Press Web site at
http://www.crcpress.com

Preface

The global burden of diabetes and diabetes related complications is growing rapidly. In many ways it is a "perfect storm" that reflects the combined effects of aging, obesity and change of lifestyles around the world. Lower extremity complications are an obvious part of the diabetes epidemic. It has been estimated that every 30 seconds a leg is lost due to diabetes somewhere in the world. These amputations by themselves have been shown to lead to increased risk of further complications such as additional amputations, chronic wounds, hospital admissions and death.

Though feared by patients and doctors alike, amputations are not the only lower extremity complication of diabetes. Amputations are usually preceded by ulcers and wounds with a low tendency to heal. These chronic wounds can be a source of infection and further decay. There are several factors associated with the development of these skin lesions such as: peripheral vascular disease, numbness of the foot caused by peripheral symmetric polyneuropathy, foot deformities and ill fitting shoes. Patients at risk for foot complications can be identified by screening for these risk factors. In this book, we will try to shed light on the complex interaction of these risk factors and on their sequelae.

It was not long ago that recommendations about the evaluation and treatment of diabetic foot complications were solely based on expert opinion or small case series. Much of the work in this text references the level of medical evidence that is currently available. The authors applied the system used by the UK National Health Service to grade the level of evidence factored into recommendations for treatments or interventions. These recommendations will be present throughout the book and can be summarized by:

- **Level A:** Systematic reviews, consistent randomised controlled clinical trial, cohort study, clinical decision rule validated in different populations.
- **Level B:** Consistent retrospective cohort, exploratory cohort, ecological study, outcomes research, case-control Study; or extrapolations from level A studies.
- **Level C:** Case-series study or extrapolations from level B studies
- **Level D:** Expert opinion without explicit critical appraisal, or based on physiology, bench research or first principles.

This book provides guidelines for the recognition, diagnosis and treatment of the high-risk diabetic foot. The diabetic foot is preferably treated by a multidisciplinary team of caregivers. This book is specifically written for these caregives, which include physicians, surgeons, nurses, podiatrists, physiotherapists, radiologists, health care managers and potentially many more specialists. Ultimately, we hope that this book will help reduce the number of amputations in diabetic patients.

Lawrence A. Lavery
Edgar J. G. Peters
Ruth L. Bush

Contents

Contributors

Sicco A. Bus Department of Rehabilitation, Academic Medical Center, University of Amsterdam, Amsterdam, The Netherlands Diabetic Foot Unit, Department of Surgery, Ziekenhuisgroep Twente, location Almelo, The Netherlands

Ruth L. Bush Texas A&M College of Medicine, Scott & White Memorial Hospital, Temple, Texas, U.S.A.

Mark G. Davies Department of Surgery, University of Rochester Medical Center, Rochester, New York, U.S.A.

Daniel T. Ginat Department of Imaging Science, University of Rochester Medical Center, Rochester, New York, U.S.A.

R. J. Hinchliffe St. Georges Vascular Institute, St. George's Hospital, London, U.K.

Nathan A. Hunt* Scott & White Memorial Hospital and Clinic, Temple, Texas, U.S.A.

K. G. Jones St. Georges Vascular Institute, St. George's Hospital, London, U.K.

Javier La Fontaine Texas A&M Health Science Center, Scott & White Memorial Hospital, Temple, Texas, U.S.A.

Lawrence A. Lavery Department of Plastic Surgery and Department of Orthopaedic Surgery, University of Texas Southwestern Medical Center, Dallas, Texas, U.S.A.

George T. Liu Department of Orthaopaedics, University of Texas Southwestern Medical Center, Dallas, Texas, U.S.A.

Jason Maggi Department of Surgery, New York University School of Medicine, New York, New York, U.S.A.

Rajesh Malik Division of Vascular Surgery, Mount Sinai School of Medicine, New York, New York, U.S.A.

Rayaz A. Malik Division of Cardiovascular Medicine, Central Manchester Foundation Trust, and University of Manchester, Manchester, UK

Current affiliation: Orthopaedic Center of the Rockies, Fort Collins, Colorado, U.S.A.

Christopher J. Marrocco Texas A&M College of Medicine, Scott & White Memorial Hospital, Temple, Texas, U.S.A.

Douglas P. Murdoch Scott & White Memorial Hospital and Clinic, Temple, Texas, U.S.A.

Firas F. Mussa Division of Vascular and Endovascular Surgery, New York University School of Medicine, New York, New York, U.S.A.

Joseph J. Naoum Weill-Cornell Medical College, The Methodist Hospital, Division of Vascular Surgery, Cardiovascular Surgery Associates, Houston, Texas, U.S.A.

Agor Ndip Manchester Diabetes Centre, Manchester Academic Health Science Centre, Manchester NIHR Biomedical Research Centre, Central Manchester University Hospitals NHS Foundation Trust, and Cardiovascular Research Group, School of Laboratory and Clinical Sciences, University of Manchester, Manchester, U.K.

I. M. Nordon St. Georges Vascular Institute, St. George's Hospital, London, U.K.

Eric K. Peden Weill-Cornell Medical College, The Methodist Hospital, Division of Vascular Surgery, Cardiovascular Surgery Associates, Houston, Texas, U.S.A.

Edgar J. G. Peters Department of Internal Medicine and Infectious Diseases, University Medical Center Utrecht, Utrecht, The Netherlands

Lee C. Rogers Amputation Prevention Center, Valley Presbyterian Hospital, Los Angeles, California, U.S.A.

Wael E. A. Saad Department of Imaging Science, University of Rochester Medical Center, Rochester, New York, U.S.A.

Hans H. Savelberg Maastricht University Medical Centre, Maastricht, The Netherlands

Nicolaas C. Schaper Maastricht University Medical Centre, Maastricht, The Netherlands

Kristien Van Acker H. Familie Hospital, Rumst; Sint Maarten, Mechelen and Centre Sante des Fagnes, Chimay, Belgium

1 Peripheral arterial disease

Christopher J. Marrocco and Ruth L. Bush

EPIDEMIOLOGY OF PERIPHERAL ARTERIAL DISEASE

Peripheral vascular disease of the lower extremity can be due to either arterial or venous disease, with arterial being by far the most common cause. Peripheral arterial disease (PAD) more specifically refers to disease located in the lower extremity. PAD may be asymptomatic, but when symptoms arise they range from intermittent claudication to limb-threatening ischemia. It is estimated that 10 to 12 million people in the United States (1,2) have PAD and 4 million have intermittent claudication (2). These entities may be looked at as a continuum, bearing in mind, however that acute limb ischemia may be representative of a systemic or distant process such as atrial fibrillation with distal embolization. This usually results in the "blue toe" syndrome seen as ischemic toes, but larger emboli can cause more damage and greater tissue loss. Intermittent claudication or functional limb ischemia is the cardinal symptom of PAD of the lower extremity, though the majority of the patients are asymptomatic with as less than 20% reporting typical symptoms (3).

The ankle brachial pressure index (ABI) is an effective screening tool for PAD. A diminished ABI (<0.9) is a definite sign of PAD (3,4). The term claudication comes from the Latin root *clauicatio*, which literally means to limp. The clinical definition of claudication is pain in one or both legs occurring in a functional muscle group while walking (primarily affecting the calves) that does not go away with continued walking and is relieved only by rest (5). Critical limb ischemia, or limb-threatening ischemia, is the most severe manifestation of PAD (5) and occurs when there is tissue loss associated with ischemic pain in the distal foot, ischemic ulceration, or gangrene (5). A patient with critical limb ischemia who has the lowest ABI values will have an annual mortality rate of 25% (5).

PAD is most commonly caused by atherosclerosis (3–5), which results in progressive arterial occlusion. Importantly, PAD is an important surrogate marker of systemic atherosclerosis. A patient with a history of PAD has the same relative risk of death, even in the absence of a history of myocardial infarctions or ischemic stroke, as patients with cerebrovascular or coronary artery disease (5). Moreover, the severity of PAD is closely associated with the risk of myocardial infarction, ischemic stroke, and death from vascular causes. The lower the ABI, the greater is the risk of a cardiovascular event (5,6). Overall, 1% to 3% of claudicants ever require major surgery or amputation over a five-year period; only approximately one-fourth of patients significantly deteriorate, and that deterioration occurs most frequently during the first year after diagnosis (6–9%) compared with the 2% to 3% per annum (6). However, the mortality rate in claudicants is 30% at 5 years, 50% at 10 years, and 70% at 15 years, mainly due to the increased risk of stroke and heart disease (6).

THE ANKLE BRACHIAL INDEX

The ankle brachial index, or ABI, is the ratio of systolic pressure at the ankle to that in the arm. This simple noninvasive test can be performed in an office setting with a standard blood pressure cuff and a continuous wave Doppler. Its relative ease of use has made it a mainstay in the diagnosis and confirmation of lower extremity vascular disease. Many health care providers use the ABI as a predictive value to estimate the severity of vascular occlusive disease. Further, more detailed information can be gathered by performing segmental pressure measurements and pulse volume recordings (or plethysmography) in a noninvasive vascular laboratory (Fig. 1). For this test, additional cuffs are placed just below the knee and one large cuff or two narrow cuffs are placed above the knee and at the upper thigh. A significant drop in pressure between two adjacent cuffs indicates a narrowing of the artery or blockage along the arteries in a specific arterial segment. Plethysmography will measure changes in blood flow and is useful in patients with noncompressible vessels (see in the following text).

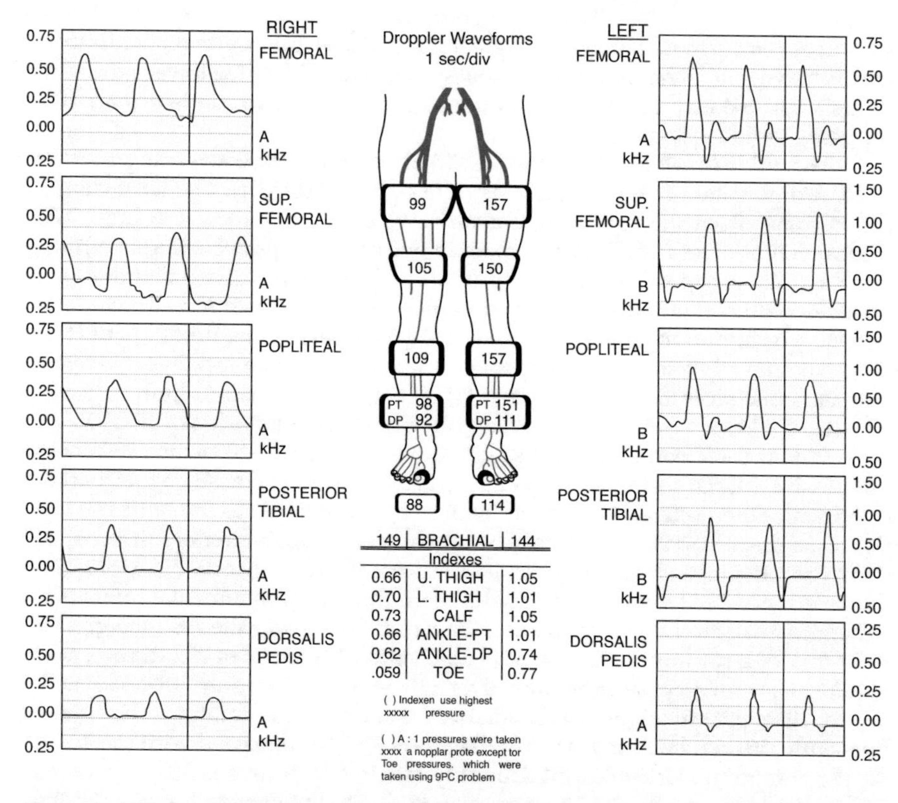

Figure 1 This is an example of a report that may be obtained from a noninvasive vascular laboratory. The segmental blood pressures as well as waveforms (plethysmography) are given. Biphasic or triphasic waveforms in general indicate adequate blood flow whereas monophasic, or flat waveforms, indicate greatly decreased flow. In these cases, further imaging may be required to see if intervention is possible to improve flow to heal a wound.

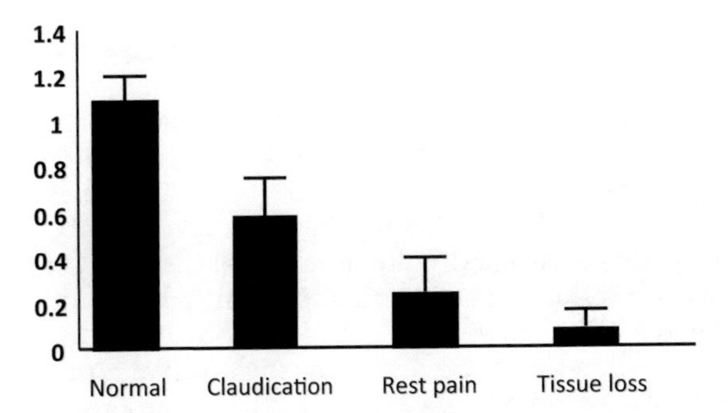

Figure 2 The chart in the figure shows the association of ABI with clinical symptoms. These are only estimates as each individual patient may vary in tolerance to ischemia.

In addition to PAD, the ABI is also an indicator of generalized atherosclerosis because lower levels have been associated with higher rates of concomitant coronary and cerebrovascular disease, and with the presence of cardiovascular risk factors (7). An ABI of greater than 1.1 is considered normal, whereas an ABI <0.9 is considered abnormal. An ABI of 0.4 to 0.9 is in the claudication range while an ABI of less than 0.4 is in the critically ischemic range (Fig. 2).

Interestingly, the ABI is now being considered as a tool in the assessment of a patient's cardiovascular risk as previously mentioned. There are many cardiac risk assessment scales used by researchers, but perhaps the most famous is the Framingham Risk Score (FRS), which is calculated by taking into account age, gender, total cholesterol, high-density cholesterol, smoking status, and systolic blood pressure. In a recent study reported in JAMA, the FRS was combined with the ABI. They concluded that: measurement of the ABI may improve the accuracy of cardiovascular risk predication beyond FRS (7).

RISK FACTORS FOR PAD

The risk factors for PAD are similar to those for coronary artery disease and cerebrovascular disease (2) as these are all felt to be part of the continuum of atherosclerotic disease. They include age, gender, race, hypertension, hyperhomocysteinemia, dislipidemia, diabetes mellitus, and smoking status. These risk factors have been the subjects of intense research over the past half a century and have ultimately defined our daily activities from diet to habits and exercise. The two most important risk factors for the development and progression of PAD are cigarette smoking and diabetes mellitus (1,3–5). Both of these factors are related to heart disease and stroke, but are even more specifically linked to PAD and will be discussed later (2).

Risk factors for PAD can be divided into those thought of as "traditional risk factors" such as smoking and diabetes and hyperlipidemia (8) and newer risk factors that have come to light via ongoing research such as elevated homocystine levels and c-reactive protein. The American Heart Association outlines traditional risk factors that can be altered, such as smoking, diabetes mellitus, obesity, physical inactivity, high cholesterol, and high blood pressure. These risk factors are important because they can be modified, unlike genetics and personal or family history of cardiovascular diseases. Risk factor modification is believed to decrease the chances of initial disease development and to slow the progression of PAD once it has been established.

PAD is also often divided into large and small vessel atherosclerotic disease (8). This definition, although overly simplifying the disease process, helps to further delineate the disease processes conceptually. Large vessel disease is defined as the vessels proximal to the ankle and its progress is followed by the ABI. A decline in the ABI is therefore associated with large vessel disease. On the other hand, small vessel disease is defined as the vessels distal to the ankle and is followed with the toe brachial index, similar to the ABI but using toe pressure (normal greater than 0.7). Therefore, a decline in the toe brachial index while maintaining an ABI is indicative of small vessel disease (8). It is important to note that these definitions do not take into account factors important in the development of PAD in the diabetic patient such as vessel permeability and changes in the basement membrane associated with microvascular dysfunction (8). The ABI is also unreliable in ruling out the presence of PAD in diabetic patients due to the well-known medial calcification that artificially elevates the ABI (8). This leads either to inability to obtain the ABI or to very high values (9). Medial artery calcinosis is due to the deposition of large amounts of calcium in the medial layer of arteries and results in the artery becoming stiff and noncompressible with cuff inflation. Risk factors for this condition are not clearly understood but the role of diabetes is strong. Furthermore, since the ABI cannot be used to diagnose PAD in the presence of stiff arteries, the relationship between medial calcinosis and concomitant PAD is unknown (9).

AGE OF ONSET OF PAD

The prevalence of PAD is highly age dependent with age cut off varying from 45 years of age in a veteran administration study to 60 years of age in a more recent evaluation of the National Health and Nutritional Survey taken from 1999 to 2002 (1,10,11). The veterans study, a prospective analysis of 51 Caucasian men, referred to a single vascular surgery service, showed an astonishing amount of disease. In this relatively young population, 41% of vascular referrals required multiple vascular interventions or amputations, 30% demonstrated progression of their coronary disease, and the study had a 17% mortality rate within 5 years (10). Similarly, the National Health and Nutritional Survey taken from 1999 to 2002 study showed that there is an increased risk for the development of PAD in patients younger than 60 years old with coexisting coronary disease (1), further demonstrating the connection between PVD as a manifestation of systemic atherosclerotic disease (5) and the considerable overlap between PAD, coronary artery disease, and cerebrovascular disease (2).

SMOKING

The World Health Organization (WHO) report on the tobacco epidemic released in 2008 attributes 100 million deaths due to tobacco in the 20th century (12). There are currently 5.4 million deaths per year worldwide and they estimate 1 billion deaths during the 21st century will be due to tobacco exposure (12). In this report, WHO claims that tobacco is the only legal consumer product that can harm everyone exposed to it and that it kills up to half of those who use it (12). Tobacco is a very interesting risk factor for the development of PAD. It is the *only* risk factor that is completely controlled by the individual and thus, fully modifiable.

Multiple studies have been done over the past few decades that show consistent and overwhelming evidence that cigarette smoking plays a significant role in cerebrovascular disease (13), cardiovascular disease (14), and peripheral vascular disease (15) as well as oral, esophageal, tracheal, and lung cancers. Tobacco is considered the most important preventable risk factor for vascular disease and has stronger associations with PAD than it does with CAD (15,16).

The diagnosis of PAD was made a decade earlier in smokers than in nonsmokers and the amputation rate of smokers is nearly double versus those that never smoked (16). PAD is 2.3 fold more common in current smokers and up to 2.6 fold higher in former smokers, with a high dose–response relationship demonstrated in heavy smokers (15). In counties where approximately 30% of the population are smokers, 50% of PAD can be attributed to smoking (15). The age that one starts smoking also seems to play a role, with a starting age of 16 years or less more than doubling the risk of symptomatic PAD regardless of amount of cigarette smoke exposure (17). A recent study in the Journal of the American Medical Association addressed smoking cessation and risk reduction: 665 publications were screened and 20 studies were included for analysis. Results showed a 36% reduction in crude relative risk (RR) of mortality for patients with coronary heart disease (CHD) who quit smoking compared with those who continued [RR, 0.64; 95% confidence interval (CI), 0.58–0.71] (18). Results from the individual studies did not vary greatly despite many differences in patient characteristics, such as age, gender, type or cause of heart disease, and the years in which studies took place. The authors concluded in JAMA that the smoking cessation is associated with a substantial reduction in risk of all-cause mortality among patients with CHD. This risk reduction appears to be consistent regardless of age, sex, index cardiac event, country, and year of study commencement (18).

DIABETES MELLITUS

Diabetes mellitus affects approximately 100 million people worldwide (19). Diabetes is broken down into type 1 juvenile, early onset or insulin-dependent diabetes, and type 2, late onset or insulin-independent diabetes. There is another entity that has been noticed in the more recent literature, known as insulin resistance and linked to the syndrome X, or the metabolic syndrome. The 'Metabolic Syndrome' (MetS) is a clustering of components that reflect overnutrition, sedentary lifestyles, and resultant excess adiposity. The MetS includes the clustering of abdominal obesity, insulin resistance, dyslipidemia, and elevated blood pressure, and is associated with other comorbidities including the prothrombotic state, proinflammatory state, nonalcoholic fatty liver disease, and reproductive disorders (20).

Most diabetic patients are adult onset type 2 (90–95%) with only 5% to 10% being type 1. It is, however, believed that the incidence of type 2 diabetes is on the rise; mainly due to sedentary lifestyle and the epidemic of obesity. Obesity has reached epidemic proportions globally, with more than 1 billion adults overweight—at least 300 million of them clinically obese—and is a major contributor to the global burden of chronic disease and disability (21). There has also been another disturbing trend noticed recently, which has been described as early onset type 2 diabetes in obese children—normally an adult disease (22,23). Type 2 diabetes mellitus has emerged as a diagnosis among adolescents in the United States, particularly among minority groups and concurrent with the well-documented epidemic of overweight and obesity (24). Recent studies have revealed the presence of components of the MetS in children and adolescents. Obesity has a central role in the syndrome. There is an increasing amount of data to show that being overweight during childhood and adolescence is significantly associated with insulin resistance, abnormal lipids, and elevated blood pressure in young adulthood (25).

Diabetes affects the macrovascular system manifesting as medial artery calcinosis (MAC) and atherosclerosis (9,26). This disease pattern results in retinopathy and nephropathy, which are the leading causes of blindness and end-stage renal disease in the United States. Microvascular injuries also result in PAD of the lower extremities, as well as the whole broad spectrum of disease related to atherosclerosis including heart disease and stroke. Diabetic microvascular disease contributes to diabetic neuropathy, foot ulcers, and ultimately amputations leading to limb loss and further contributing to immobility and the progression of the atherosclerotic process.

PATHOPHYSIOLOGY OF VASCULAR DISEASE IN THE DIABETIC PATIENT

The pathological processes that contribute to the development of vascular disease in the diabetic patient are related to those that affect the average person, only they are accelerated and the consequences of unchecked risk factors are much greater. The endothelial cell is believed to be a major player in vascular health. In the diabetic patient endothelial dysfunction is believed to be a key factor leading to the development of vascular disease. The endothelial cell is believed to play a central role in vascular homeostasis and to facilitate smooth blood flow across the vessel wall as well as participate in nutritional delivery to the vessel and surrounding structures. The endothelial cell is also thought to prevent smooth muscle and white blood cell migration, proliferation, and thrombosis. The key substance nitric oxide (NO) is believed to be the mediator of healthy vascular function, and the loss of NO, also known as endothelial-derived relaxation factor because off its ability to cause vessel dilation, is believed to be the key component in endothelial dysfunction. Studies have found that endothelium-dependent vasodilation is abnormal in patients with type 1 or type 2 diabetes (26–30). Thus, decreased levels of NO in diabetes may underlie its atherogenic predisposition (26–30). The decrease in the production of endothelial NO allows for an increased production of leukocyte adhesion molecules, which then allows for monocyte and smooth muscle cell migration into the intima of the vessel wall producing the macrophage foam cells characteristic of atherosclerosis. Many of the metabolic derangements known to occur in diabetes, including hyperglycemia, excess free fatty acid liberation, and insulin resistance, mediate abnormalities in endothelial cell function by affecting the synthesis or degradation of NO (26).

PROGRESSION OF PAD

The nonoperative treatment of PAD includes so-called conservative management with the general aim being the limitation of disease progression. Controlling the risk factors discussed earlier such as hyperglycemia of diabetes as well as smoking cessation along with others not discussed (lipid control, hypertension, weight loss) is the first line of therapy in a patient without critical limb ischemia. Although risk factor management, behavioral modification, and pharmacologic agents are important also in those with critical limb ischemic, surgical intervention may become a first-line therapy in these cases.

REFERENCES

1. Lane JS, Vittinghoff E, Lane KT, et al. Risk factors for premature peripheral vascular disease: Results for the National Health and Nutritional Survey, 1999–2002. J Vasc Surg 2006; 44(2):319–324; discussion 24–25.
2. Criqui MH. Peripheral arterial disease—Epidemiological aspects. Vasc Med 2001; 6(3 suppl):3–7.
3. White C. Clinical practice. Intermittent claudication. N Engl J Med 2007; 356(12): 1241–1250.
4. Diehm C, Kareem S, Lawall H. Epidemiology of peripheral arterial disease. Vasa 2004; 33(4):183–189.
5. Hiatt WR. Medical treatment of peripheral arterial disease and claudication. N Engl J Med 2001; 344(21):1608–1621.
6. Dormandy J, Heeck L, Vig S. The fate of patients with critical leg ischemia. Semin Vasc Surg 1999; 12(2):142–147.
7. Fowkes FG, Murray GD, Butcher I, et al. Ankle brachial index combined with Framingham Risk Score to predict cardiovascular events and mortality: A meta-analysis. JAMA 2008; 300(2):197–208.
8. Aboyans V, Criqui MH, Denenberg JO, et al. Risk factors for progression of peripheral arterial disease in large and small vessels. Circulation 2006; 113(22):2623–2629.
9. Aboyans V, Ho E, Denenberg JO, et al. The association between elevated ankle systolic pressures and peripheral occlusive arterial disease in diabetic and nondiabetic subjects. J Vasc Surg 2008; 48(5):1197–1203.
10. Valentine RJ, Jackson MR, Modrall JG, et al. The progressive nature of peripheral arterial disease in young adults: A prospective analysis of white men referred to a vascular surgery service. J Vasc Surg 1999; 30(3):436–444.
11. Selvin E, Erlinger TP. Prevalence of and risk factors for peripheral arterial disease in the United States: Results from the National Health and Nutrition Examination Survey, 1999–2000. Circulation 2004; 110(6):738–743.
12. WHO. WHO Report on The Global Tobacco Epidemic, 2008: The MPOWER Package. http://apps.who.int/bookorders/anglais/detart1.jsp?sesslan=1&codlan=1&codcol=93&codcch=220.
13. Jonas MA, Oates JA, Ockene JK, et al. Statement on smoking and cardiovascular disease for health care professionals. American Heart Association. Circulation 1992; 86(5):1664–1669.
14. van Domburg RT, Meeter K, van Berkel DF, et al. Smoking cessation reduces mortality after coronary artery bypass surgery: A 20-year follow-up study. J Am Coll Cardiol 2000; 36(3):878–883.
15. Willigendael EM, Teijink JA, Bartelink ML, et al. Influence of smoking on incidence and prevalence of peripheral arterial disease. J Vasc Surg 2004; 40(6):1158–1165.
16. Management of peripheral arterial disease (PAD). TransAtlantic Inter-Society Consensus (TASC). Section D: Chronic critical limb ischaemia. Eur J Vasc Endovasc Surg 2000;19(suppl A):S144–S243.
17. Planas A, Clara A, Marrugat J, et al. Age at onset of smoking is an independent risk factor in peripheral artery disease development. J Vasc Surg 2002; 35(3):506–509.
18. Critchley JA, Capewell S. Mortality risk reduction associated with smoking cessation in patients with coronary heart disease: A systematic review. JAMA 2003; 290(1):86–97.
19. Amos AF, McCarty DJ, Zimmet P. The rising global burden of diabetes and its complications: Estimates and projections to the year 2010. Diabet Med 1997;14(suppl 5): S1–S85.
20. Cornier MA, Dabelea D, Hernandez TL, et al. The metabolic syndrome. Endocr Rev 2008; 29(7):777–822.

21. Global Strategy on Diet, Physical Activity and Health. 2008. http://www.who.int/dietphysicalactivity/publications/facts/obesity/en/
22. Chiarelli F, Marcovecchio ML. Insulin resistance and obesity in childhood. Eur J Endocrinol 2008; 159(suppl 1):S67–S74.
23. Lee JM. Why young adults hold the key to assessing the obesity epidemic in children. Arch Pediatr Adolesc Med 2008; 162(7):682–687.
24. Mayer-Davis EJ. Type 2 diabetes in youth: Epidemiology and current research toward prevention and treatment. J Am Diet Assoc 2008; 108(4 suppl 1):S45–S51.
25. Steinberger J. Diagnosis of the metabolic syndrome in children. Curr Opin Lipidol 2003; 14(6):555–559.
26. Luscher TF, Creager MA, Beckman JA, et al. Diabetes and vascular disease: Pathophysiology, clinical consequences, and medical therapy: Part II. Circulation 2003; 108(13):1655–1661.
27. McVeigh GE, Brennan GM, Johnston GD, et al. Impaired endothelium-dependent and independent vasodilation in patients with type 2 (non-insulin-dependent) diabetes mellitus. Diabetologia 1992; 35(8):771–776.
28. Williams SB, Cusco JA, Roddy MA, et al. Impaired nitric oxide-mediated vasodilation in patients with non-insulin-dependent diabetes mellitus. J Am Coll Cardiol 1996; 27(3):567–574.
29. Clarkson P, Celermajer DS, Donald AE, et al. Impaired vascular reactivity in insulin-dependent diabetes mellitus is related to disease duration and low density lipoprotein cholesterol levels. J Am Coll Cardiol 1996; 28(3):573–579.
30. Johnstone MT, Creager SJ, Scales KM, et al. Impaired endothelium-dependent vasodilation in patients with insulin-dependent diabetes mellitus. Circulation 1993; 88(6):2510–2516.

2 Clinical and vascular laboratory assessment of peripheral vascular disease

Daniel T. Ginat, Wael E. A. Saad, and Mark G. Davies

INTRODUCTION

Diabetic patients have at least a four times greater risk for developing peripheral vascular disease (PVD) than does the general population (1). Indeed, an estimated 45% of individuals with diabetes mellitus will acquire clinically significant PVD after 20 years of disease onset (2). Diabetic individuals have an 11 times greater risk than the general population for developing critical limb ischemia (1). Indeed, PVD tends to manifest with greater severity in diabetes mellitus compared with other etiologies of PVD, such as smoking, hyperlipidemia, and hypertension (3).

There is a significantly greater prevalence of complete occlusion of the infrapopliteal vessels in diabetic patients compared with those who do not have diabetes (4). The extent of collateral circulation varies widely in diabetic patients with PVD, even those with foot gangrene (5). Distal vessels typically become tortuous and develop microaneurysms in diabetic patients with PVD (6). Another characteristic feature of PVD resulting from diabetes mellitus is medial arterial (Monkeberg) calcification, which produces the "lead-pipe" appearance and decreased compliance of intermediate diameter vessels (1). This makes direct imaging evaluation of the infragenicular vessels paramount, given that anticipated non–imaging- and non–invasive-based studies may be inaccurate below the knee.

INDICATIONS

The distribution of lower extremity PVD involvement is characteristic in diabetic patients. The disease is typically bilateral and multisegmental. The iliac arteries are relatively spared in diabetic patients, whereas most distal arteries are preferentially involved, even during the incipient asymptomatic course of arterial disease (2,7). In particular, the popliteal, anterior tibial, peroneal, posterior tibial, and profunda femoris are the most common arteries affected in diabetic patients, regardless of the type (3).

The severity of PVD correlates with amputation rate, which is at least five times higher in the diabetic population compared with the non–diabetic population (3,8). Similarly, the degree of PVD in diabetic patients is a major prognostic indicator for the outcome of amputation (9). Detailed evaluation of the location, length, vessel morphology, severity of stenoses, and runoff vessel patency is necessary for planning revascularization procedures (9). In addition, distal surgical bypass reconstruction requires identification of suitable target vessels. Thus, successful treatment depends on accurate preintervention imaging.

Table 1 TASC II Inter-Society Consensus on Peripheral Arterial Disease Classification

Lesion category	Description
Type A	Single stenosis $\leq$ 10 cm
	Single occlusion $\leq$ 5 cm
Type B	Multiple lesions (stenoses or occlusions) each $\leq$ 5 cm
	Single stenosis or occlusion $\leq$ 15 cm not involving the infrageniculate popliteal artery
	Single or multiple lesions in the absence of continuous tibial vessels to improve inflow for a distal bypass
	Heavily calcified occlusion $\leq$ 5 cm
	Single popliteal stenosis
Type C	Multiple stenoses or occlusions totaling $>$ 15 cm with or without heavy calcification
	Recurrent stenoses or occlusions that need treatment after two endovascular interventions
Type D	Chronic total occlusions of CFA or SFA ($>$ 20 cm, involving the popliteal artery)
	Chronic total occlusion of popliteal artery and proximal trifurcation vessels

Several classification systems that can be used to describe the imaging appearance of PVD lesions have been formulated. For femoropopliteal PVD lesions, the TASC II Inter-Society Consensus on Peripheral Arterial Disease has devised a classification scheme detailed in Table 1 (10): TASC guidelines grades help delineate management of PVD. For example, TASC A lesions are generally treated with intraluminal angioplasty, whereas TASC D lesions require surgical intervention.

A commonly implemented grading system for characterizing peripheral arterial stenoses and occlusions on imaging studies was described by Bollinger et al. in 1981 (11). According to this grading system, lesions are classified into four categories (Table 2).

For the purpose of imaging, the distribution of lower extremity lesions can be categorized in terms of three "stations." Station 1 extends from the abdominal aorta to the iliac arteries (inflow), station 2 encompasses the femoral and popliteal arteries, and station 3 includes the calf and foot arteries (runoff). Station 3 must be accurately depicted, particularly in diabetic patients. This poses spacial and temporal resolution constraints for direct imaging studies, which include (1) conventional x-ray angiography, (2) computed tomographic angiography (CTA), and (3) magnetic resonance angiography (MRA). The techniques and performance of these modalities are described in the following sections.

Table 2 Hemodynamically Significant Versus Non–Hemodynamically Significant Lesions

Non–hemodynamically significant	Hemodynamically significant
Stenosing plaques $\leq$ 25% of artery diameter	Stenosing lesions with $>$ 50% lumen narrowing[a]
Stenosing lesions with between 25% and 50% narrowing	Occlusive lesions

[a] Some authors cite a threshold of $>$70%.

GENERAL CONSIDERATIONS FOR CONTRAST ADMINISTRATION

Iodinated Contrast Media

The most widely utilized contrast materials for x-ray angiography and CTA are radiopaque nonionic iso-osmolar iodine-based media, which are often prepared at a concentration of 300 mg of iodine per milliliter. Adverse reactions to iodinated contrast agents range from mild to severe and can be acute or delayed. Mild acute reactions occur in about 3% of patients receiving nonionic contrast and include nausea, vomiting, pain at injection site and urticaria (12). Severe acute reactions occur at an overall rate of 0.04% with nonionic contrast and consist of severe bronchospasm, laryngeal edema, vagal reaction, anaphylactic reaction, and hypotension with bradycardia (12). Complications of contrast administration occur with greater frequency with ionic agents. Predisposing factors adverse reactions include renal disease, asthma, heart disease, and history of allergy (12).

Perhaps the most significant delayed reaction is contrast-induced nephrotoxicity, which is reported to occur in up to 50% of patients with known diabetic nephropathy (12). To minimize the occurrence of this adverse reaction, it is essential to evaluated renal function tests before performing a contrast-enhanced study. It is generally contraindicated to administer iodinated contrast in patients with creatinine levels that exceed 1.5 mg/dL. Another contraindication to contrast angiography is hypergammaglobulinemia (13).

Numerous prophylactic measures are available for contrast-induced nephropathy in high-risk patients (glomerular filtration rate < 60 mL/min/ 1.73 m^2). Hydration by using 0.45% or 0.9% normal saline at a rate of 0.5 to 1 mL/ kg/hr beginning 6 to 12 hours before the examination and 4 to 12 hours after administering contrast is generally recommended (14,15). Some advocate the addition of sodium bicarbonate infusion to normal saline hydration at a rate of 1 to 1.5 mg/kg body weight for 9 to 26 hours prior to contrast injection (16,17). The proposed mechanism of action remains uncertain but may be related to reduction in free radical production. There is also conflicting evidence for the effectiveness of intravenous sodium bicarbonate in preventing contrast-induced nephropathy and potential negative effects of this treatment including alkalosis (15,18). *N*-acetylcysteine (Mucomyst) administered in 600 mg or 1200 mg doses before and after a contrast examination is also proposed to confer renal protection to iodinated contrast material (15). However, there is no conclusive evidence as of yet that establishes the effectiveness of this agent in preventing contrast medium–induced nephropathy (19).

Diuretics and angiotensin inhibitors should be discontinued the day before and the day of the contrast examination. Of particular concern in the diabetic patients treated with metformin is the risk of lactic acidosis after contrast administration. Metformin should be discontinued 24 to 48 hours after contrast angiography (1,12). An insulin sliding scale can be instituted as a temporary measure until laboratory testing demonstrates intact renal function (1).

It is considered good practice to minimize the amount of contrast utilized for any examination. Contrast dose can be reduced by implementing saline chaser techniques, which consists of administering a small bolus of saline, such as 25 mL, following the contrast injection. This method decreases the amount of contrast pooling near the injection site and has the potential to improve vascular enhancement in CT angiography (20). If possible, prolonging the interval between contrast studies as much as possible is certainly helpful. Similarly, non–contrast-imaging modalities should be considered when feasible.

Gadolinium and carbon dioxide are alternative contrast agents that can be used for x-ray angiography examinations, especially in patients with renal failure. However, contrast and spatial resolution of carbon dioxide digital subtraction angiography (DSA) of the lower extremity arteries is inferior to angiography with iodinated contrast (21).

Gadolinium Contrast

Contrast-enhanced MRA utilizes gadolinium-based agents, of which numerous types exist. Recent multicenter clinical trials have demonstrated superior clinical efficacy and safety of gadobenate dimeglumine compared with conventional gadolinium agents for the evaluation of peripheral artery disease (22). This agent displays higher T1 relaxivity, which produces higher intravascular signal than conventional agents (22). As a result, a smaller dose of contrast is necessary compared with other forms of gadolinium contrast media. However, certain conventional gadolinium agents, particularly gadodiamide (Omniscan), have been implicated in the development of nephrogenic systemic fibrosis (19,23,24). Consequently, the U.S. Food & Drug Administration issued a public health advisory that magnetic resonance imaging (MRI) or MRA utilizing gadolinium-based contrast agents be avoided in patients with moderate to end-stage renal disease (glomerular filtration rate [GFR] < 60 mL/min/1.73 m^2) (25). If such examinations are to be conducted in this patient population, immediate hemodialysis is recommended (25). The American College of Radiology (ACR) guidelines indicate that patients with GFR > 60 mL/min/1.73 m^2 do require particular precautions, whereas gadolinium-based MRI should not be conducted in individuals with acute renal injury or GFR < 60 mL/min/1.73 m^2 unless the benefit clearly outweighs the potential risk (17). The ACR also recommends that any patient with renal disease should not receive Omniscan for contrast-enhanced MRI. For patients with GFR < 30 mL/min/1.73 m^2 or patients who are on hemodialysis, it may be prudent to consult nephrology services to investigate the risks and benefits of gadolinium-enhanced MRI/MRA. Recommended dosages for contrast-enhanced MRA consist of a maximum of 0.1 mmol/kg for patients with GFR < 30 mL/min/1.73 m^2, up to 0.2 mmol/kg for patients with GFR between 30 and 60 mL/min/1.73 m^2, and an upper limit of 0.3 mmol/kg for all other patients (26).

CONVENTIONAL AND DIGITAL SUBTRACTION X-RAY ANGIOGRAPHY

Techniques

Conventional catheter angiography of the lower extremity has been the gold standard by which other techniques are measured. Images are acquired via fluoroscopy units that incorporate a movable patient table. Small focal-spot fluoroscopic systems are employed to provide the high resolution necessary for detailed visualization of distal vessels.

Catheter angiography of the lower extremity normally consists of accessing the common femoral artery with a Seldinger needle (18-gauge puncture needle).

Table 3 Laterality of the Femoral Approach and Its Advantages Relative to Subsequent Diagnostic and Therapeutic Maneuvers[a]

Femoral approach relative to lower limb symptoms	Diagnostic angiography		Endoluminal interventions	
	Ipsilateral	Contralateral	Ipsilateral	Contralateral
Antegrade ipsilateral	Yes	No	Yes[b]	No
Retrograde ipsilateral	Yes[c]	Yes[c]	No	Yes
Antegrade contralateral[d]	No	No	No	No
Retrograde contralateral[e]	Yes[c]	Yes[c]	Yes	No

[a] The laterality of the approach is relative to the presenting symptoms/the more symptomatic lower limb unless otherwise specified.
[b] The primary indication for an antegrade ipsilateral approach is ipsilateral diagnostic angiogram with the intention of endoluminal antegrade endoluminal intervention on the same side.
[c] Retrograde approach (whether ipsilateral or contralateral to the presenting symptoms) allows bilateral lower extremity angiography providing that the iliac arteries ipsilateral to the femoral access are patent.
[d] Antegrade contralateral approach is not resorted to because it has no diagnostic or therapeutic value to the operator to resolve the ipsilateral arterial disease.
[e] Retrograde contralateral approach is preferred by the authors, as many others, because it provides the option of a bilateral diagnostic angiogram as well as "a first crack" at the more symptomatic side (ipsilateral to presenting side) without adding additional injury or obstruction to the ipsilateral arteries at the inguinal and infrainguinal level (avoiding adding insult to injury to the ipsilateral limb).

A single wall (anterior femoral artery wall puncture) or a double wall access (puncturing the femoral artery through-and-through and pulling back from the posterior wall into the femoral artery lumen) can be utilized to access the femoral artery. Needle puncture can be guided by palpation, or real-time imaging guidance such as ultrasound and/or fluoroscopy. Accessing the femoral artery can be performed in a retrograde manner (directed against arterial flow toward the aortic bifurcation) or in an antegrade manner (directed in the direction of the arterial flow toward the feet). Ipsilateral common femoral artery antegrade approach is resorted to when antegrade endoluminal interventions are contemplated subsequent to the initial diagnostic angiogram. Diagnostic and subsequent endoluminal therapeutic options based on antegrade versus retrograde femoral approaches and ipsilateral versus contralateral approaches are summarized in Table 3.

If common femoral artery access is not feasible (occluded femoral arteries), other approaches, such as transaxillary, transbrachial, and translumbar, can be attempted. However, these approaches are less desirable due to increased access complications, reduced sheath sizes when interventions are contemplated, and more technically challenging for access and subsequent selective diagnostic angiograms and/or interventional procedures.

Subsequently, a 4- or 5-French catheter system is introduced using the modified Seldinger technique, with exchange performed over soft-tipped guidewires. Once a catheter is positioned several centimeters above the aortic bifurcation, a runoff is performed via manual or power injection of contrast. Suitable injection rates for a lower extremity examination using an aortic injection and bolus-chase technique are 10 to 20 mL/sec for a total of 20 to 40 mL. If the catheter is positioned within the pelvis, the injection rate can be reduced to 5 to 10 mL/sec for a total of 10 to 20 mL. Overall, catheter angiography examinations of the entire bilateral lower extremities may require on the order of 150 to 200 mL of contrast.

The amount of contrast utilized may be reduced by using a selective examination, which is performed by advancing the catheter into the specific vessel of interest before injecting the contrast. Road-mapping techniques can be used to facilitate passage of guidewires into the smaller vessels for selective examinations. This technique involves superimposing live fluoroscopy over a saved fluoroscopic image with contrast material lining the vessels in the same region of interest.

Digital subtraction is routinely performed to generate images that are used for final interpretation of the lower extremity vasculature. This method consists of acquiring a fluoroscopic mask image without contrast that is subtracted from subsequent images obtained in the same region of interest by using intravascular contrast. DSA produces images that have superior detail of the vascular anatomy compared with conventional fluoroscopy due to postprocessing amplification of vessel contrast without distracting background structures. Thus, with DSA, inherently low-contrast objects can be more easily detected despite the use of less contrast material.

Anteroposterior views are generally sufficient for imaging station 2 and 3 vessels. Supplemental 15° to 30° views may be obtained for station 1. Excluding significant iliofemoral tortuousity, contralateral obliques are utilized so that the internal and external iliac arteries do not superimpose. Images are typically acquired by using 17- to 35-cm field-of-view image intensifiers and 1024 × 1024 matrix sizes. The entire procedure can be completed within approximately 30 minutes.

The imaging quality of a catheter angiography examination is considered adequate upon demonstration of at least one distal runoff vessel or visualization of angiographic blush in the soft tissues of small caliber peripheral arteries. Technical success rates for lower extremity examinations approaches 99% (11).

Once the examination is completed, point pressure is applied to the puncture site for 10 to 20 minutes, unless a closure device has been used. Subsequently, patients are monitored for 4 to 6 hours or are admitted for brief hospitalization (rarely necessary for a diagnostic examination). The authors of this chapter do not routinely admit patients following uncomplicated diagnostic angiography only. However, they do admit patients after complicated diagnostic angiograms or after all therapeutic interventions whether successful or not.

Clinical Applications

Catheter DSA is indicated for demonstrating occlusive disease in symptomatic patients with palpable pulses or normal ankle-brachial index measurement, who otherwise would have been considered to have neuropathic feet (13). DSA scoring of PVD in diabetic patients with foot ulcers correlates with the rate of eventual major amputation surgery (13). For example, the presence of one occluded infrapopliteal vessel corresponds to major amputation in less than 5% of patients, whereas more than 80% of diabetic patients with foot ulcers underwent major amputation if they had three or more occluded arteries on x-ray DSAs (13). In addition, infrapopliteal x-ray angiographic scores correlate with the occurrence of foot ulcer healing, treated either with or without amputation (13). Nevertheless, it is to be cautioned that, by itself, the scoring should not be used for selecting patients for primary amputation (27).

Similarly, attempts to devise x-ray DSA foot scoring as a predictor of bypass patency show limited potential (27). Although there appears to be an association between foot score and bypass patency, high patency rates were achieved in patients with unfavorable foot scores. Thus, relying on catheter DSA findings could deny diabetic patients with PVD a potentially limb salvaging procedure. Furthermore, although conventional DSA has traditionally been considered the gold standard for imaging infrapopliteal arteries, it does not accurately depict potential target vessels for anastomosis in distal bypass (28). Figure 1 shows a lower extremity DSA in which the anatomic detail is well depicted; however, there is a minimal contrast reaching within the distal foot.

Another drawback to catheter DSA is that this technique is associated with a relatively high complication rate, ranging from 1.7% to 7% for a transfemoral approach (11,29,30). Complication rates associated with transaxillary and translumbar puncture sites are substantially higher. The most common complications include hemorrhage, hematoma arterial obstruction/thrombosis, and pseudoaneurysm formation. Acute contrast-induced nephropathy occurs in an estimated 5% to 8% of patients who undergo lower extremity DSA (31–33).

COMPUTED TOMOGRAPHY

Techniques

The advent of multidetector or multidetector CT (MDCT) has facilitated rapid, high-resolution imaging. As a result, long segments of vasculature can be scanned to reveal small arterial branches during a single breath hold. Indeed, with 16- and 64-slice CT, lower extremity angiograms can be completed within approximately 30 to 60 seconds after a scan delay of 10 to 30 seconds, producing 0.75- to 2-mm wide sections and 0.4- to 1-mm reconstructions (34). Such scans require 75 to 150 mL of contrast, which is generally less than that used for comparable x-ray DSAs. Similarly, effective doses are smaller for lower extremity CTA than for DSA (35). Typical scan parameters include 120 kVp and variable current setting ranging from 50 to 300 mA (34). Considerable radiation dose reductions can be achieved using the newer iterative reconstruction algorithms for CT.

In addition to being able to view the vascular tree through axial sections, CTA data can be reconstructed as maximal intensity projection (MIP), volume rendering, surface display, and curved multiplanar reformations (MPR). MIP provides higher contrast-to-noise ratio than does volume rendering and surface display modes (25). Therefore, MIP is better suited for interpreting areas of high-grade stenosis. To achieve optimal diagnostic accuracy, vascular segments should be interrogated in two orthogonal MIP views, such as sagittal and coronal. For heavily calcified segments, curved MPR and axial sections yield more accurate quantification of stenosis (35). While dual-energy CTA is not yet widely available for clinical use, this modality has the potential to further facilitate interpretation of stenoses in segments that contain abundant calcification, through automatic removal algorithms (36).

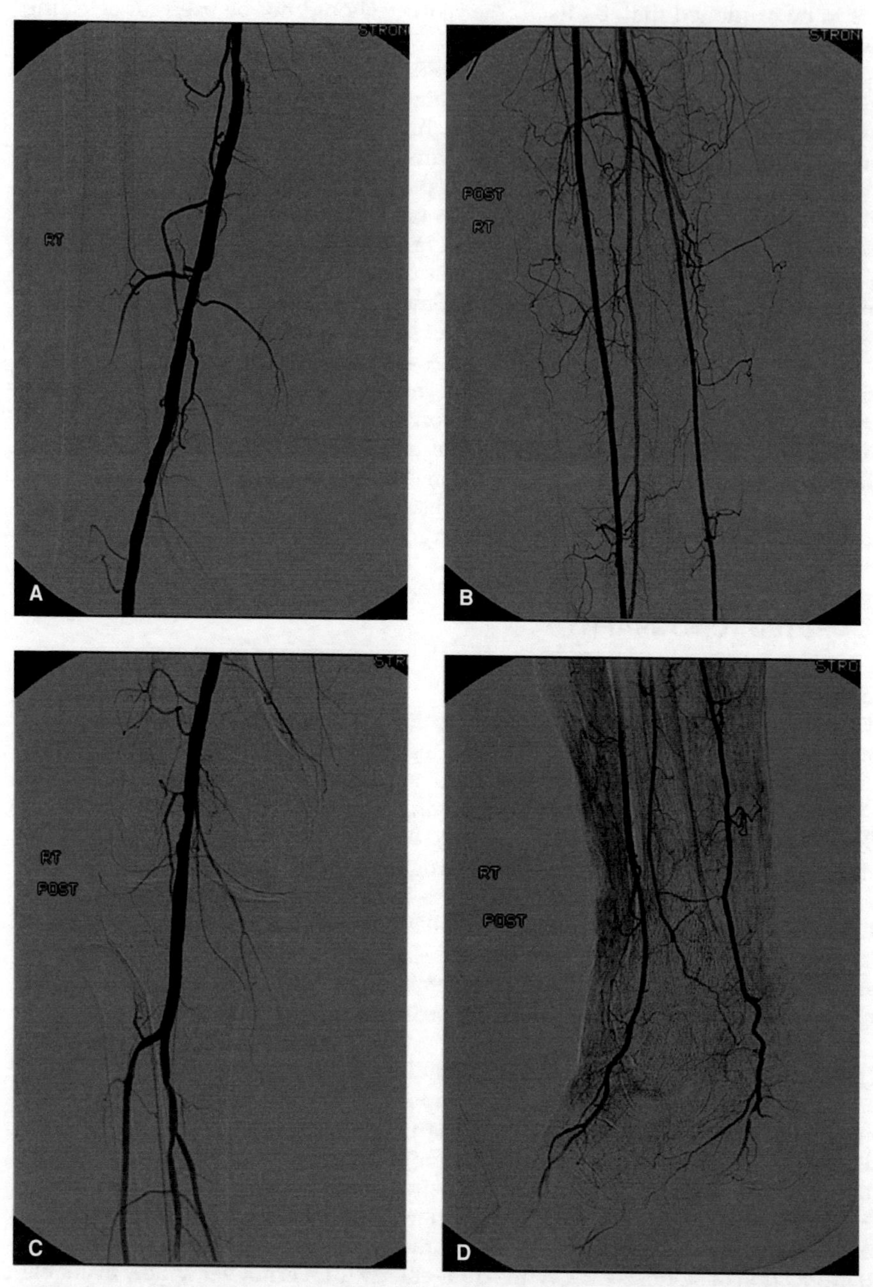

Figure 1 Digital subtraction angiography (DSA) of the stations 2 and 3 was performed in a 71-year-old woman with atherosclerotic disease. Mild to moderate stenosis is noted within the superficial femoral and the popliteal artery (**A–C**). Although the DSA provides fine anatomic detail, there is a faint amount of contrast filling the distal foot (**D**).

Clinical Applications

MDCT angiography is a highly sensitive and specific modality for imaging hemodynamically significant stenoses. In comparison with x-ray DSA, CTA demonstrates average overall sensitivity and specificity for significant lower extremity on the order of 92% and 93%, respectively, and sensitivities, specificities and accuracies of 91%, 85%, and 87%, respectively, for assessing stenoses in infrapopliteal arteries (34,37). However, for infrapopliteal lesions with hemodynamically significant stenoses, sensitivity, specificity, accuracy, positive predictive, and negative predictive values as high as 98.3%, 99.8%, 98.1%, 99.3%, and 99.4%, respectively, have been achieved by multidetector CTA (38). In fact, CTA appears to yield fewer nondiagnostic calf and pedal artery segments compared with catheter DSA (36,39). Similar performance characteristics are achieved in other arterial levels and degrees of stenosis (Table 4). In addition, assessment of number and length of lesions are comparable between CTA and DSA (38). This information is important for therapeutic decision making using TASC guidelines, as described earlier. Figure 2 shows an example of popliteal artery occlusion with distal reconstitution on CTA.

In general, diagnostic accuracy improves with increasing number of detectors and smaller slice-thickness. However, these performance characteristics are somewhat marred by the presence of abundant calcifications, with sensitivity, specificity, and accuracy on the order of 95%, 89.7%, and 91.8%, respectively, for lesions with more than 50% stenosis (40,41). Regarding data representation, axial reconstruction provides higher sensitivity and specificity than does MIP but requires more time for interpretation (38).

Since soft tissues can also be evaluated in CTA, it has the potential to provide an alternative diagnosis for patients' symptoms (42). However, there is a tendency for clinicians to order a greater number of follow-up examinations after CTA compared with that after catheter DSA (42). In addition, no studies to date have assessed the utility of CTA in an exclusively diabetic population. Nevertheless, MDCT angiography appears to be a cost-effective alternative to x-ray DSA for diagnosis and treatment planning in patients with lower extremity arterial disease (42,43).

MAGNETIC RESONANCE IMAGING

Techniques

Numerous MRA techniques have been devised and applied to evaluating peripheral artery disease in the lower extremity, including non–gadolinium contrast-based (phase-contrast and time-of-flight MRA), gadolinium contrast-enhanced MRA (CE MRA). Thus, MRA is a versatile modality in which a myriad of special sequences and techniques can be tailored to specific clinical situations.

Phase Contrast MRA

Phase contrast MRA consists of detecting phase shifts produced by flowing blood and bipolar gradients. This technique is quantitative, providing an estimate of mean blood flow velocity. Phase contrast MRA also allows the use of large field-of-view coronal or sagittal slices in the direction of the vessel of interest (44). In addition, phase contrast MRA can be acquired in two dimensions or three dimensions (3D).

Table 4 Performance Characteristics of MDCT Angiography for Evaluation of Lower Extremity Arterial Stenosis

Arterial segment	Sensitivity (%)			Specificity (%)			Accuracy (%)	Positive predictive value (%)	Negative predictive value (%)
	>50% Stenosis	>70% Stenosis	Occluded	>50% Stenosis	>70% Stenosis	Occluded	>70% Stenosis	>70% Stenosis	>70% Stenosis
Iliac	97	100	89–96	98–100	99.5	82–98	99.5	97.6	100
Femoropopliteal	97.5–100	97.4		95–96	99		96.5	98.5	99.6
Calf	96.5–100	98.3		95.5–100	99.8		98.1	99.3	99.9

Abbreviation: MDCT, multidetector computed tomography.

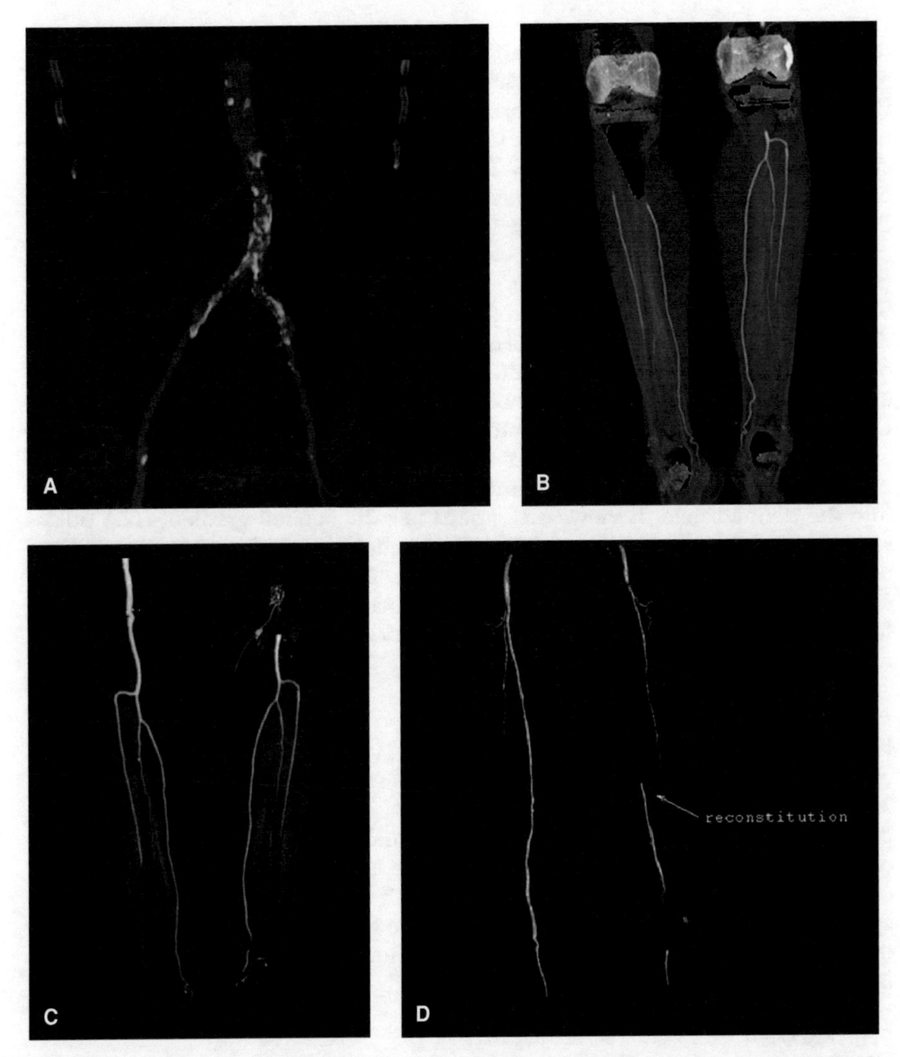

Figure 2 Computed tomographic angiography maximal intensity projection of station 1 (**A**) and portions of stations 2 and 3 (**B–D**), coronal projection, and volume rendering are shown for a 70-year-old woman with left lower extremity pain. There is complete occlusion of the left superficial femoral artery at its takeoff with reconstitution at the mid-thigh from a distal branch of the deep femoral artery. In addition, there is complete occlusion of the left popliteal artery with reconstitution below the knee by the lateral geniculate artery. There is a metallic artifact from the knee replacement hardware (**B**).

Time-of-Flight MRA

Time-of-flight (TOF) MRA, unlike phase contrast, is nonquantitative. This technique consists of tagging moving blood via saturation, inversion, or relaxation to distinguish it from stationary structures. Imaging acquisition is relatively time-consuming, and vessel intensities can vary along different planes. In particular, this technique is not well suited for imaging tortuous distal arteries. Other drawbacks of TOF include motion artifacts on MIP and the inability to depict retrograde arterial flow due to venous saturation pulses and in plane saturation (45). Pulsation artifacts result from triphasic flow, which is not sufficiently mitigated using electrocardiogram triggering (8). In addition, rapid saturation of flowing spins limits the utility of 3D TOF. This effect is not a concern with contrast-enhanced MRA. Overall, non–contrast-enhanced MRA demonstrate lower signal and contrast-to-noise ratios than do gadolinium-enhanced techniques.

Standard bolus-chase MRA

Standard bolus-chase MRA consists of several preparatory steps including obtaining nonenhanced localizer images of all three stations, followed by administering a small (1 mL) test bolus to estimate timing and generating a mask image for eventual subtraction. Commercial bolus timing algorithms are available, such as CARE bolus software (Siemens, Forchheim, Germany). These programs incorporate real-time triggering schemes that use automatic bolus detection or MR fluoroscopic triggers. Imaging is initiated upon detection of the bolus arrival into the defined field of view. A standard fast 3D spoiled gradient-echo pulse sequence is typically implemented for bolus-chase MRA. Fat saturation is also used to increase contrast between vessels and surrounding tissues. Dynamic k-space-filling techniques, in which acquisition occurs from the edge to the center for stations 1 and 2 and in reverse order for station 3, minimize contrast dose and motion artifacts (46,47).

Hybrid MRA

Hybrid MRA is a variant of CE MRA, designed to provide superior resolution of calf and foot vessels. This is accomplished via sagittal acquisition with parallel 3D CE MRA imaging of station 3. This allows initial imaging of distal vessels prior to possible venous contamination. Alternatively, a two-stage examination can be performed. This involves coronal plane acquisition of station 3 by using one contrast bolus, followed by station 1 and 2 imaging, using another dose of contrast (48). In general, imaging quality of the foot is optimized by positioning the lower extremity in maximum external rotation such that the length of the foot is parallel to the phased-array coil.

TRICKS MRA

Contrast-enhanced time-resolved imaging of contrast kinetics (TRICKS) MRA requires repeated acquisition of multiple images in rapid succession (every 1 to 2 seconds) during transit of the contrast bolus. This precludes slice encoding and provides high temporal resolution. In addition, pure arterial phase imaging can be obtained without relying on bolus timing or triggering (48). Thus, TRICKS MRA yields information regarding distal vessel patency and blood flow, such as retrograde filling of obstructed arteries (45,49). TRICKS sequences can be performed with less than 10 mL of contrast material.

The high temporal resolution of TRICKS MRA compromises spatial resolution to some extent as a result of decreased sampling of high spatial frequency data (less edge information). Refinements such as undersampled projection reconstruction (PR) hyper TRICKS, preferentially fills higher-frequency k-space domains without prolonging scan times. However, near-isotropic resolution is not achieved. Rather, parallel imaging assessment techniques, which use several

Table 5 Performance of TOF MRA Compared to DSA for Calf Vessels

Sensitivity (%)	Specificity (%)	Accuracy (%)	Positive predictive value (%)	Negative predictive value (%)
3.7–47.9	63.8–75.3	47.8–64.1	3.6–33.6	64.5–76.9

Abbreviations: TOF, time of flight; MRA, magnetic resonance angiography, DSA, digital subtraction angiography.

receiver coils and provide isotropic resolution in the sub-millimeter range. To maintain a minimum scan time, fewer k-space samples are also acquired. Although this results in a reduction of the signal-to-noise ratio, this is mitigated by the inherently high contrast of this technique (48).

Clinical Applications

Many of the MRA techniques described earlier are useful for evaluating lower extremity PVD and planning percutaneous and surgical interventions. For example, CE MRA has an estimated 1.4% technical failure rate (22). In fact, failed attempts of DSA to cross the occluded segments can often be successfully assessed with CE MRA (50). However, TOF MRA is associated with a 6% to 18% technical failure rate (22). In addition, this method is affected by artifacts such as pseudostenosis, step-ladder motion artifacts, and pseudo-opacification (51). Furthermore, TOF MRA demonstrates mitigated clinical performance, even for imaging calf stenoses, as summarized in Table 5.

In general, CE MRA (Fig. 3) provides higher-quality images and requires less time for interpretation than does TOF MRA. In particular, CE MRA is superior to TOF MRA and other noncontrast techniques for the identification of patent calf and foot tibial runoff vessels, which is necessary for interventional planning (52). Performance characteristics for standard bolus-chase MRA and TRICKS MRA

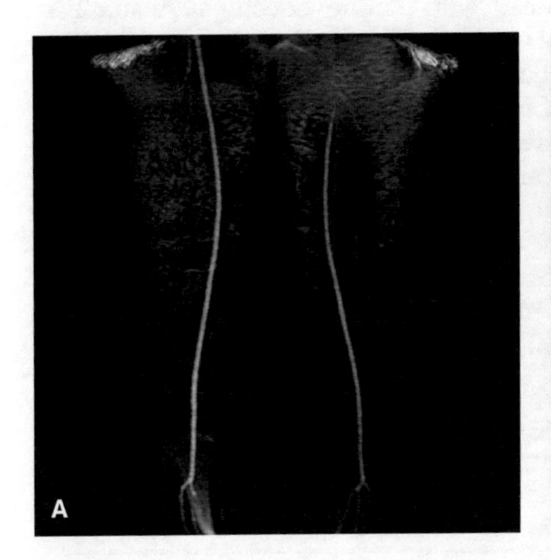

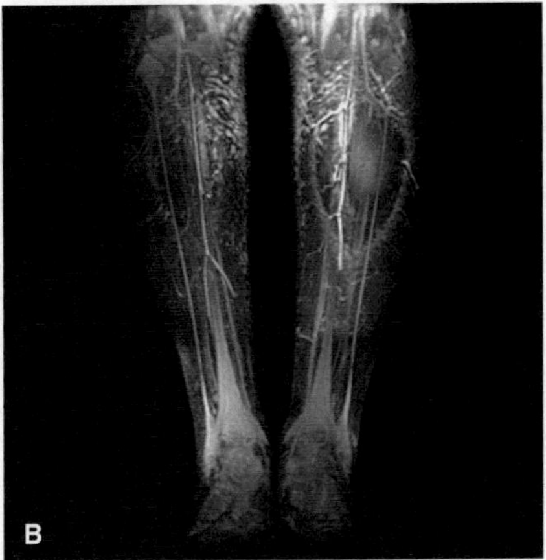

Figure 3 Magnetic resonance angiography performed by using a 1.5-T magnet with intravenous administration of gadolinium contrast in a 43-year-old male patient with atherosclerotic disease. Coronal maximal intensity projection of stations 2 (**A**) and 3 (**B**) demonstrate mild atherosclerotic plaque in the right posterior tibial and left mid-peroneal arteries.

Table 6 Performance of Bolus-Chase and TRICKS MRA

Modality	Significant stenosis				
Bolus-chase MRA	Sensitivity (%)	Specificity (%)	Accuracy (%)	Positive predictive value (%)	Negative predictive value (%)
Femoropopliteal arteries	92	94	93	88	96
Infrapopliteal arteries	93	91	86	88	93

	Stenosis		Occlusion	
TRICKS MRA	Sensitivity (%)	Specificity (%)	Sensitivity (%)	Specificity (%)
Lower extremity overall	89	97	87	90
Calf arteries	84	94	89	95
Foot arteries	79	71	79	86
Popliteal arteries	94	92		

are shown in Table 6 (49,53,54). The diagnostic accuracy for these techniques varies with the use of coils, specific contrast injection protocols, and moving bed technologies (49,55,56).

Dedicated calf imaging techniques can significantly improve the accuracy of distal target vessels, although this may require an additional dose of contrast when performed in conjunction with standard bolus-chase MRA (57). For calf vessels, hybrid MRA techniques have sensitivity and specificity as high as 100% and 91%, respectively (9).

Clinical trials that contrast-enhanced MRA more effectively visualizes patent distal calf and foot vessels affected by severe PVD in diabetic patients than does DSA (28,58,59). Indeed, contrast-enhanced MRA detects 38% more potential distal target arteries for surgical bypass than does DSA (28). As a result, some institutions rely on contrast-enhanced MRA to find suitable distal bypass vessels when initial DSA examination is unrevealing (59). Among CE MRA techniques investigated in diabetic patients, TRICKS MRA in particular has superior diagnostic performance compared with bolus-chase MRA for calf and foot vessel imaging (Table 7) (58). Excellent diagnostic performance is reported for hybrid MRA in diabetic patients (9). For example, the sensitivity for detecting lower extremity stenoses that are hemodynamically significant is 95.5% and 98%, respectively.

Table 7 Performance of Bolus-Chase and TRICKS MRA in Diabetic Patients

	TRICKS MRA		Bolus-chase MRA	
Segment	Sensitivity (%)	Specificity (%)	Sensitivity (%)	Specificity (%)
Calf	82–86	91–93	78–80	90
Foot	58–66	88–90	NA	NA

Abbreviations: TRICKS, time-resolved imaging of contrast kinetics; MRA, magnetic resonance angiography; NA: not available.

Similarly, the sensitivity and specificity for demonstrating occlusions in lower extremity vessels are 92.5% and 98.5%, respectively.

MRA has several drawbacks. For example, MRA demonstrates a limited ability to image segments containing stents due to excess signal loss. Also, overestimation of lesion size is estimated at 3%, whereas underestimation of size occurs in 19% of lesions (60). Diagnostic costs associated with MRA are higher than those for CTA (61). Thus, factors such as cost, availability, experience, and patient comorbidities may influence the choice of modality in the initial evaluation of lower extremity arterial occlusive disease, particularly in the diabetic population.

SUMMARY

- Use of iodine- or gadolinium-based contrast media requires special precautions in the diabetic population, particularly those with already-compromised renal function.

Table 8 Advantages and Disadvantages of DSA, CTA, and MRA for Evaluating Lower Extremity PVD

Modality	Advantages	Disadvantages
X-ray DSA	• Dynamic procedure • Good anatomic detail • Traditionally considered the gold standard for diagnosis • Access can be used for therapy	• Invasive with higher complication rate • Relatively high ionizing radiation exposure • Does not adequately demonstrate potential distal anastomotic site for surgical bypass
CTA	• Noninvasive • Widely available • Rapid scan time • 3D volumetric display capability • Fewer artifacts from metallic clips, stents, and prostheses than with MRA • Reveals more calf vessels than does DSA • Cost-effective. • Reproducible—good for follow-up	• May result in greater number of follow-up studies than by DSA • Difficult to interpret with abundant calcifications • Ionizing radiation exposure and use of iodinated contrast (lower than with x-ray DSA)
MRA	• Noninvasive • Detects slow flow and angiographically occult runoff vessels • 3D imaging enables reconstruction of an infinite number of planes and orientations • Calcifications do not cause artifacts	• Not widely available • Contraindicated in patients with spinal stimulators, pacemakers, cochlear implants, and intracranial clips and shunts • Stents and clips produce artifacts

Abbreviations: DSA, digital subtraction angiography; CTA, computed tomographic angiography; MRA, magnetic resonance angiography; PVD, peripheral vascular disease.

- X-ray DSA evaluation of the distal lower extremities can serve as a supplementary diagnostic and prognostic indicator of the likelihood of major amputation and ulcer healing in diabetic patients with foot ulcers.
- X-ray DSA is an invasive test associated with an overall complication rate of 1.7% to 7%.
- MSCT angiography provides comparable, or perhaps superior, assessment of distal lower extremity arteries compared with DSA.
- MSCT angiography is cost-effective for therapeutic decision making in patients with lower extremity arterial disease.
- Because of longer acquisition time and greater artifacts, non–contrast-enhanced MRA has fallen out of favor compared with CE MRA techniques.
- Diagnostic costs associated with MRA are higher than for CTA.
- Ultimately, factors such as cost, availability, and familiarity with each imaging modality influence which one is selected for anatomic localization of peripheral artery occlusive disease. Advantages and disadvantages are listed in Table 8.

REFERENCES

1. Dyet JF, Nicholson AA, Ettles DF. Vascular imaging and intervention in peripheral arteries in the diabetic patient. Diabetes Metab Res Rev 2000; 16(suppl 1):S16–S22.
2. Van Der Feen C, Neijens FS, Kanters SD, et al. Angiographic distribution of lower extremity atherosclerosis in patients with and without diabetes. Diabet Med 2002; 19(5):366–370.
3. Jude EB, Oyibo SO, Chalmers N, et al. Peripheral arterial disease in diabetic and nondiabetic patients: A comparison of severity and outcome. Diabetes Care 2001; 24(8):1433–1437.
4. Ciavarella A, Silletti A, Mustacchio A, et al. Angiographic evaluation of the anatomic pattern of arterial obstructions in diabetic patients with critical limb ischaemia. Diabete Metab 1993; 19(6):586–589.
5. Hietala SO, Lithner F. Foot angiography in diabetic patients with gangrene. Acta Med Scand Suppl 1984; 687:61–67.
6. Chomel S, Douek P, Moulin P, et al. Contrast-enhanced MR angiography of the foot: Anatomy and clinical application in patients with diabetes. AJR Am J Roentgenol 2004; 182(6):1435–1442.
7. Rubba P, Leccia G, Faccenda F, et al. Diabetes mellitus and localizations of obliterating arterial disease of the lower limbs. Angiology 1991; 42(4):296–301.
8. Hoch JR, Kennell TW, Hollister MS, et al. Comparison of treatment plans for lower extremity arterial occlusive disease made with electrocardiography-triggered two-dimensional time-of-flight magnetic resonance angiography and digital subtraction angiography. Am J Surg 1999; 178(2):166–172.
9. Lapeyre M, Kobeiter H, Desgranges P, et al. Assessment of critical limb ischemia in patients with diabetes: Comparison of MR angiography and digital subtraction angiography. AJR Am J Roentgenol 2005; 185(6):1641–1650.
10. Norgren L, Hiatt WR, Dormandy JA, et al. TASC II Working Group: Inter-Society Consensus for the Management of Peripheral Arterial Disease (TASC II). J Vasc Surg 2007; 45(suppl S):S5–S67.
11. Bollinger A, Breddin K, Hess H, et al. Semiquantitative assessment of lower limb atherosclerosis from routine angiographic images. Atherosclerosis 1981; 38(3/4):339–346.
12. Namasivayam S, Kalra MK, Torres WE, et al. Adverse reactions to intravenous iodinated contrast media: A primer for radiologists. Emerg Radiol 2006; 12(5):210–215.

13. Faglia E, Favales F, Quarantiello A, et al. Angiographic evaluation of peripheral arterial occlusive disease and its role as a prognostic determinant for major amputation in diabetic subjects with foot ulcers. Diabetes Care 1998; 21(4):625–630.
14. Merten GJ, Burgess WP, Gray LV, et al. Prevention of contrast-induced nephropathy with sodium bicarbonate: A randomized controlled trial. JAMA 2004; 291(19):2328–2334.
15. Thomsen HS, Morcos SK. Contrast-medium-induced nephropathy: Is there a new consensus? A review of published guidelines. Eur Radiol 2006; 16(8):1835–1840.
16. Ozcan EE, Guneri S, Akdeniz B, et al. Sodium bicarbonate, N-acetylcysteine, and saline for prevention of radiocontrast-induced nephropathy: A comparison of 3 regimens for protecting contrast-induced nephropathy in patients undergoing coronary procedures: A single-center prospective controlled trial. Am Heart J 2007; 154(3):539–544.
17. Kanal E, Barkovich AJ, Bell C, et al. ACR Blue Ribbon Panel on MR Safety: ACR guidance document for safe MR practices: 2007. AJR Am J Roentgenol 2007; 188(6):1447–1474.
18. Schmidt P, Pang D, Nykamp D, et al. N-acetylcysteine and sodium bicarbonate versus N-acetylcysteine and standard hydration for the prevention of radiocontrast-induced nephropathy following coronary angiography. Ann Pharmacother 2007; 41(1):46–50.
19. Stenstrom DA, Muldoon LL, Armijo-Medina H, et al. N-acetylcysteine use to prevent contrast medium-induced nephropathy: Premature phase III trials. J Vasc Interv Radiol 2008; 19(3):309–318.
20. Auler MA, Heagy T, Aganovic L, et al. Saline chasing technique with dual-syringe injector systems for multi-detector row computed tomographic angiography: Rationale, indications, and protocols. Curr Probl Diagn Radiol 2006; 35(1):1–11.
21. Bees NR, Beese RC, Belli AM, et al. Carbon dioxide angiography of the lower limbs: Initial experience with an automated carbon dioxide injector. Clin Radiol 1999; 54(12):833–838.
22. Thurnher S, Miller S, Schneider G, et al. Diagnostic performance of gadobenate dimeglumine enhanced MR angiography of the iliofemoral and calf arteries: A large-scale multicenter trial. AJR Am J Roentgenol 2007; 189(5):1223–1237.
23. Sadowski EA, Bennett LK, Chan MR, et al. Nephrogenic systemic fibrosis: Risk factors and incidence estimation. Radiology 2007; 243(1):148–157.
24. Broome DR, Girguis MS, Baron PW, et al. Gadodiamide-associated nephrogenic systemic fibrosis: Why radiologists should be concerned. AJR Am J Roentgenol 2007; 188(2):586–592.
25. http://www.fda.gov/Drugs/DrugSafety/PublicHealthAdvisories/ucm124344.htm.
26. Bongartz G, Mayr M, Bilecen D. Magnetic resonance angiography (MRA) in renally impaired patients: When and how. Eur J Radiol 2008; 66(2):213–219.
27. Toursarkissian B, D'Ayala M, Stefanidis D, et al. Angiographic scoring of vascular occlusive disease in the diabetic foot: Relevance to bypass graft patency and limb salvage. J Vasc Surg 2002; 35(3):494–500.
28. Dorweiler B, Neufang A, Kreitner KF, et al. Magnetic resonance angiography unmasks reliable target vessels for pedal bypass grafting in patients with diabetes mellitus. J Vasc Surg 2002; 35(4):766–772.
29. AbuRahma AF, Robinson PA, Boland JP, et al. Complications of arteriography in a recent series of 707 cases: Factors affecting outcome. Ann Vasc Surg 1993; 7(2):122–129.
30. Hessel SJ, Adams DF, Abrams HL. Complications of angiography. Radiology 1981; 138(2):273–281.
31. Srodon P, Matson M, Ham R. Contrast nephropathy in lower limb angiography. Ann R Coll Surg Engl 2003; 85(3):187–191.
32. Gomes AS, Baker JD, Martin-Paredero V, et al. Acute renal dysfunction after major arteriography. AJR Am J Roentgenol 1985; 145(6):1249–1253.
33. Parfrey PS, Griffiths SM, Barrett BJ, et al. Contrast material-induced renal failure in patients with diabetes mellitus, renal insufficiency, or both: A prospective controlled study. N Engl J Med 1989; 320(3):143–149.

34. Sun Z. Diagnostic accuracy of multislice CT angiography in peripheral arterial disease. J Vasc Interv Radiol 2006; 17(12):1915–1921.
35. Heuschmid M, Wiesinger B, Tepe G, et al. Evaluation of various image reconstruction parameters in lower extremity stents using multidetector-row CT angiography: Initial findings. Eur Radiol 2007; 17(1):265–271.
36. Albrecht T, Foert E, Holtkamp R, et al. 16-MDCT angiography of aortoiliac and lower extremity arteries: Comparison with digital subtraction angiography. AJR Am J Roentgenol 2007; 189(3):702–711.
37. Heijenbrok-Kal MH, Kock MC, Hunink MG. Lower extremity arterial disease: Multidetector CT angiography meta-analysis. Radiology 2007; 245(2):433–439.
38. Schernthaner R, Stadler A, Lomoschitz F, et al. Multidetector CT angiography in the assessment of peripheral arterial occlusive disease: Accuracy in detecting the severity, number, and length of stenoses. Eur Radiol 2008; 18(4):665–671.
39. Martin ML, Tay KH, Flak B, et al. Multidetector CT angiography of the aortoiliac system and lower extremities: A prospective comparison with digital subtraction angiography. AJR Am J Roentgenol 2003; 180(4):1085–1091.
40. Ota H, Takase K, Igarashi K, et al. MDCT compared with digital subtraction angiography for assessment of lower extremity arterial occlusive disease: Importance of reviewing cross-sectional images. AJR Am J Roentgenol 2004; 182(1):201–209.
41. Ouwendijk R, Kock MC, van Dijk LC, et al. Vessel wall calcifications at multi-detector row CT angiography in patients with peripheral arterial disease: Effect on clinical utility and clinical predictors. Radiology 2006; 241(2):603–608.
42. Kock MC, Adriaensen ME, Pattynama PM, et al. DSA versus multi-detector row CT angiography in peripheral arterial disease: Randomized controlled trial. Radiology 2005; 237(2):727–737.
43. Willmann JK, Baumert B, Schertler T, et al. Aortoiliac and lower extremity arteries assessed with 16-detector row CT angiography: Prospective comparison with digital subtraction angiography. Radiology 2005; 236(3):1083–1093.
44. Reimer P, Boos M. Phase-contrast MR angiography of peripheral arteries: Technique and clinical application. Eur Radiol 1999; 9(1):122–127.
45. Hahn WY, Hecht EM, Friedman B, et al. Distal lower extremity imaging: Prospective comparison of 2-dimensional time of flight, 3-dimensional time-resolved contrast-enhanced magnetic resonance angiography, and 3-dimensional bolus chase contrast-enhanced magnetic resonance angiography. J Comput Assist Tomogr 2007; 31(1):29–36.
46. Lee HM, Wang Y. Dynamic k-space filling for bolus chase 3D MR digital subtraction angiography. Magn Reson Med 1998; 40(1):99–104.
47. Huber A, Heuck A, Baur A, et al. Dynamic contrast-enhanced MR angiography from the distal aorta to the ankle joint with a step-by-step technique. AJR Am J Roentgenol 2000; 175(5):1291–1298.
48. Tongdee R, Narra VR, McNeal G, et al. Hybrid peripheral 3D contrast-enhanced MR angiography of calf and foot vasculature. AJR Am J Roentgenol 2006; 186(6):1746–1753.
49. Swan JS, Carroll TJ, Kennell TW, et al. Time-resolved three-dimensional contrast-enhanced MR angiography of the peripheral vessels. Radiology 2002; 225(1):43–52.
50. Mell M, Tefera G, Thornton F, et al. Clinical utility of time-resolved imaging of contrast kinetics (TRICKS) magnetic resonance angiography for infrageniculate arterial occlusive disease. J Vasc Surg 2007; 45(3):543–548, discussion 548.
51. Sharafuddin MJ, Stolpen AH, Sun S, et al. High-resolution multiphase contrast-enhanced three-dimensional MR angiography compared with two-dimensional time-of-flight MR angiography for the identification of pedal vessels. J Vasc Interv Radiol 2002; 13(7):695–702.
52. Lee HM, Wang Y, Sostman HD, et al. Distal lower extremity arteries: Evaluation with two-dimensional MR digital subtraction angiography. Radiology 1998; 207(2):505–512.
53. Huegli RW, Aschwanden M, Bongartz G, et al. Intraarterial MR angiography and DSA in patients with peripheral arterial occlusive disease: Prospective comparison. Radiology 2006; 239(3):901–908.

54. Koelemay MJ, Lijmer JG, Stoker J, et al. Magnetic resonance angiography for the evaluation of lower extremity arterial disease: A meta-analysis. JAMA 2001; 285(10):1338–1345.
55. Zhang HL, Khilnani NM, Prince MR, et al. Diagnostic accuracy of time-resolved 2D projection MR angiography for symptomatic infrapopliteal arterial occlusive disease. AJR Am J Roentgenol 2005; 184(3):938–947.
56. Loewe C, Schoder M, Rand T, et al. Peripheral vascular occlusive disease: Evaluation with contrast-enhanced moving-bed MR angiography versus digital subtraction angiography in 106 patients. AJR Am J Roentgenol 2002; 179(4):1013–1021.
57. Binkert CA, Baker PD, Petersen BD, et al. Peripheral vascular disease: Blinded study of dedicated calf MR angiography versus standard bolus-chase MR angiography and film hard-copy angiography. Radiology 2004; 232(3):860–866.
58. Andreisek G, Pfammatter T, Goepfert K, et al. Peripheral arteries in diabetic patients: Standard bolus-chase and time-resolved MR angiography. Radiology 2007; 242(2):610–620.
59. Kreitner KF, Kalden P, Neufang A, et al. Diabetes and peripheral arterial occlusive disease: Prospective comparison of contrast-enhanced three-dimensional MR angiography with conventional digital subtraction angiography. AJR Am J Roentgenol 2000; 174(1):171–179.
60. Davis CP, Schöpke WD, Seifert B, et al. MR angiography of patients with peripheral arterial disease before and after transluminal angioplasty. AJR Am J Roentgenol 1997; 168(4):1027–1034.
61. Ouwendijk R, de Vries M, Pattynama PM, et al. Imaging peripheral arterial disease: A randomized controlled trial comparing contrast-enhanced MR angiography and multi-detector row CT angiography. Radiology 2005; 236(3):1094–1103.

3 Endovascular treatment of infrainguinal arterial disease

Jason Maggi, Rajesh Malik, and Firas F. Mussa

INTRODUCTION

Endovascular treatment of arterial occlusive disease has been widely accepted because of its low morbidity and mortality, patient comfort, and cost. Anecdotal reports and retrospective reviews of case series have expanded the indications of this therapeutic modality to include those with nondisabling intermittent claudication, which was traditionally treated by risk-factor modifications and progressive exercise regimen. Percutaneous techniques have largely replaced open bypass surgery for patients with critical limb ischemia. Furthermore, recent advances in vascular imaging have been instrumental in selecting patients with anatomically suitable lesions for percutaneous management. This chapter reviews the endovascular options in the treatment of infrainguinal arterial occlusive disease.

TASC CLASSIFICATION

Lesion location, length, calcification, and occlusion have each posed significant challenges to the successful and enduring endovascular treatment of peripheral arterial disease (PAD). In 2000, the Trans Atlantic Inter-Society Consensus (TASC) guidelines were published to help standardize treatment algorithms for patients with PAD of the lower extremity that considered severity and distribution of the lesions (1). The anatomical guidelines of TASC were revised in 2007, in the TASC II document, to reflect significant advances in diagnosis and multidisciplinary treatment of PAD (2). As compared with TASC I, TASC II strongly favors endovascular therapy for type B and surgery for type C lesions. Although the lesion classification within the TASC system provides a consensus of best practice to guide physicians in their choice of therapy, individualized approach is recommended on the basis of patients' comorbidities and interventionalists' scope of practice and training.

ENDOVASCULAR OPTIONS FOR INFRAINGUINAL OCCLUSIVE ARTERIAL DISEASE

Endovascular therapy in infrainguinal occlusive arterial disease can improve symptoms, quality of life, and, in selected patients, avoid limb loss (3). The choice of percutaneous technique is dependent on lesion morphology (length of lesion and the presence of occlusion versus stenosis). While technical success is high with endovascular treatment, enthusiasm for this mode of therapy has been tempered by the long-term clinical results. The bypass versus angioplasty in severe ischemia of the leg (BASIL) trial, which was a multicenter, randomized controlled trial, showed that a bypass-surgery-first and a balloon-angioplasty-first strategy are associated with broadly similar outcomes in terms of amputation-free survival; and in the short term, surgery is more expensive than angioplasty (4). Late failure of balloon angioplasty may be attributed to elastic recoil, dissection, or disease progression (3), whereas stents in the lower extremity are associated with late deformation and mechanical compression leading to fatigue, stent fracture, and re-stenosis.

PERFORMING THE BEST ANGIOGRAM

Although several diagnostic imaging modalities are currently being utilized in the diagnosis of infrainguinal occlusive arterial disease, the angiogram remains the gold standard. The angiogram provides detailed visualization of the arterial distribution and is essential for planning any revascularization by endovascular or open techniques. Furthermore, it allows for hemodynamic measurements across the lesion of interest. Although an invasive technique, in most cases, it can be performed under local anesthesia; the pain and discomfort that had been associated with contrast injection in the past have been greatly abated with the use of low-osmolarity, nonionic agents.

Several points are worth mention about the use of the contrast power injector. Understanding the rate of contrast injection and its relation to the timing of image capture enhances the quality of the angiogram. This understanding allows for reduction in the total volume of contrast media used when compared with the traditional method of manual contrast injection. In addition, it reduces the variability in rate of injection associated with manual injection. Using the contrast injector will deliver the contrast at the selected rate until the maximum pressure is reached; at this maximal pressure, the contrast will be injected at a lesser rate until the total preselected volume is reached. Therefore, the choice of catheter and contrast agent is significant, as the resistance of the catheter and the viscosity of the contrast agent will limit flow. Finally, having nursing and support staff familiar with the equipment is essential, allowing for intraoperative adjustments as needed.

The choice of catheter used for contrast delivery is critical to performing an adequate angiogram. The length of the catheter, the amount of distal taper, and the number of side holes all affect contrast flow. Ideally, a catheter should be as short as possible with the largest feasible lumen to eliminate resistance. Reducing the amount of taper in the catheter and maximizing the number of side holes will also decrease the pressure and resistance to contrast flow.

Reducing motion artifact during image acquisition maximizes angiographic images' quality. Even the slightest motion will distort images and affect planning for intervention. The procedure should be performed in a suite equipped for interventional procedures, eliminating the possibility for structural interference in imaging. Finally, optimal imaging relies on good cooperation between the physician and the patient. This reduces patient anxiety and provides a comfortable, cooperative, and pain-free setting.

PERCUTANEOUS TRANSLUMINAL ANGIOPLASTY

The use of percutaneous transluminal angioplasty (PTA) to revascularize the superficial femoral artery (SFA) can result in initial technical success rates of more than 95%, with a low risk of complications. However, restenosis occurs in 40% to 60% of treated segments after 1 year (5). Successful femoropopliteal angioplasty is influenced by several factors including the severity of presenting symptoms (e.g., claudication vs. rest pain and/or tissue loss), lesion length (proximal short lesions yield better results), stenosis versus occlusion, runoff status (2- and 3-vessel runoff consistently associated with better outcomes than 0- and 1-vessel runoff), and the presence or absence of diabetes mellitus (6,7). In 2006, a randomized study by Schillinger et al. (8) demonstrated superior results of primary stenting of the SFA by using a self-expanding nitinol stent to those treated by balloon angioplasty with optional secondary stenting. At 6 months, the rate of restenosis on angiography was 24% in the stent group and 43% in the angioplasty group ($P = 0.05$). At 1 year, the rates of re-stenosis on duplex ultrasound examination of the two groups were 37% and 63%, respectively ($P = 0.01$) (8). Despite the lack of conclusive evidence, PTA as the sole endovascular option is currently reserved for those with short segment disease ($\leq$3 cm) and stenosis rather than total arterial occlusion.

CUTTING BALLOON ANGIOPLASTY

The idea of mounting cutting blades (atherotomes) on an angioplasty balloon is adapted from the coronary circulation where overinflation of the balloon may lead to detrimental arterial injury, recoil, and distal dissection. As the balloon expands, the atherotomes cut into and score the stenotic plaque, allowing lower balloon inflation pressures and resulting in less distension, vessel stretch, and barotrauma compared with conventional angioplasty. Cutting balloons are primarily used to treat restenosis subsequent to a previous endovascular (in-stent restenosis), or anastamotic or in-graft stenoses after open bypass procedures. This modality has largely replaced patch angioplasty revisions after bypass surgery (9).

SUBINTIMAL ANGIOPLASTY

Subintimal angioplasty was first described by Bolia et al. (10) and is indicated to treat long occlusions ($\geq$15 cm), highly calcified occlusions, diffuse tandem lesions, and flush SFA occlusions. Briefly, a flexible hydrophilic guidewire is used to create a subintimal dissection plane; the wire tip is looped to form a blunt end while traversing the occluded segment to just beyond the occlusion. Ideal reentry into the true lumen should be controlled and placed at the distal extent of the occlusion. The most feared complication of subintimal angioplasty results from uncontrolled reentry and potential compromise of surgical options by encroachment into vessels that can serve as future distal target for bypass such as the popliteal or tibial arteries. Although technical success with subintimal angioplasty may be more than 90%, it is highly dependant on the interventionist's skill and comfort with this technique, the 1-year primary patency rates in the treatment of infrainguinal disease range from 53% to 94% (11,12).

CRYOPLASTY BALLOON DILATATION

Endovascular cryoplasty induces cold thermal injury to the arterial wall while delivering mechanical dilatation force of angioplasty. Both effects are achieved by inflating the catheter with nitrous oxide and experimentally have been shown to induce apoptosis in smooth muscle cells altering the immediate response to injury and reducing negative remodeling after balloon angioplasty. In a preliminary study, Fava et al. (13) used cryoplasty in 15 patients with femoropopliteal arterial lesions. Technical success was achieved in 93% of patients (defined as

<30% residual stenosis or minimal and non–flow-limiting arterial dissection). Immediate follow up at 1 and 3 months with ankle brachial indices measurement demonstrated improvement from baseline. Similarly, angiographic follow up at 14 months demonstrated primary patency in 83% of treated vessels (13). In one multicenter study, cryoplasty was used to treat 102 patients with claudication and lesions of the femoropopliteal segment less than 10 cm in length. Overall, the technical success rate was 85%, with a primary patency rate of 70%, as defined by duplex ultrasound with a systolic velocity ratio of more than 2.0. Sixteen of the 102 patients required target lesion revascularization during the 9-month follow-up (14). The 6-month outcome from a prospective multicenter study investigating the use of cryoplasty to treat below-knee occlusive disease in patients with critical limb ischemia (BTK-CHILL) trial demonstrated technical success in 97%, with 0.9% rate of clinically significant dissections. During the 6-month follow-up, only 88 of the original 108 (81.5%) patients with 91 (82.0%) treated limbs were available for assessment. The rate of freedom from major amputation was 93.4%. Amputation-free survival was 89.3% (15).

EXCISIONAL ATHERECTOMY

The concept is not novel, in which removing plaque burden from the arterial wall has traditionally been associated with prohibitively high re-stenosis rates. With recent advances in device development, this modality had witnessed renewed enthusiasm. This therapy may be particularly useful in ostial disease of the SFA and the popliteal artery (16). In a study by Kandzari et al. (16), 69 patients underwent percutaneous atherectomy for chronic limb ischemia with almost universal technical success. Complete or partial limb salvage was obtained in 92% of patients at 30 days and in 82% at 6 months. A major risk from using this technique, however, is the increased risk of distal embolization, and few investigators have suggested the use of distal embolization protection devices for such intervention.

PTFE-COVERED (STENT-GRAFT) ENDOPROSTHESES

The concept behind using stent-graft in the SFA is to "reline" the diseased segment with the functional equivalent of an endoluminal prosthetic bypass. Excluding the diseased plaque from the bloodstream is believed to decrease the likelihood of re-stenosis via intimal hyperplasia and tissue in-growth (17). The Viabahn endoprosthesis (W.L. Gore & Associates, Flagstaff, Arizona) is a self-expanding nitinol stent with polytetrafluoroethylene (PTFE) in-lining. It is the only currently FDA-approved stent-graft for treatment of SFA disease. Primary patency rates of 90% ± 3% and 79% ± 5% at 6 and 12 months, respectively, were reported for femoral arteries (80 limbs) treated in an international safety and efficacy study (17). The 2-year clinical results were published from single center experience in which 28 patients suffering from claudication referable to femoropopliteal stenoses or occlusions were prospectively randomized to receive PTA alone or PTA in combination with a PTFE-covered endoprosthesis (18). The primary patency rate was 87% among patients in the combination treatment group versus 25% for those treated with PTA alone ($P = 0.002$). The extent of advanced disease in the study group was reportedly responsible for the poor patency rate for PTA. Citing concerns of increased risk of embolization, thigh pain, and cost factors, Saxon et al. (18) concluded that the improvements in long-term patency and clinical outcome warranted further evaluation. An additional concern is that collaterals in the excluded segment are sacrificed, possibly leading to more severe ischemia should the revascularization fail. A randomized comparison of the Viabahn endoprosthesis and standard open femoropopliteal bypasses with prosthetic conduit was undertaken by Kedora et al. (19). Eighty-six patients with symptoms ranging from claudication to rest pain, with or without tissue loss, were included in the study. The median follow-up was 18 months. Primary patencies at 3, 6, 9, and 12 months were 84%, 82%, 75.6%, and 73.5%, respectively, for the stent group and 90%, 81.8%, 79.7%, and 74.2%, respectively, for the surgical group. Secondary patency rates were also identical. The rate of required reinterventions between the groups was interestingly comparable. Kedora et al. (19) concluded that for at least 12 months, percutaneous treatment with Viabahn of femoropopliteal disease was comparable with surgical revascularization with conventional femoral to above-knee popliteal artery bypass using synthetic conduit.

MANAGING COMPLICATIONS

Distal Embolization

Clinically significant embolization during endovascular intervention is unusual but may lead to catastrophic outcome. High-risk lesions include those with irregular or ulcerated plaque, those with occlusions, those who present with embolization, and those associated with fresh thrombus. Distal embolization may be evident intraoperatively as filling defect distal to the intervention site or may present as pain experienced by the patient in the involved extremity. Management of such complication starts by full anticoagulation with heparin systemically as well as locally through the existing intra-arterial sheath. Maintenance of distal guidewire access is the key. Further treatment depends on the cause of embolization. Occasionally, stabilization of the angioplasty site with stent or stent-graft placement may prevent further embolization. Placement of multi-side-hole catheter to administer and infuse tissue plasminogen activator in the distal vascular bed along with vasodilators may help expedite recovery.

Acute Arterial Dissection

Any percutaneous intervention anywhere in the arterial system may lead to dissection. Dissection tends to occur at branch points, in the presence of bulky or circumferential plaque especially if heavily calcified. It could also result from overdilatation with balloon angioplasty. Prior to the widespread use of intravascular stents, dissection used to be feared as a devastating complication with potential limb loss. Since stents became readily available, a bailout option is readily available in case of arterial dissections during endovascular intervention.

Arterial Rupture

Arterial rupture usually presents with acute and sharp pain experienced by the patient at the site of intervention, and contrast extravasation is immediately evident on angiogram. Hemodynamic instability may indicate rupture in patients who cannot express pain because of heavy sedation or anesthesia. Contained rupture that is localized may heal with no consequences or may form a pseudoaneurysm. Significant rupture may result from overdilatation and may be salvaged by advancing the balloon into the location of rupture and inflating it to its nominal diameter. This maneuver will tamponade the bleeding until definitive therapy is performed with open surgery or stent-graft. Another consequence of arterial rupture is acute occlusion, which may lead to limb-threatening ischemia. To avoid rupture, careful consideration of the diameter of the balloon in relation to the size of the artery is paramount. Similarly, accepting less than perfect angiographic results and knowing when to stop or convert to open surgery may avoid the patient a potentially life-threatening complication.

Acute Occlusion

Acute occlusion usually results from dissection and becomes apparent on completion angiogram. While guidewire access is in place, the dissection is treated with a single stent at the dissection site (site of intervention). If needed, a second stent is placed just proximal to the first stent until patency is resorted.

CONCLUSION

With the expanding field of endovascular therapy and recent advances in technology, a paradigm shift is ongoing toward treating more complex lesions in patients who would otherwise receive best medical therapy as the sole treatment. Despite the lack of level 1 evidence, immediate, intermediate, and long-term results have been encouraging. Thromboembolism and uncontrolled dissection are intraoperative risks, whereas intimal hyperplasia, late device failure, and disease progression have plagued the long-term results. Further investigation is warranted, and careful patient selection remains the most critical factor in determining the proper utilization of these modalities.

REFERENCES

1. Dormandy JA. Management of peripheral arterial disease (PAD): TASC Working Group: TransAtlantic Inter-Society Consensus (TASC). J Vasc Surg 2000; 31(suppl): S1–S296.
2. Norgren L, Hiatt WR, Dormandy JA, et al. Inter-society consensus for the management of peripheral arterial disease (TASC II). J Vasc Surg 2007; 45(suppl):S5–S67.
3. Laird JR. Limitations of percutaneous transluminal angioplasty and stenting for the treatment of disease of the superficial femoral and popliteal arteries. J Endovasc Ther (Phoenix) 2006; 13(suppl II):II30–II40.
4. Adam DJ, Beard JD, Cleveland T, et al. Bypass versus angioplasty in severe ischaemia of the leg (BASIL): Multicentre, randomised controlled trial. Lancet 2005; 366(9501):1925–1934.
5. Krepel VM, van Andel GJ, van Erp WF, et al. Percutaneous transluminal angioplasty of the femoropopliteal artery: Initial and long-term results. Radiology 1985; 156:325–328.
6. Johnston KW. Femoral and popliteal arteries: Reanalysis of results of balloon angioplasty. Radiology 1992; 183:767–771.
7. Capek P, McLean GK, Berkowitz HD. Femoropopliteal angioplasty: Factors influencing long-term success. Circulation 1991; 83:170–180.
8. Schillinger M, Sabeti S, Loewe C, et al. Balloon angioplasty versus implantation of nitinol stents in the superficial femoral artery. N Engl J Med 2006; 354:1879–1888.
9. Schneider PA, Caps MT, Nelken N. Infrainguinal vein graft stenosis: Cutting balloon angioplasty as the first-line treatment of choice. J Vasc Surg 2008; 47(5):960–966.
10. Bolia A, Fishwick G. Recanalization of iliac artery occlusion by subintimal dissection using the ipsilateral and the contralateral approach. Clin Radiol 1997; 52(9):684–687.
11. Loftus IM, Hayes PD, Bell PR. Subintimal angioplasty in lower limb ischaemia. J Cardiovasc Surg (Torino) 2004; 45:217–229.

12. McCarthy RJ, Neary W, Roobottom C, et al. Short-term results of femoropopliteal subintimal angioplasty. Br J Surg 2000; 87:1361–1365.
13. Fava M, Loyola S, Polydorou A, et al. Cryoplasty for femoropopliteal arterial disease: Late angiographic results of initial human experience. J Vasc Interv Radiol 2004; 15:1239–1243.
14. Laird J, Jaff MR, Biamino G, et al. Cryoplasty for the treatment of femoropopliteal arterial disease: Results of a prospective, multicenter registry. J Vasc Interv Radiol 2005; 16:1067–1075.
15. Das T, McNamara T, Gray B, et al. Cryoplasty therapy for limb salvage in patients with critical limb ischemia. J Endovasc Ther 2007; 14(6):753–762.
16. Kandzari DE, Kiesz RS, Allie D, et al. Procedural and clinical outcomes with catheter-based plaque excision in critical limb ischemia. J Endovasc Ther (Phoenix) 2006; 13(1):12.
17. Lammer J, Dake MD, Bleyn J, et al. Peripheral arterial obstruction: Prospective study of treatment with a transluminally placed self-expanding stent-graft: International Trial Study Group. Radiology 2000; 217:95–104.
18. Saxon RR, Coffman JM, Gooding JM, et al. Long-term results of ePTFE stent-graft versus angioplasty in the femoropopliteal artery: Single center experience from a prospective, randomized trial. J Vasc Interv Radiol 2003; 14:303–311.
19. Kedora J, Hohmann S, Garrett W, et al. Randomized comparison of percutaneous Viabahn stent grafts vs. prosthetic femoral-prosthetic bypass in the treatment of superficial femoral arterial occlusive disease. J Vasc Surg 2007; 45:10–16.

4 Open arterial reconstruction of the diabetic foot

Joseph J. Naoum and Eric K. Peden

INTRODUCTION

In the United States, approximately 20.6 million people 20 years or older have diabetes. Among these, 10.3 million are older than 60 years. In 2005, 1.5 million new patients were diagnosed as having diabetes, and approximately 30% of people 40 years or older have impaired sensation in their feet or neuropathy. More than 60% of nontraumatic lower-limb amputations occur in people with diabetes as a result of peripheral neuropathy, infections, ulcers, or peripheral arterial disease (1). Ramsey and colleagues (2) reviewed a cohort of patients with diabetes and observed that over a 3-year period, 5.8% developed a foot ulcer, 15% of those had osteomyelitis and an equal number required amputation. Survival at 3 years was lower for patients with foot ulcers compared with those without ulceration. The incidence of foot ulceration was nearly 2% to 3% per year with a lifetime incidence of approximately 15% (2,3). It comes as no surprise that major complications of diabetes are associated with a worse health-related quality of life (4).

Diabetes mellitus increases the risk of lower extremity peripheral arterial disease by two- to fourfold (5–9) and is present in 12% to 20% of persons with lower extremity peripheral arterial disease (6,8). In the Framingham Heart Study, diabetes increased the risk of intermittent claudication by 3.5- and 8.6-fold in men and women, respectively (10). The risk of developing lower extremity peripheral arterial disease is proportional to the severity and duration of diabetes (9,11). The risk of developing chronic limb ischemia is also greater in those with diabetes than in those without diabetes (12,13). Diabetic patients with lower extremity peripheral arterial disease are 7- to 15-fold more likely to undergo a major amputation than are non–diabetic patients with lower extremity peripheral arterial disease (13–15).

The estimated direct medical cost for treatment of diabetes in the United States in 2002 was approximately $92 billion. An additional $40 billion was attributed to disability, work loss, and premature mortality (16). The health care expenditures associated with diabetic foot ulceration amount to $18.9 billion and amount to $11.7 billion for lower extremity amputations (17). Medicare expenditures for lower extremity ulcer patients were 3 to 5.4 times higher than those for the rest of the patients in general, and only a quarter of that was spent on outpatient treatment (3,18). Interestingly, total ulcer-related costs were 27% higher for patients younger than 65 years than for those older than 65 years (18).

MANAGEMENT

Evaluation of the diabetic patient with foot ulceration begins with a detailed history and physical examination. A thorough vascular examination aimed at detecting other potential causes of cardiac and vascular morbidity such as heart, carotid, or aneurysmal disease is essential. If open surgical revascularization or bypass is contemplated, addressing and resolving those comorbidities first may be necessary.

The evaluation of the extremity with peripheral arterial disease is first done by noninvasive methods. Bilateral Doppler ultrasound with multilevel segmental pressures and measurement of the ankle brachial index for each leg is performed. When vessels are severely calcified and the Doppler waveforms are not sufficient to delineate the extent of disease, arterial duplex of the affected limb can provide further details relating to the extent of lesions and patency of potential runoff vessels. These early noninvasive studies provide a set point to which one can compare the results following therapy or revascularization.

Computed tomography angiography (CTA) or magnetic resonance angiography (MRA) can be used to delineate or map the vascular anatomy and help therapeutic planning. The latter can overestimate the extent of disease, especially when flow is severely compromised, hence failing to expose a potential open infrapopliteal target vessel. Diagnostic digital subtraction angiography is preferred as the gold standard for the evaluation of the ischemic or at-risk extremity. A complete examination should include an abdominal aortogram, imaging of the iliac or pelvic vessels, and serial images of the lower extremity, including the foot to the toes.

Endovascular approaches are attempted for arterial revascularization. However, if this is not successful, an effort should be made to clearly identify a target vessel and its runoff in preparation for open surgical revascularization. This often will require additional contrast dye injections and images focusing on the distal leg and foot runoff. According to the authors, a detailed angiographic search will demonstrate a patent distal infrapopliteal vessel adequate for bypass. If uncertainty exists, at the time of surgery, an open on-table angiogram using a 21- to 23-gauge angiocatheter placed into the target vessel can help better delineate or even change the operative plan. On-table prebypass angiography has been shown to alter the operative plan and extend operability (19). When performing a femoral to distal infrapopliteal artery bypass, there is a preference to tunnel the graft in a subcutaneous or subfascial manner and not necessarily in anatomical position, using a Gore Tunneler (W.L. GORE & Associates, Flagstaff, Arizona). It is important to make a counter-incision at or above the knee in order to achieve proper placement of the conduit. According to the authors, failing to do so can lead to kinks of the conduit, entrapment, or compression of the graft by the fascia with movement of the knee joint. When the peroneal artery is the target vessel, it is one of the author's preferences to expose this artery through a medial approach instead of the lateral approach that necessitates excision of a portion of fibula. This medial approach provides the ability to extend the incision more distal or proximal and thus achieve greater exposure of the peroneal artery. The authors also perform a completion on-table arteriogram evaluating the entire length of the graft, the distal anastomosis, and the runoff to the foot at the end of the procedure (Fig. 1).

Limb salvage in patients with diabetes requires more than just adequate revascularization. Aggressive wound care, debridement, and the appropriate use of antibiotics are also part of the cornerstone of treatment. It has been proposed that one of the keys to achieving high salvage rates following bypass is the quality of perioperative wound care and the timing or selection of soft tissue coverage

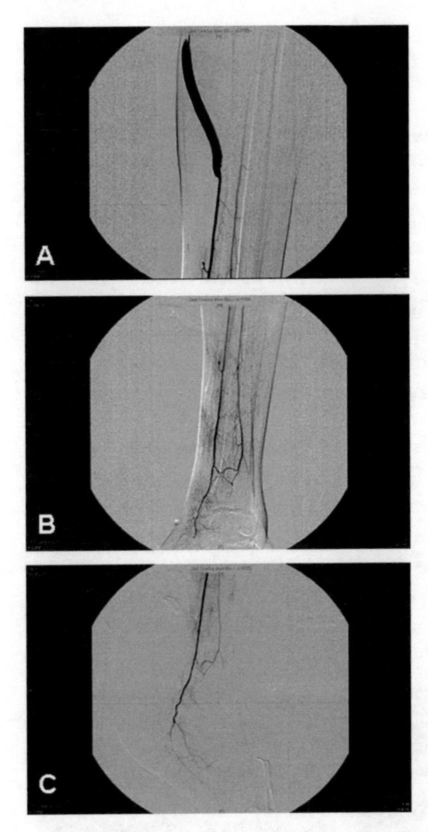

Figure 1 Completion on table arteriogram (**A**). The distal anastomosis is to the left posterior tibial artery (**B** and **C**). The run-off to the left foot also showing filling of the left peroneal artery through collaterals.

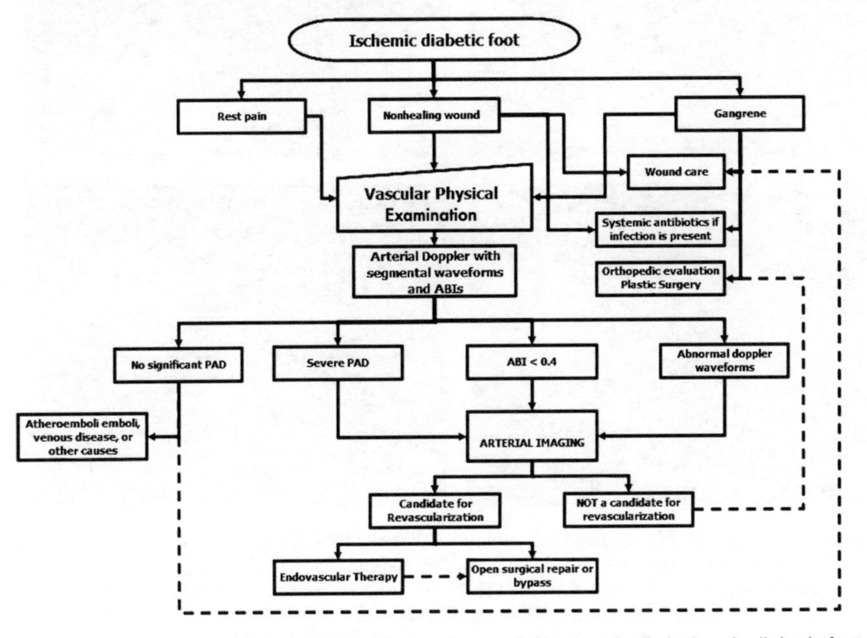

Figure 2 Algorithm for the evaluation and treatment of the chronically ischemic diabetic foot.

when needed (20). The authors involve infectious disease specialists to address the appropriate and targeted use of antibiotics. Orthopedic surgeons specializing in the foot and ankle are also involved to address the foot wounds and determine the extent of necessary wound care, debridements, and even amputations (Fig. 2). The authors also seek the input from reconstructive plastic surgeons to address the needs for wound coverage and reconstruction as the needs arise. In general, wounds achieve closure with simple primary closure techniques, wound vacuum assisted closure (V.A.C.) (KCI Medical, San Antonio, Texas), skin grafts, or local flaps (20) (Fig. 3). In the outpatient setting, close follow-up and evaluation by a podiatrist helps ensure proper foot examinations, footwear, and the care of the diabetic foot.

According to the authors, patients with diabetes present with four characteristic distributions of disease (Fig. 4). The first common presentation involves proximal disease involving the iliac and proximal femoral vessels, sparing the profunda or deep femoral artery. The second common presentation involves multiple foci of calcific obstructive disease in the superficial femoral artery and popliteal or infrapopliteal vessels. This is often amenable to endovascular techniques. The third common presentation involves diffuse disease of the

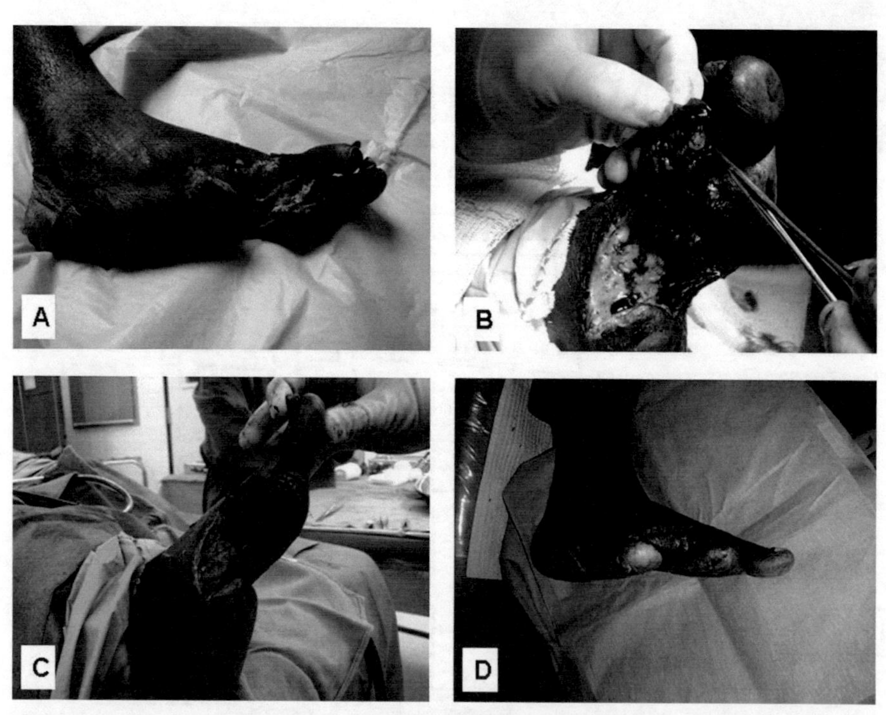

Figure 3 Multidisciplinary approach to salvage a diabetic foot with a large nonhealing wound. (**A**) The patient had undergone initial femoral-tibial bypass by vascular surgeons followed by amputation of necrotic and infected tissues by orthopedic surgeons. (**B**) Sharp debridement of the wound bed in preparation for tissue flap and skin graft reconstruction by plastic surgeons. (**C**) Mobilized tissue flap with partial wound coverage (**D**) Covered and healed wound following skin grafting.

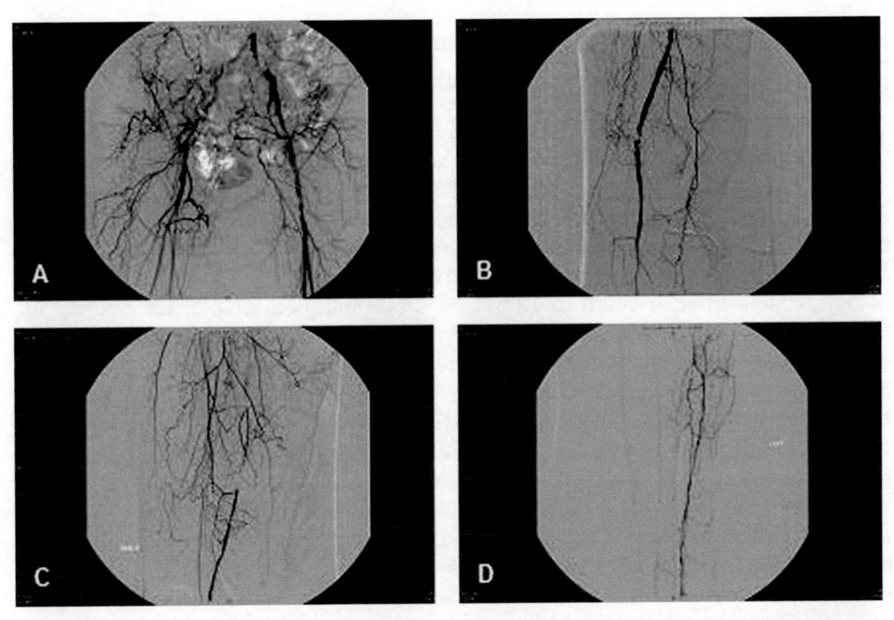

Figure 4 General arterial disease distribution in diabetics. (**A**) Proximal disease involving the iliac and proximal femoral vessels, sparing the profunda or deep femoral artery. (**B**) Focal calcific obstructive disease in the right popliteal artery. (**C**) Diffuse disease of the right superficial femoral artery. (**D**) Diffuse disease of their infrapopliteal vessels with occlusion of the posterior tibial artery, severe disease of the peroneal artery, a diseased but patent left anterior tibial artery.

superficial femoral artery extending into the popliteal artery, which could well progress or present as complete vessel occlusion. The fourth common presentation involves, more characteristically, diabetic patients with diffuse disease of their infrapopliteal vessels that include the anterior tibial, posterior tibial, and peroneal arteries. The latter artery often remains patent distally despite disease or occlusion of the other two infrapopliteal vessels. Revascularization to the distal third of the peroneal artery is an important target that can achieve adequate bypass patency and limb salvage rates (21).

AUTOGENOUS VENOUS CONDUITS FOR BYPASS

The use of autogenous vein has characteristically been the most favored conduit for bypass. Some authors have advocated the preferential use of in situ greater saphenous vein (GSV). Harris and associates (22) used in situ GSV in 71 patients for limb salvage. The patency rate at 1 year was 80% when the anastomosis was done to the popliteal artery and 75% when done to the infrapopliteal vessel. Limb salvage at 1 year was 91%. In a study of 440 consecutive in situ GSV bypasses, Donaldson and colleagues (23) achieved a primary revised patency (revised while still functioning) of 78% and limb salvage of 88% at 5 years. Eighteen grafts were identified during surveillance and revised while still patent. The presence of diabetes in 38% of patients did not diminish graft patency.

The use of autogenous reversed veins can be performed by using a variety of techniques, including the use of arm veins, lesser saphenous veins, and spliced veins. In a report by Taylor and associates (24), 110 bypasses were performed by using reversed autogenous veins, and they achieved a primary patency of 90%, 85%, and 85% at 1, 3, and 5 years, respectively. Limb salvage at 5 years was 93%. In this report, 55% of patients had diabetes. Similarly, Davidson and Callis (25) reported 75 bypasses for arterial reconstruction of the foot and ankle. A total of 77% of patients had diabetes, 56% had gangrene, 28% had nonhealing ulceration, and 16% had rest pain. Davidson and Callis (25) used in situ GSV, reversed GSV (RGSV), lesser saphenous vein, and arm vein for reconstruction. The recipient vessel or target artery was the dorsalis pedis in 57%, posterior tibial in 24%, distal anterior tibial in 12%, and distal peroneal or plantar arteries in the remainder. Their cumulative primary patency, secondary patency, and limb salvage rates were 79%, 82%, and 88%, respectively, at 36 months. Rosenbloom and colleagues (26) retrospectively reviewed a series of 49 bypasses performed in patients in whom three-fourths had tissue loss. The primary patency rates were 83%, 62%, and 41% at 1, 3, and 5 years, respectively. Sixty-nine percent of limbs were salvaged. In a randomized study by Schulman and coauthors (27), superficial femoropopliteal vein (SFPV) and RGSV were compared for primary femoropopliteal bypass. Forty-five percent of the patients who received RGSV had diabetes with critical limb ischemia, compared with 63% with SFPV. The primary patency at 3 years was 60% for RGSV recipients and was 64% for those with SFPV. Secondary patency rates were also similar. However, the use of deep veins or SFPV has been associated with an increase of venous stasis and edema (28). Edwards and Wright (29) described the use of RGSV in 97 bypasses to the posterior tibial, peroneal, or anterior tibial arteries. The authors reported a 72% primary patency rate at 1 year. Of interest, there were 11 cases of perioperative in-hospital failures underscoring the technical complexities of reconstruction even in the face of high-quality preoperative angiograms for the selection of target vessels to receive the bypass.

POLYTETRAFLUOROETHYLENE CONDUITS FOR BYPASS

There are a group of patients in whom autogenous vein is not available or is not adequate. Other patients may have severe comorbid conditions in whom an expeditious operation that avoids the time and trauma of harvesting vein may be of benefit. Last, surgeon preference or judgment may be another consideration to use a conduit other than a vein. Polytetrafluoroethylene (PTFE) grafts are commonly used prosthetic materials for peripheral bypass. Eagleton and associates (30) performed 74 femoral to infrapopliteal bypass with expanded PTFE for limb salvage. The primary patency, assisted primary patency, and secondary patency rates at 24 months were 40% ± 10%, 48% ± 11%, and 52% ± 11%, respectively. Limb salvage was successful in 62% ± 10% cases. Forty-six percent of bypasses were performed with a distal arteriovenous fistula, 35% with an end-to-side distal anastomosis, and 19% with a vein patch distal anastomosis.

The creation of a distal arteriovenous fistula is an attempt to improve graft patency results of prosthetic bypasses to infrapopliteal arteries. Ascer and colleagues (31) performed this technique with an adjunct vein interposition graft at the distal anastomosis to improve compliance mismatch. Their cumulative 3-year assisted primary patency was between 62% and 78%. The 3-year limb salvage rate was 78%. Of interest, all patients received heparin anticoagulation postoperatively and were continued on chronic anticoagulation.

In contrast to these results, others have demonstrated that creation of an arteriovenous fistula at the distal anastomotic site of a tibial bypass augments flow only in the postoperative period without the added effectiveness or graft patency (32).

The interposition of a venous segment at the distal anastomosis has been advocated to improve the results of prosthetic grafts to tibial arteries. Neville and associates (33) treated 79 patients with a PTFE bypass graft with a distal vein interposition patch. Half of the patients had tissue loss and the other had rest pain. Fifty-three percent had diabetes. The peroneal artery was the most common distal target. The 4-year primary patency and limb salvage rates were 63% ± 10.6% and 79% ± 8.5%, respectively. The authors concluded that the technique of interposition vein patch at the distal anastomosis of the tibial arteries has an acceptable long-term patency and limb salvage rate. In a multicenter randomized study designed to examine the effect of a Miller vein cuff at the distal anastomosis of femoral to above- or below-knee popliteal artery PTFE bypasses, 120 patients received a Miller cuff and 115 did not. The cumulative 5-year patency rate for above-knee bypasses with or without a Miller cuff was similar. However, the cumulative 3-year patency rate for below-knee bypasses with a Miller cuff was significantly better compared with noncuffed bypasses (34).

The patency of expanded PTFE (ePTFE) as a femoropopliteal bypass alternative was evaluated in a prospective randomized trial that compared it with GSV. Forty-nine patients with occlusion of the superficial femoral artery and limb-threatening ischemia were enrolled. At 54-month follow-up, the patency rate for the expanded PTFE group was 37% as compared with 70% for patients who had GSV. This study concluded that GSV is far superior to PTFE (35). In a study by Bergan and colleagues (36), 446 femoral distal reconstructions were performed. Patients were divided into groups depending on whether the distal insertion site was the popliteal or infrapopliteal artery; the patient received a randomized vein or PTFE graft, or an obligatory PTFE graft. The 30-month patency for randomized GSV bypass to infrapopliteal arteries was significantly better than the patency of randomized or obligatory PTFE graft to the same level (36). In another study, PTFE was used only when GSV was unsuitable or unavailable. The cumulative patency rate at 30 months was similar at 54% for GSV and 45% for PTFE. The authors concluded that PTFE is a suitable alternative when GSV is unavailable (37).

The Gore Propaten (W.L. GORE & Associates, Flagstaff, Arizona) vascular graft is an ePTFE with heparin covalently bonded to its luminal surface, which is designed to impart thromboresistant properties to the graft conduit for a period of 12 weeks (38). In a prospective nonrandomized study using heparin-bonded ePTFE, 55 above-knee and 44 below-knee bypasses were performed with an overall 1-year primary and secondary patency rates of 82% and 97%, respectively. The primary patency rate for the infrapopliteal bypass subgroup was the lowest at 74%. Twenty-eight percent of patients had diabetes, and approximately half of patients had at least one adequate vessel runoff (39). In another study by Walluscheck and colleagues (40), 43 patients were bypassed using the heparin-bonded graft. The indication for bypass grafting was limb-threatening ischemia in 88% of the patients. The 2-year primary patency rate for above-knee bypass grafts was 68% and that for below knee bypasses was 81%. In contrast to these encouraging results, Battaglia and associates (41) compared 37 infragenicular bypass procedures using 6-mm ePTFE Propaten graft with 37 RGSV bypasses and found no significant difference in patency, suggesting that when autologous vein is not available, the Propaten graft represents a valid alternative for conduit (41,42).

CRYOPRESERVED HOMOGRAFT CONDUITS FOR BYPASS

Cryopreserved saphenous vein homografts have served as an alternative for femoral distal bypass conduits when adequate autologous vein is not available. Reasons for reduced patency of cryopreserved vein grafts have been attributed to the destruction of the cellular components and fibrosis as a result of cryopreservation and also to poor distal runoffs in the treated patients (43). It is the authors' preference to use instead single or spliced superficial femoropopliteal artery homografts in patients with unsuitable veins and unavailable leg or arm veins and especially in patients with open distal foot wounds, gangrene, or evidence of infection. According to the authors, this conduit may obviate the potential risk of infection or colonization that can potentially occur with a PTFE conduit in this setting. The authors believe arterial homografts to be a viable alternative for revascularization in patients with diabetic foot wounds. However, it is clear that further studies and reports of long-term patency are necessary.

RISK FACTORS FOR BYPASS FAILURE

A stenosis of 20% proximal to the origin of the bypass posses a significant risk for graft failure (26). However, if these morphologic alterations can be corrected preoperatively or intraoperatively, a bypass can be performed with satisfactory patency (44). For instance, percutaneous angioplasty with or without stenting proximal to the intended origin of a bypass graft has proven as a useful strategy to secure the inflow and guarantee patency in selected patients with significant atherosclerotic disease and limited length of autogenous conduit. When a bypass is performed within 30 days of intervention, a 58% primary patency was achieved with a 70% limb salvage rate (28).

Vein diameters less than 3.5 mm and composite graft types have been associated with early graft failures (45). Therefore, performing a preoperative vein mapping by using ultrasound can assist in identifying the presence of adequate venous conduits whether in the legs or in the arms. Predictors of limb loss include early graft failure before 3 months, previous ipsilateral vascular procedure, and tobacco use (46). The importance of stressing smoking cessation to patients can not be emphasized enough.

The availability of adequate runoffs can help assure graft patency and success. However, the absence of runoff vessels in the foot should not be used to exclude patients from revascularization. Successful results can occur in the face of limited runoff (25). When comparing patients undergoing blind bypass with bypass with at least one patent outflow vessel, no differences in patency rates at 13 months were found; however, the limb salvage rate at 2 years in limbs with blind outflow was significantly worse than that in limbs with at least one outflow vessel (47).

Overt calcification of the recipient distal artery has been considered a poor prognostic factor for femoral distal artery bypass patency. In a study by Rubin and colleagues (48), 33 patients underwent 36 femoral distal tibial bypasses to calcified recipient artery. Eighty-six percent of the operations were performed by using in situ GSV. Limb salvage was achieved in 31 of 36 limbs. The authors concluded that femoral distal bypass can be successfully accomplished even in the presence of overt calcific arterial disease.

ORIGIN OF THE ARTERIAL INFLOW

The use of inflow sources distal to the common femoral artery (CFA) for bypass to infrapopliteal arteries is usually a compromise measure when the length of the autologous vein is not enough. Ballotta and associates (49) randomized 80 patients with inflow arising from the CFA and 80 patients with inflow arising distal to the CFA. Gangrene as an indication for surgery was more frequent in the first group, and nonhealing ulcer or rest pain were more common in the latter. Patency and limb salvage were similar for both groups at 1-, 3-, and 5-year follow-up. Of interest, the authors noted that in selected patients, procedures arising distal to the CFA required fewer graft revision to maintain patency of failing grafts. Similarly, other authors have shown equal patency rates for infrapopliteal bypasses originating from the CFA and those originating distal to it (50).

The viability of popliteal-to-distal artery bypass for limb salvage has been documented. Wengerter and colleagues (51) performed 153 popliteal-to-distal artery bypasses over a 12-year period. Limb salvage was the indication for all procedures, and 87% of the patients had diabetes. The primary and secondary 5-year patency rates were 55% and 60%, respectively. The authors pointed out that when a stenosis of 35% to 53% developed proximal to the origin of the bypass, this adversely affected its 2-year patency. The authors used percutaneous transluminal angioplasty to treat stenoses and improve overall graft patency. In a similar study, Galaria and associates (46) performed 92 popliteal–distal bypasses for chronic limb ischemia in 86% of patients and followed them for 5 years. Cumulative patency rates were 74% at 6 months, 70% at 2 years, and 63% at 5 years. In their report, limb salvage rates paralleled patency rates.

Quinones-Baldrich and associates (52) reported results of 46 bypass grafts to tibial arteries distal to the ankle, with various inflow origins. The CFA was the inflow in 11%, the popliteal artery in 54%, and the mid-tibial arteries in 35% cases. All patients had gangrene or nonhealing foot wounds, and 80% had diabetes. All reconstructions were performed with autologous GSV in situ, reversed, or nonreversed. The overall 2-year patency rate was 72%, and the limb salvage rate was 89%. No significant differences were noted when comparing the site of origin of the bypass.

Sequential femoropopliteal to tibial artery bypass has been recommended for the treatment of lower limb ischemia in patients with multisegmental arterial disease. The preservation of proximal graft patency after distal segmental occlusion and the augmentation of the outflow runoff (53,54) have been suggested as potential benefits of such technique. Flinn and associates (55) performed sequential femoropopliteal to tibial artery bypass in which half the patients had either distal ulceration or gangrene. A salvage rate was achieved in 76% of patients.

POTENTIAL COMPLICATIONS

Patients with diabetes often have other associated comorbidities, such as coronary artery disease, renal insufficiency, and hypertension among others. This places them at a high operative morbidity and mortality. Addressing and optimizing those risks factor preoperatively is advantageous. However, survival rates for this patient population vary between 65% at 5 years (28) and 24% at 6 years (26). Patency rates have been already discussed, and as such, graft failure or occlusion can occur either in the immediate postoperative period as a result of poor inflow or outflow vessel selection, poor conduit, technical errors, and even hypercoagulable states. When bypasses fail, amputations are not necessary the norm but a more likely occurrence. However, amputation of a part of a distal limb even in the face of a functioning bypass is not inevitable. Control of the wound bed down to viable tissue is necessary to achieve healing and avoid persistent infection.

Wound infections need to be addressed immediately because they can compromise the integrity of the bypass reconstruction. Aggressive wound management with control of infection is necessary. Lymphatic leaks especially after redo reconstruction in the groin can lead to increased morbidity. Often these resolve spontaneously with drainage; however, when persistent, wound reexploration with ligation of the lymphatic leak or muscle flap coverage with wide drainage may be necessary.

Postreconstructive edema can develop independently of postoperative hyperemia or disturbances in venous outflow. The severity and duration of edema has been reported to correlate with the degree and duration of the postoperative hyperemia. However, Eickhoff and Engell (54) have concluded that postbypass edema is a result of lymphedema due to surgical trauma rather than the result of microvascular derangement. Leg elevation and light compression therapy can achieve improvement in symptoms.

BYPASS GRAFT SURVEILLANCE

Early bypass graft failure within 30 days is usually due to technical error, poor arterial inflow, inadequate distal runoff, hypotension, or hypercoagulable conditions. Yet, there is a growing awareness that postoperative graft surveillance can detect early signs of failure that can be addressed by either endovascular or open interventions.

A graft at risk of failure is defined as having a peak systolic flow velocity less than 45 cm/sec (Fig. 5). The ratio of the peak systolic velocity at the site of a stenosis or lesion (PSVS) to the peak systolic velocity proximal to it at an area of normal conduit (PSVN) can help define the degree of stenosis. A ratio of PSVS to PSVN of 2, 3, and 4 correlate with a less than 50% stenosis, 50% to 75% stenosis, and more than 75% stenosis, respectively. During surveillance duplex examination, any irregularities such as inflow/outflow problems, graft dilatation, or arteriovenous fistula are also sought.

The initial duplex graft examination is performed 4 weeks after the surgical scars have healed. This time allows for a decrease in tissue edema and better visualization of the bypass conduit especially of the proximal and distal anastomoses. Thereafter, continued graft surveillance examinations are performed at 3, 6, and 12 months. For those grafts that have remained patent over 1 year, surveillance is performed at every 6-month interval. However, if a patient develops clinical signs of a failing graft, such as onset of disabling claudication, ischemic pain, ischemic ulcers, or a decrease in ankle brachial index, the duplex examination graft surveillance is performed much sooner. In general, the overall length and frequency of follow-up examinations remain largely unknown.

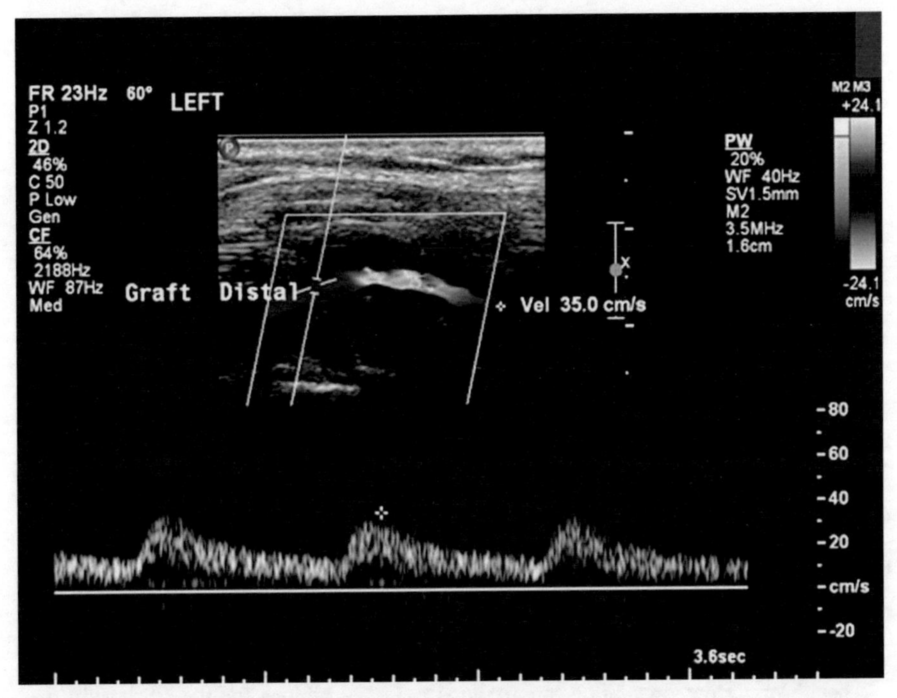

Figure 5 Graft surveillance duplex ultrasound examination showing a failing graft a peak systolic flow velocity proximal to a distal anastomotic stricture of 35 cm/sec.

CONCLUSIONS

Diabetic patients are a group with peripheral arterial disease and high risk for foot wound complications and limb loss even in the face of proper preventive measures. A multidisciplinary approach is necessary to evaluate these patients once these complications occur. An aggressive approach to wound management and revascularization is necessary to achieve limb salvage or prevent further limb loss. The choice of conduit for bypass is determined by the availability of autogenous vein. When arm or leg veins are not available, the use of PTFE or homograft provides an adequate alternative.

REFERENCES

1. Centers for Disease Control and Prevention. National Diabetes Fact Sheet: General Information and National Estimates on Diabetes in the United States, 2005. Atlanta, GA: U.S. Department of Health and Human Services, Centers for Disease Control and Prevention, 2005.
2. Coffey JT, Brandle M, Zhou H, et al. Valuing health-related quality of life in diabetes. Diabetes Care 2002; 25:2238–2243.
3. Ramsey SC, Newton K, Blough D, et al. Incidence, outcomes, and costs of foot ulcers in patients with diabetes. Diabetes Care 1999; 22:382–387.
4. Tockl K, Tafesse E, Vanderplas A, et al. Costs of lower-extremity ulcers among patients with diabetes. Diabetes Care 2004; 27:2129–2134.
5. Criqui MH, Denenberg JO, Langer RD, et al. The epidemiology of peripheral arterial disease: Importance of identifying the population at risk. Vasc Med 1997; 2:221–226.

6. Meijer WT, Hoes AW, Rutgers D, et al. Peripheral arterial disease in the elderly: The Rotterdam Study. Arterioscler Thromb Vasc Biol 1998; 18:185–192.
7. Newman AB, Siscovick DS, Manolio TA, et al. Ankle-arm index as a marker of atherosclerosis in the Cardiovascular Health Study: Cardiovascular Heart Study (CHS) Collaborative Research Group. Circulation 1993; 88:837–845.
8. Hiatt WR, Hoag S, Hamman RF. Effect of diagnostic criteria on the prevalence of peripheral arterial disease: The San Luis Valley Diabetes Study. Circulation 1995; 91:1472–1479.
9. Beks PJ, Mackaay AJ, de Neeling JN, et al. Peripheral arterial disease in relation to glycemic level in an elderly Caucasian population: The Hoorn study. Diabetologia 1995; 38:86–96.
10. Kannel WB, McGee DL. Update on some epidemiologic features of intermittent claudication: The Framingham Study. J Am Geriatr Soc 1985; 33:13–18.
11. Katsilambros NL, Tsapogas PC, Arvanitis MP, et al. Risk factors for lower extremity arterial disease in non–insulin-dependent diabetic persons. Diabet Med 1996; 13: 243–246.
12. Bowers BL, Valentine RJ, Myers SI, et al. The natural history of patients with claudication with toe pressures of 40 mm Hg or less. J Vasc Surg 1993; 18:506–511.
13. McDaniel MD, Cronenwett JL. Basic data related to the natural history of intermittent claudication. Ann Vasc Surg 1989; 3:273–277.
14. Dormandy JA, Murray GD. The fate of the claudicant—A prospective study of 1969 claudicants. Eur J Vasc Surg 1991; 5:131–133.
15. Most RS, Sinnock P. The epidemiology of lower extremity amputations in diabetic individuals. Diabetes Care 1983; 6:87–91.
16. Rogers LC, Lavery LA, Armstrong DG. The right to bear legs—An amendment to healthcare: How preventing amputations can save billions for the US health-care system. J Am Podiatr Med Assoc 2008; 98(2):166–168.
17. Harrington C, Zagari MJ, Corea J, et al. A cost analysis of diabetic lower-extremity ulcers. Diabetes Care 2000; 23:1333–1338.
18. Stockl K, Tafesse E, Vanderplas A, et al. Costs of lower extremity ulcers among patients with diabetes. Diabetes Care 2004; 27:2129–2134.
19. Ricco JB, Pearce WH, Yao JST, et al. The use of operative prebypass arteriography and Doppler ultrasound recordings to select patients for extended femoro-distal bypass. Ann Surg 1983; 198(5):646–653.
20. Attinger CE, Ducic I, Neville RF, et al. The relative roles of aggressive wound care versus revascularization in salvage of the threatened lower extremity in the renal failure diabetic patient. Plast Reconstr Surg 2002; 109(4):1281–1290.
21. Ballotta E, Da Giau G, Gruppo M, et al. Infrapopliteal arterial revascularization for critical limb ischemia: Is the peroneal artery at the distal third a suitable outflow vessel? J Vasc Surg 2008; 47(5):952–959.
22. Harris RW, Andros G, Dulawa LB, et al. The transition to "in situ" vein bypass grafts. Surg Gynecol Obstet 1986; 163(1):21–28.
23. Donaldson MC, Mannick JA, Whittemore AD. Femoral-distal bypass with in situ greater saphenous vein. Ann Surg 1991; 213(5):457–464.
24. Taylor LM, Edwards JM, Porter JM, et al. Reversed vein bypass to infrapopliteal arteries—Modern results are superior to or equivalent to in situ bypass for patency and for vein utilization. Ann Surg 1987; 205(1):90–97.
25. Davidson JT, Callis JT. Arterial reconstruction of vessels in the foot and ankle. Ann Surg 1993; 217(6):699–710.
26. Rosenbloom MS, Walsh JJ, Schuler JJ, et al. Long-term results of infragenicular bypasses with autogenous vein originating from the distal superficial femoral and popliteal arteries. J Vasc Surg 1988; 7(5):691–696.
27. Schulman ML, Badhey MR, Yatco R. Superficial femoral-popliteal veins and reversed saphenous veins as primary femoropopliteal bypass grafts: A randomized comparative study. J Vasc Surg 1987; 6(1):1–10.

28. Coburn M, Ashworth C, Francis W, et al. Venous stasis complications of the use of the superficial femoral and popliteal veins for lower extremity bypass. J Vasc Surg 1993; 17(6):1005–1009.
29. Edwards WH, Wright RS. Tibial and peroneal bypass in severe occlusive disease of the lower extremities. Ann Surg 1976; 183(6):710–718.
30. Eagleton MJ, Ouriel K, Shortell C, et al. Femoral-infrapopliteal bypass with prosthetic grafts. Surgery 1999; 126(4):759–765.
31. Ascer E, Gennaro M, Pollina RM, et al. Complementary distal arteriovenous fistula and deep vein interposition: A five year experience with a new technique to improve infrapopliteal prosthetic bypass patency. J Vasc Surg 1996; 249(1):134–143.
32. Snyder So, Wheeler JR, Gregory RT, et al. Failure of arteriovenous fistulas at distal tibial bypass anastomotic sites. J Cardiovasc Surg (Torino) 1985; 26(2):137–142.
33. Neville RF, Tempesta B, Sidway AN. Tibial bypass for limb salvage using polytetrafluoroethylene and a distal vein patch. J Vasc Surg 2001; 33(2):266–271.
34. Griffiths GD, Nagy J, Black D, et al. Randomized clinical trial of distal anastomotic interposition vein cuff in infrainguinal polytetrafluoroethylene bypass grafting. Br J Surg 2004; 91(5):560–562.
35. Tilanus HW, Obertop H, Van Urk H. Saphenous vein or PTFE for femoropopliteal bypass—A prospective randomized trial. Ann Surg 1985; 202(6):780–782.
36. Bergan JJ, Veith FJ, Bernhard VM, et al. Randomization of autogenous vein and polytetrafluoroethylene graft in femoral-distal reconstruction. Surgery 1982; 92(6): 921–930.
37. Hobson RW, O'Donnell JA, Jamil Z, et al. Below-knee bypass for limb salvage: Comparison of autogenous saphenous vein, polytetrafluoroethylene, and composite Dacron-autogenous vein grafts. Arch Surg 1980; 115(7):833–837.
38. Begovac PC, Thomson RC, Fisher JL, et al. Improvements in GORE-TEX vascular graft performance by Carmeda bioactive surface heparin immobilization. Eur J Vasc Endovasc Surg 2003; 25(5):432–437.
39. Bosiers N, Deloose K, Verbist J, et al. Heparin-bonded expanded polytetrafluoroethylene vascular graft for femoropopliteal and femorocrural bypass grafting: 1-year results. J Vasc Surg 2006; 43:313–319.
40. Walluscheck KP, Beirkandt S, Brandt M, et al. Infrainguinal ePTFE vascular graft with bioactive surface heparin bonding: First clinical results. J Cardiovasc Surg (Torino) 2005; 46(4):425–430.
41. Battaglia G, Tringale R, Monaca V. Retrospective comparison of a heparin bonded ePTFE graft and saphenous vein infragenicular bypass: Implications for standard treatment protocol. J Cardiovasc Surg (Torino) 2006; 47(1):41–47.
42. Peeters P, Verbist J, Deloose K, et al. Results with heparin bonded polytetrafluoroethylene grafts for femorodistal bypasses. J Cardiovasc Surg (Torino) 2006; 47(4):407–413.
43. Sellke FW, Meng RL, Rossi NP. Cryopreserved saphenous vein homografts for femoral-distal vascular reconstruction. J Cardiovasc Surg (Torino) 1989; 30(5):838–842.
44. Probst H, Saucy F, Dusmet M, et al. Clinical results of autologous infrainguinal revascularization using grafts originating distal to the femoral bifurcation in patients with mild inflow disease. J Cardiovasc Surg (Torino) 2006; 47(4):437–443.
45. Schanzer A, Hevelone N, Owens CD, et al. Technical factors affecting autogenous vein graft failure: Observations from a large multicenter trial. J Vasc Surg 2007; 46(6): 1180–1190.
46. Galaria II, Surowiec SC, Tanski WJ, et al. Popliteal-to-distal bypass: Identifying risk factors associated with limb loss and graft failure. Vasc Endovascular Surg 2005; 39(5):393–400.
47. Desai, TR, Meyerson SL, Skelly CL, et al. Patency and limb salvage after infrainguinal bypass with severely compromised ("blind") outflow. Arch Surg 2001; 136(6):635–642.
48. Rubin JR, Persky J, Lukens MC, et al. Femoral-tibial bypass for calcific arterial disease. Am J Surg 1989; 158(2):146–150.
49. Ballotta E, Renon L, De Rossi A, et al. Prospective randomized study on reversed saphenous vein infrapopliteal bypass to treat limb-threatening ischemia: Common

femoral artery versus superficial femoral or popliteal and tibial arteries inflow. J Vasc Surg 2004; 40(4):732–740.

50. Veith F, Gupta SK, Samson RH, et al. Superficial femoral and popliteal arteries as inflow sites for distal bypasses. Surgery 1981; 90(6):980–990.
51. Wengerter KR, Yang PM, Veith FJ, et al. A twelve-year experience with the popliteal-to-distal artery bypass: The significance and management of proximal disease. J Vasc Surg 1992; 15(1):143–151.
52. Quinones-Baldrich WJ, Colburn MD, Ahn SS, et al. Very distal bypass for salvage of the severely ischemic extremity. Am J Surg 1993; 166(2):117–123.
53. Jarrett F, Berkoff HA, Crummy AB. Sequential femoral-tibial bypass grafting for limb salvage. Ann Surg 1978; 188(5):685–688.
54. Eickhoff JH, Engell HC. Local regulation of blood flow and the occurrence of edema after arterial reconstruction of the lower limbs. Ann Surg 1982; 195(4):474–478.
55. Flinn WR, Flanigan DP, Verta MJ, et al. Sequential femoral-tibial bypass for severe limb ischemia. Surgery 1980; 88(3):357–365.

5 Diabetic neuropathy and the lower extremity

Nicolaas C. Schaper and Hans H. Savelberg

INTRODUCTION

Diabetic foot ulcers pose a great burden to both the patient and the health care system. These ulcers have a poor tendency to heal and can result in infection and gangrene, leading to long-term in-hospital treatment and/or amputation (1). Foot ulcers have major negative effects on the quality of life due to morbidity, loss of work, loss of mobility, and reduction of social activities (2). As summarized by Boulton (3), the commonest component causes in the pathway to ulceration include diabetic neuropathy, foot deformity, external trauma, peripheral vascular disease, and peripheral edema. The vast majority of patients with a diabetic foot ulcer will have signs of sensory loss in their feet, although sensation can be present in some patients with pure ischemic foot ulcers (4). Because of the loss of protective sensation, acute trauma or chronic repetitive biomechanical stress caused by elevated foot pressures and/or ill-fitting shoes are perceived less well, and finally an ulcer develops (3,5). In addition, in most patients, foot ulceration is a sign of multiple and extensive changes that occur in the lower extremity as a consequence of diabetes. These changes include loss of normal anatomic integrity, loss of function, impaired tissue perfusion, and enhanced susceptibility to tissue damage and infection (6). In many patients, these processes develop with signs or symptoms that are not easily recognized by the patient and the health care workers involved. Moreover, many of the underlying pathologies are not limited to the foot but are a sign of widespread disease. In this chapter, current views on the clinical presentation, epidemiology, pathogenesis of diabetic neuropathy, and its consequences for the lower extremity have been summarized .

THE DEFINITION AND EPIDEMIOLOGY OF DIABETIC NEUROPATHY

Distal (or peripheral) polyneuropathy is characterized by a chronic and slowly progressive sensory-motor loss in both legs. *Clinical neuropathy* can be defined as "the presence of symptoms and/or signs of peripheral nerve dysfunction in people with diabetes after exclusion of other causes." Clinical neuropathy can be further subdivided as painful and painless neuropathies. *Subclinical neuropathy* refers to patients without demonstrable signs or symptoms and can be detected with diagnostic procedures such as electrophysiological or (semi-) quantitative sensory tests (7). Diabetic neuropathy can also be classified into large fiber and small fiber neuropathy. Large fiber damage results in slowing of nerve conduction and is characterized by symptoms and signs such as paresthesia, impairment of sensation, joint position, touch and pressure sensations, loss of muscle strength, and loss of ankle reflexes. Small fiber neuropathy, on the other hand, is characterized by symptoms such as burning or stabbing pain, impaired temperature

Table 1 Diagnostic Tools in Diagnosing Distal Neuropathy

Clinical symptoms
Clinical signs
Electrophysiological procedures
Quantitative sensory testing
Symptoms, signs and tests for autonomic neuropathy

sensation, and autonomic neuropathy (8). In Table 1, the diagnostic strategies are summarized that can be used to define distal neuropathy. Neuropathy is frequently accompanied by distal autonomic neuropathy, which leads to diminished sweat secretion and increased thermoregulatory shunt blood flow, resulting in a dry and warm foot (3).

Unfortunately, there is no gold standard to diagnose distal neuropathy. As summarized in a report by the American Academy of Neurology in 2006, the highest likelihood of neuropathy occurs with a combination of multiple symptoms, multiple signs, and abnormal electrophysiological studies. In epidemiological studies, there is a modest likelihood of neuropathy when it is diagnosed by a combination of multiple symptoms and multiple signs (9). Unfortunately, most epidemiological studies in diabetes have used different definitions and diagnostic criteria in different patient populations. Data on the prevalence of neuropathy in unselected groups of diabetic patients are therefore relatively scarce, but ranges between 13% and 45% have been reported in population-based studies. In study of U.K. patients by Kumar et al. (10), approximately 40% of patients with type 2 diabetes and a mean age of 65 years had clinical neuropathy. Interestingly, less than half of these patients reported neuropathic symptoms (10). In another large U.K. study, in patients with both type 1 and 2 diabetes and a mean age of 61 years, the prevalence of neuropathy was 22% (11). Cabezas-Cerrato reported a prevalence of 21% in primary care, and an Australian study found a prevalence of 13% in patients with known diabetes in the general population (12, 12a). Data on the incidence of neuropathy are even scarcer; in one prospective study, new neuropathy developed in 33.5 % of the patients 10 years after the diagnosis of type 2 diabetes (13). In type 1 diabetes, the large-scale EURODIAB study found a prevalence rate of 28% and a 7-year incidence of neuropathy of 23.5% (14,15).

In summary, approximately one in four of each diabetic patient will have clinical neuropathy; in the elderly population, which is at particular risk for diabetic foot ulceration, almost one in two will have neuropathy. Many of these patients do not report symptoms spontaneously, but as discussed below, they frequently have complaints such as tiredness, dizziness, cramps, or pain that are not recognized by both the patient and health care worker as being related to the underlying neuropathy. Painful neuropathy is sometimes seen as a relatively rare complication of neuropathy, but recent studies suggest that it is more prevalent than perhaps previously thought. Two community-based studies report a prevalence of painful neuropathy as around 16% to 26%, and in one study, 80% of these people had moderate or severe pain (16,17). In one U.K. population-based study, almost 40% of people with painful neuropathy reported that they had never received any treatment and 12.5% had never reported their pain to their treating physician (16). Similar findings of inadequate treatment were seen in two more recent European and American studies (18,19).

Table 2 Risk Factors for Neuropathy

Level and duration of hyperglycemia
Age
Height
Male sex
Potential risk factors
Hypertension
Smoking
Dyslipidemia
Ethnicity

Diabetic neuropathy has several modifiable and nonmodifiable risk factors, which include age, male sex, height, the severity of hyperglycemia, the duration of diabetes, and perhaps ethnicity (as shown in Table 2) (7). Moreover, neuropathy is closely associated with other microvascular complications such as microalbuminuria and retinopathy, suggesting a common underlying pathogenetic mechanism. Longer axons are thought to be more prone to the toxic effects of hyperglycemia, which could explain the association between the height and neuropathy (20). In addition, differences in height might contribute to the higher prevalence of neuropathy in men than in women.

In the Diabetes Control and Complications Trial (DCCT), intensive insulin therapy in patients with type 1 diabetes resulted in a marked reduction of neuropathy, stressing the importance hyperglycemia. After 5 years, 5% of the intensive therapy group had neuropathy compared with 13% of the conventional therapy group, a reduction of 64% (21). In contrast, tight glycemic control was only marginally effective in preventing neuropathy in the type 2 patients of the United Kingdom Prospective Diabetes Study (22). However, the differences between these two studies could be related to differences in diagnostic procedures and/or the degree of metabolic control. Recent studies also suggest that cardiovascular risk factors, such as hypertension, low level of high-density lipoprotein cholesterol, body mass index, and smoking, could also be risk factors for neuropathy (15,23–25). Interestingly, intensive multifactorial treatment in patients with type 2 diabetes and microalbuminuria resulted in a reduced risk for the development of autonomic neuropathy (odds ratio, 0.32) (26). Moreover, also a lifestyle intervention in patients with impaired glucose tolerance and painful neuropathy resulted in a reduction in symptoms (27). These data suggest that in addition to hyperglycemia, diabetic neuropathy could be associated with several other modifiable risk factors, which could open up new avenues for the development of more effective preventive or treatment strategies.

PATHOLOGY AND PATHOGENESIS

In biopsies of the sural nerve, diabetic peripheral neuropathy is characterized by axon loss, which is frequently patchy or multifocal, and usually both large and small fibers are involved (28). Other abnormalities include segmental demyelinization and multiple abnormalities in the nerve microvessels, such as basement membrane thickening, pericyte degeneration, endoneurial capillary closure, and thrombosis, suggesting that neural microangiopathy might play a role in the development of diabetic neuropathy (28,29). These alterations in the nerve microvasculature have several similarities to the changes that can be observed in the microvasculature of the retina in diabetic retinopathy. Already early in the course of type 2 diabetes, loss of intraepidermal nerve fibers (IENFs) can be observed in punch biopsies of the skin, which is an index of small fiber neuropathy (30). As reported by Malik and coworkers (31), small fiber abnormalities can also be detected in diabetic patients noninvasively with confocal microscopy of the cornea. In a subsequent study, the small fiber damage measured with confocal corneal microscopy was correlated with neuropathic symptoms, IENF abnormalities, and temperature detection thresholds, suggesting that this technique could be a useful clinical tool in diagnosing small fiber neuropathy (32).

The pathogenesis of diabetic neuropathy is complex and only partly unravelled. In summary, it is likely that because of the chronic hyperglycemia, several metabolic pathways are activated, which result in inflammation and increased oxidative stress in neurons and microvessels (33). These pathways include increased production of free radicals by the mitochondria, the production of advanced glycation end products, excessive flow of glucose through the polyol and hexosamine pathways, and activation of poly-ADP ribose polymerase and protein kinase C (28,33). Several of these pathways closely interact and augment each other, resulting in a further increase in oxidative stress and stimulation of inflammatory responses (34). In addition, cardiovascular risk factors, such as smoking, hypertension, and dyslipidemia, might further increase the oxidative stress in endoneurial microvessels (35). These abnormalities could result in both structural and functional changes in the nerve microvasculature, resulting in reduced nerve perfusion and endoneurial hypoxia (35). In many animal models of diabetic neuropathy, therapeutic interventions aimed at one or more of these pathways were successful in preventing or improving experimental diabetic neuropathy. Unfortunately, the translation of these concepts to diabetic patients is up to now largely unsuccessful, and currently there is no effective long-term treatment for diabetic neuropathy (7).

NEUROPATHY AND MOBILITY

Neuropathy is one of the major factors affecting mobility in diabetes. *Mobility* can be defined as the ability to move around independently; it involves the capacity to walk, to stand, and to change from sitting to standing. Moreover, one needs to apply these capabilities under different, often challenging conditions, such as walking on uneven or slippery surfaces. Mobility is a determinant of independence and self-care, and consequently, an important determinant of the quality of life. Gregg et al. (36) found in a community-based survey that 32% of the women and 15% of men with diabetes who where 60 years or older experienced major problems to walk one-fourth of a mile, climb a stairs, or do housework (36). In diabetic women 65 years or older, neuropathy, peripheral arterial disease (PAD), and depression were the main factors explaining this relation between diabetes and disability (37). Recently, we performed a community-based study on mobility in 100 patients with type 2 diabetes, who were asked to wear a validated pedometer for 1 week. Those with diabetes took around 6500 steps/day and after correction for other factors affecting mobility, patients with neuropathy took almost 30% steps/day less compared with patients without neuropathy (van Sloten T, unpublished data). These values resemble "sedentary lifestyle" and "low activity" and are considerably below the public health advice of 10,000 steps/day

(38). Several different factors, such as sensory impairment, muscle coordination, and muscle strength, are probably involved in the impaired mobility in patients with neuropathy, as discussed in the following paragraphs.

POSTURAL STABILITY AND GAIT

As summarized in a recent review by van Schie, several authors observed reduced postural stability in patients with diabetic neuropathy. Typically, patients with diabetic neuropathy have a slower walking speed and a greater step variability (39–42). Moreover, under challenging conditions, such as walking on an uneven surface or during low illumination, patients with diabetic neuropathy walk less stable (43,44). This impaired postural stability is probably the consequence of a loss of proprioception, such as muscle spindle function and other sensory modalities in the lower extremity (45–48). Clinically, this loss of sensory-motor feedback can be observed as a positive Romberg test, when closing eyes patients have difficulties in remaining in a stable standing position. Postural instability has a major impact on the quality of life and peripheral neuropathy as well as instability during walking are associated with a marked risk of falls (44,49) and, as recently shown by Vileikyte et al. (50), unsteadiness is an important predictor of depression in patients with diabetic neuropathy (50). In one small randomized study of 20 diabetic patients with neuropathy, a 3-week exercise program did improve balance, but further evidence for the efficacy of such interventions is scarce (51) and clearly there is a need for the development of interventions programs to improve balance and walking stability in diabetic patients with neuropathy.

MUSCLE FUNCTION AND STRENGTH

The effort of specific muscle groups involved in walking can be estimated by calculating net joint moments from information on ground reaction forces, accelerations of body segments, and inertial characteristics of the involved body segments. Two studies revealed that patients with diabetic neuropathy had a lower plantar flexion moment and, in one study, also had a reduced knee joint extension compared with healthy participants (52,53). However, these results were not confirmed in two other studies (54,55). A methodological problem with most of the aforementioned studies is that they did not standardize gait velocity, which is a major determinant of almost all gait parameters and doubtlessly affects joint moments and ground reaction forces. In a recent, velocity-controlled study, we found that patients with diabetic neuropathy displayed higher ankle plantar flexion moments during the first half of the stance phase and at the same time decreased knee joint extension moments (56). Although sometimes technically challenging, more research is needed on the dynamic aspects of gait to improve our understanding of the impact of neuropathy in diabetic patients.

Quantitative data on the effect of neuropathy on muscle volumes and strength have resulted in a clearer picture. Although clinically less apparent, quantitative measurements of muscle strength and magnetic resonance imaging (MRI) data indicate that distal neuropathy is associated with diminished muscle strength and atrophy in the foot and the lower leg (57–60). Two MRI studies found an approximately 50% to75% reduction of the volume of intrinsic foot muscles in diabetic patients with neuropathy compared with patients without neuropathy (61,62). Also a more proximal reduction of muscle mass in the lower limb has been reported. Andersen and coworkers (63) found that patients with diabetic neuropathy had 32% smaller plantar and dorsal flexors of the ankle joint compared with patients without neuropathy (63). Moreover, muscle strength was reduced by 41% in the neuropathic patients and the authors concluded that muscle atrophy was a major cause of the muscle weakness around the ankle joint. Andreassen and coworkers (64) concluded that this muscle weakness is a result of an increased rate of muscle wasting (64). Whereas control patients lost about 0.8% of their muscle strength of ankle plantar and dorsal flexors each year, muscle strength decreased by 3.2% per year in patients with symptomatic neuropathy, and this loss was related to the severity of neuropathy. Muscle weakness in diabetic neuropathy is not limited to distal lower limb muscles but extends—at a lower degree—to knee extensors and flexors and is also present in upper limb muscles (58).

ALTERED BIOMECHANICS OF THE FOOT

Loss of proprioception, altered gait, and impaired muscle function could contribute to an increase in plantar pressures during walking. Cross-sectional and prospective studies have shown that elevated peak plantar pressures can predict future ulceration in patients with diabetic neuropathy (65,66). Several mechanisms are probably involved in the development of altered biomechanics in the feet of patients with neuropathy. Changes in walking pattern could result in increased plantar pressures. In normal walking, the centre of pressure under the foot transfers gradually from the heel to the forefoot. Several authors found that in diabetic patients with neuropathy, the pressures under the forefoot are relatively increased compared with those under the heel and the forefoot-to-rear foot plantar pressure ratio predicted ulceration (67,68). One explanation of this early and prolonged loading of the forefoot could be a reduced capacity to control forward velocity at heel strike. Because of muscle weakness and/or an imbalance of the lower leg muscles, patients with neuropathy seem less capable of braking the foreword movement of their body during walking, resulting in a rise in forefoot pressures (56).Theoretically, loss of sensation could also contribute to the rise in plantar pressure. But in one study, a reduction of plantar sensation by intradermal injections of an anesthetic did not result in a rise of plantar pressures in healthy patients (69). Loss of proprioception might also contribute to an abnormal walking pattern with abnormal loading of the foot, but this remains to be further explored.

Elevated plantar pressures are usually observed in a limited subset of individuals with neuropathy, suggesting that additional factors besides neuropathy play a role (70). Moreover, in the aforementioned studies, plantar pressures were usually measured during barefoot walking using pressure-platforms, and it is debatable whether the laboratory conditions under which the measurements were performed allow generalization of these results to daily life. When in-shoe pressures were measured during daily life activities, Guldemond et al. (71) observed that patients with diabetic neuropathy, but without major deformities, had about 10% lower plantar pressures compared with diabetic patients without neuropathy. These lower pressures could have been caused by a slower walking speed in the neuropathic patients, but walking speed was not measured in this study (71). It is likely that, besides the functional abnormalities in the lower extremities, structural abnormities such as foot deformities can have a major impact on plantar pressures. Charcot disease of the foot, which in turn is closely related to neuropathy, can clearly result in mid-foot deformities with a marked increase in plantar pressure (72). Also claw and/or hammer toe deformities, reduced plantar soft tissue thickness, and limited joint mobility are associated with elevated forefoot pressures (73–75).These abnormalities seem to occur more frequently in patients with diabetic neuropathy, but the pathogenesis of these structural changes in the foot is not well understood (73). In conclusion, it is likely that in a subset of neuropathic patients, the combination of functional and structural abnormalities will result in an abnormal rise of plantar pressures. Moreover, the skin and underlying tissues are constantly at risk for excessive damage during loading of the foot, if in these patients protective sensation is also lost (76). However, our understanding of the factors that determine the loading of the foot during ambulation is limited, and in a recent study of plantar pressures in patients with neuropathy, a battery of clinical and radiological measures could explain only 39% of the variance in local forefoot plantar pressures (77).

NEUROPATHY AND TISSUE HOMEOSTASIS

Our feet and legs are the body parts most heavily used in service of support and mobility. To last a lifetime, the lower extremity must be able to cope with this biomechanical strain and to limit the tissue damage that occurs during periods of excessive biomechanical stress or after trauma. Several lines of evidence suggest that neuropathy not only contributes to impaired mobility and increased biomechanical stress on the foot but also impairs tissue responses to acute and chronic trauma. The peripheral nervous system is one of the key players in the coordinated control of tissue homeostasis and plays a major role in the integrated tissue responses to noxious stimuli (6). Afferent nerves can respond to a large range of stimuli and upon stimulation, neuropeptides are rapidly released in their microenvironment, and these nerves in the lower extremity are anatomically closely associated with various cell types of skin, bone, muscle, large and small blood vessels, and the immune system (78,79). Many of these cells express receptors for neuropeptides, and activation of these receptors can alter their function and can induce the release of a variety of mediators. As reviewed elsewhere, impaired communication of the various tissues of the lower extremity with the central nervous system and impaired cell-to-cell communication in the lower leg due to diabetic neuropathy are likely to result in abnormalities in structure and function of almost all of the lower extremity tissues (6). These abnormalities probably result in a much larger spectrum of disease than usually identified, including impaired control of local blood flow, enhanced bone resorption, and altered immune function, as summarized in the following paragraphs.

NEUROPATHY AND PAD

Peripheral arterial disease is a common finding in diabetic patients, with a prevalence of approximately 20% to 40% in patients with type 2 diabetes (80). Neuropathy could theoretically have profound effects on atherogenesis and vascular remodeling. Because of the loss of sympathetic tone, peripheral perfusion increases, thus resulting in an increase in shear stress in the arteries of the leg, contributing to endothelial activation. Neural control is also important in the regulation of smooth muscle cell growth and the large arteries of the leg are relatively richly innervated (81). This innervation probably contributes to keeping the vascular smooth muscle cells in a contractile phenotype. After chemical or surgical denervation, these cells dedifferentiate to a more synthetic phenotype, which produces growth factors, cytokines, and extracellular matrix (81). Interestingly, diabetic neuropathy, and specifically the presence of autonomic neuropathy, is associated with an increased risk of calcification of blood vessels of the lower extremity (82,83). In recent years, much has been learned about the process involved in arterial calcification, which is probably a sign of disrupted repair processes in the arterial wall and might render the vessel more susceptible to damage by cardiovascular risk factors (84). But the pathobiological processes that are responsible for the arterial calcification in patients with neuropathy remain to be further elucidated. It has been suggested that activation of the RANK-L/OPG signaling pathway might play an important role in both vascular calcification and the excessive bone resorption that can be observed in type 1 diabetic patients with neuropathy (85). Medial arterial calcification does not result in a decrease in diameter of the vessel wall and, therefore, does not obstruct local blood flow (86). However, it should be seen as a sign of generalized vascular disease, as lower extremity arterial calcification is associated with renal failure and coronary artery calcification; moreover, in prospective studies, it predicts early cardiac mortality (87–90). Calcification could also contribute to the loss of arterial elasticity in patients with neuropathy. In two studies, autonomic neuropathy was found to be associated with increased stiffness of both central and peripheral arteries, independent of classic risk factors (91,92). This loss of arterial elasticity will increase the hemodynamic burden on the heart, and as arterial stiffness predicts cardiovascular morbidity and mortality (93,94), changes in both functional and mechanical properties of the arterial vasculature could be one of the links between neuropathy and premature cardiovascular death (95).

In nondiabetic patients, PAD is usually diagnosed by the combination of typical complaints, clinical examination, and measurement of the ankle-brachial blood pressures. In diabetic patients, the clinical presentation of PAD can be different, which in part is probably due to the interaction of neuropathy and vascular disease in the lower extremity. In one cross-sectional PAD study, patients with diabetes less frequently reported classic symptoms such as claudication than did nondiabetic patients. However, the diabetic PAD patients did have poorer lower extremity functioning, which in part could be explained by the presence of neuropathy. The largest differences between diabetic and nondiabetic PAD patients were seen in measures of balance, walking endurance, and walking speed (96). Moreover, impaired tissue perfusion due to PAD in patients with neuropathy would further enhance tissue susceptibility to damage and would impair wound healing as well as local immunity. This combination of neuropathy and ischemia, which can be observed in approximately 50% of the patients with a foot ulcer, will put the patient at extra risk for a nonhealing ulcer or amputation (97). Diagnosing PAD in these patients is more complex, as medial arterial calcification can result in falsely elevated ankle and, probably, toe pressures (80). As reported in a study on the value of screening techniques to diagnose PAD, in patients without critical limb ischemia, diabetic neuropathy is associated with clinically relevant reductions in sensitivity and/or specificity of several diagnostic procedures such as palpation of foot pulses, the ankle-brachial index, and the toe-brachial index (98).

Table 3 Consequences of Neuropathy for the Lower Extremity

Loss of protective sensation
Postural instability
Muscle atrophy and loss of muscle strength
Altered gait with abnormal loading of the foot
Structural abnormalities, such as Charcot deformities, clawing of toes (?), reduced plantar thickness and bone resorption (in type 1 diabetes)
Altered biology of arterial vessel wall, calcification, and increased stiffness
Increased shunt blood flow with impaired vasodilator responses
Edema and probably increased compartmental pressures in foot
Impaired host-defense responses

NEUROVASCULAR DYSFUNCTION

As reviewed elsewhere, recent evidence suggests that denervation can result in altered capillary blood flow, oxygen delivery, fluid filtration, and inflammatory responses in the lower extremity (Table 3) (6). A warm swollen foot with distended veins upon dependency is a characteristic finding in patients with diabetic neuropathy. These abnormalities are caused by an increase in shunt blood flow due to loss of sympathetic constrictor tone (99). It is thought that this increased arteriovenous shunt blood flow results in a rise in venous pressure (and probably the distended veins upon dependency), which in turn could result in an enhanced fluid filtration and capillary leakage (99,100). Moreover, Nabuurs et al. (101) observed a reduction in supine capillary blood flow in the feet of patients with type 2 diabetes and neuropathy, suggesting that in these patients, neuropathy results in capillary hypoperfusion. Moreover, using direct pressure measurements, elevated intracompartmental pressures were observed in the feet of patients with diabetic neuropathy, which could be due to the enhanced capillary leakage (102). Such a rise in intracompartmental pressures could limit microcirculatory inflow in the deeper compartments of the foot, which might predispose deeper tissues of the foot to tissue ischemia. Tissue edema and capillary hypoperfusion will have negative consequences for the delivery of nutrients and tissue oxygenation in patients with diabetic neuropathy. Oxygen saturation in tissues of the feet was reduced in patients with diabetic neuropathy in one study, and in another study using nuclear magnetic resonance spectrometry, patients with a superficial neuropathic foot ulcer had reduced energy-rich phosphate level in plantar muscles of the foot. Moreover, the impaired energy metabolism was associated with the severity of neuropathy (103,104). Traditionally, these consequences of neurovascular dysfunction were thought to contribute to delayed wound healing, on the basis of the effects of denervation on wound healing in animal studies (105,106). However, if protected against elevated biomechanical stress, most neuropathic foot ulcers heal within weeks (107), and recently, it was reported that wound closure was unimpaired in a relatively small number of type 2 diabetic patients with neuropathy after a skin biopsy in the foot (107). It is more likely that the aforementioned changes put the neuropathic foot at an increased risk for the development of an ulcer when the foot is subjected to repetitive trauma than that it affects wound healing, but this hypothesis remains to be explored further.

Loss of neurovascular control could not only render a foot more susceptible to tissue damage but might also contribute to impaired host-defense responses once an ulcer has developed. As described earlier, basal skin blood flow is elevated in patients with diabetic neuropathy, probably due to the loss of sympathetic vasoconstrictor tone. In normal patients, local blood flow increases when tissues are stressed by noxious stimuli, but in patients with diabetic neuropathy, the vasodilator responses to various exogenous stimuli are reduced (108–111). Noxious stimuli induce release of several neuropeptides by sensory and autonomic nerves that can initiate local inflammatory responses (78,79). These neuromediators can induce vasodilatation, enhance vascular permeability, and affect the function of several cell types of the immune system. Loss of this neuronal defense system could contribute to enhanced susceptibility for infection of a diabetic foot ulcer. Approximately half of the patients with severe foot infections show few or no signs of local and systemic inflammation (e.g., redness, fever, elevated leucocytes or C-reactive protein levels), which might be related to the underlying neuropathy (112). Moreover, an intact peripheral nervous system is not only an important mediator in acute inflammatory responses but is probably also necessary for the development of immunologic memory. Elimination of nerve fibers abolishes both induction and effector stages of type 4 hypersensitivity responses without affecting the systemic immunity in mice (113).

CONCLUSION

Diabetic neuropathy is often a slow and seemingly insidious disease. There is no simple single test to diagnose neuropathy, so the clinician has to rely on careful history taking and, in particular, a standardized clinical examination that can be performed with simple techniques. Diabetic neuropathy is a diagnosis by exclusion, so causes other than diabetes have to be excluded; in the Rochester study, 10% of the diabetic patients with neuropathy had causes other than diabetes (114). In the last decades, much emphasis has been given to the pivotal role of neuropathy in the development of diabetic foot ulcers, which has resulted in the development of national and international guidelines for the prevention and treatment of these ulcers. These and other efforts have improved the outcome of diabetic foot ulcers (115), but, unfortunately, the underlying abnormalities usually remain. Given the crucial role of the peripheral nervous system in maintaining tissue homeostasis, muscle strength and coordination, control of peripheral blood flow, blood vessel wall biology, bone metabolism, and host-defense responses, it is understandable that the diabetic neuropathic limb can become severely dysfunctional with the progression of the neuropathy. These changes result in a spectrum of disease that is not easily recognized by both the patient and the health care worker. Patients may have complaints such as atypical pain, unsteadiness, falls, and tiredness, culminating in fear, depression, impaired mobility, and social isolation. Moreover, the clinical presentation and possibly the clinical course of other lower leg complications, such as PAD and foot infection, can be altered. This can lead to unnecessary patient and/or physician delay or sometimes misdiagnosis. Finally, peripheral neuropathy can be seen as a sign of generalized disease and is a harbinger of other problems to come. As there is at present no treatment for neuropathy, our aim should be to enable the patient to cope with this disease, to give support, and to prevent or treat the consequences of neuropathy, such as foot ulceration, neuropathic pain, and loss of mobility.

REFERENCES

1. Boulton AJ, Vileikyte L, Ragnarson-Tennvall G, et al. The global burden of diabetic foot disease. Lancet 2005; 366:1719–1724.
2. Nabuurs-Franssen MH, Huijberts MS, Nieuwenhuijzen Kruseman AC, et al. Health-related quality of life of diabetic foot ulcer patients and their caregivers. Diabetologia 2005; 48:1906–1910.
3. Boulton AJ. The diabetic foot: From art to science: The 18th Camillo Golgi lecture. Diabetologia 2004; 47:1343–1353.
4. Prompers L, Huijberts M, Apelqvist J, et al. High prevalence of ischaemia, infection and serious comorbidity in patients with diabetic foot disease in Europe: Baseline results from the Eurodiale study. Diabetologia 2007; 50:18–25.
5. Apelqvist J, Bakker K, van Houtum WH, et al. Practical guidelines on the management and prevention of the diabetic foot: Based upon the International Consensus on the Diabetic Foot (2007): Prepared by the International Working Group On The Diabetic Foot. Diabetes Metab Res Rev 2008; 24(suppl 1):S181–S187.
6. Schaper NC, Huijberts M, Pickwell K. Neurovascular control and neurogenic inflammation in diabetes. Diabetes Metab Res Rev 2008; 24(suppl 1):S40–S44.
7. Boulton AJ, Vinik AI, Arezzo JC, et al. Diabetic neuropathies: A statement by the American Diabetes Association. Diabetes Care 2005; 28:956–962.
8. Vinik AI, Mehrabyan A. Diabetic neuropathies. Med Clin N Am 2004; 88:947–999.
9. England JD, Gronseth GS, Franklin G, et al. Distal symmetric polyneuropathy: A definition for clinical research: Report of the American Academy of Neurology, the American Association of Electrodiagnostic Medicine, and the American Academy of Physical Medicine and Rehabilitation. Neurology 2005; 64:199–207.
10. Kumar S, Ashe HA, Parnell LN, et al. The prevalence of foot ulceration and its correlates in type 2 diabetic patients: A population-based study. Diabet Med 1994; 5:480–484.
11. Abbott CA, Carrington AL, Ashe H, et al. The North-West Diabetes Foot Care Study: Incidence of, and risk factors for, new diabetic foot ulceration in a community-based patient cohort. Diabet Med 2002; 19:377–384.
12. Cabezas-Cerrato J. The prevalence of clinical diabetic polyneuropathy in Spain: A study in primary care and hospital clinic groups: Neuropathy Spanish Study Group of the Spanish Diabetes Society (SDS). Diabetologia 1998; 41:1263–1269.

12a. Tapp RJ, Shaw JE, de Courten MP, et al. Foot complications in type 2 diabetes: An Australian population-based study. Diabet Med 2003; 20:105–113.

13. Partanen J, Niskanen L, Lehtinen J, et al. Natural history of peripheral neuropathy in patients with non-insulin-dependent diabetes mellitus. N Engl J Med 1995; 333: 89–94.
14. Tesfaye S, Stevens LK, Stephenson JM, et al. Prevalence of diabetic peripheral neuropathy and its relation to glycaemic control and potential risk factors: The EURODIAB IDDM Complications Study. Diabetologia 1996; 39:1377–1384.
15. Tesfaye S, Chaturvedi N, Eaton SE, et al. Vascular risk factors and diabetic neuropathy. N Engl J Med 2005; 352:341–350.
16. Daousi C, MacFarlane IA, Woodward A, et al. Chronic painful peripheral neuropathy in an urban community: A controlled comparison of people with and without diabetes. Diabet Med 2004; 21:976–982.
17. Davies M, Brophy S, Williams R, et al. The prevalence, severity, and impact of painful diabetic peripheral neuropathy in type 2 diabetes. Diabetes Care 2006; 29:1518–1522.
18. Gore M, Brandenburg NA, Hoffman DL, et al. Burden of illness in painful diabetic peripheral neuropathy: The patients' perspectives. J Pain 2006; 7:892–900.
19. Toelle T, Xu X, Sadosky AB. Painful diabetic neuropathy: A cross-sectional survey of health state impairment and treatment patterns. J Diabetes Complications 2006; 20:26–33.
20. Gadia MT, Natori N, Ramos LB, et al. Influence of height on quantitative sensory, nerve-conduction, and clinical indices of diabetic peripheral neuropathy. Diabetes Care 1987; 10:613–616.

21. The Diabetes Control and Complications Trial Research Group. The effect of intensive diabetes therapy on the development and progression of neuropathy. Ann Intern Med 1995; 122:561–568.
22. Intensive blood-glucose control with sulphonylureas or insulin compared with conventional treatment and risk of complications in patients with type 2 diabetes (UKPDS 33): UK Prospective Diabetes Study (UKPDS) Group. Lancet 1998; 352:837–853.
23. Forrest KY, Maser RE, Pambianco G, et al. Hypertension as a risk factor for diabetic neuropathy: A prospective study. Diabetes. 1997; 46:665–670.
24. Maser RE, Steenkiste AR, Maser RE, et al. Epidemiological correlates of diabetic neuropathy: Report from Pittsburgh Epidemiology of Diabetes Complications Study. Diabetes 1989; 38:1456–1461.
25. Mitchell BD, Hawthorne VM, Vinik AI. Cigarette smoking and neuropathy in diabetic patients. Diabetes Care 1990; 13:434–437.
26. Gaede P, Vedel P, Parving HH, et al. Intensified multifactorial intervention in patients with type 2 diabetes mellitus and microalbuminuria: The Steno type 2 randomised study. Lancet 1999; 353:606–608.
27. Smith AG, Russell J, Feldman EL, et al. Lifestyle intervention for pre-diabetic neuropathy. Diabetes Care 2006; 29:1294–1299.
28. Zochodne DW. Diabetes mellitus and the peripheral nervous system: Manifestations and mechanisms. Muscle Nerve 2007; 36:144–166.
29. Malik RA, Tesfaye S, Newrick PG, et al. Sural nerve pathology in diabetic patients with minimal but progressive neuropathy. Diabetologia 2005; 48:578–585.
30. Sumner CJ, Sheth S, Griffin JW, et al. The spectrum of neuropathy in diabetes and impaired glucose tolerance. Neurology 2003; 60:108–111.
31. Malik RA, Kallinikos P, Abbott CA, et al. Corneal confocal microscopy: A non-invasive surrogate of nerve fibre damage and repair in diabetic patients. Diabetologia 2003; 46:683–688.
32. Quattrini C, Tavakoli M, Jeziorska M, et al. Surrogate markers of small fiber damage in human diabetic neuropathy. Diabetes 2007; 56:2148–2154.
33. Figueroa-Romero C, Sadidi M, Feldman EL. Mechanisms of disease: The oxidative stress theory of diabetic neuropathy. Rev Endocr Metab Disord 2008; 9:301–314.
34. Brownlee M. The pathobiology of diabetic complications: A unifying mechanism. Diabetes 2005; 54:1615–1625.
35. Cameron NE, Eaton SE, Cotter MA, et al. Vascular factors and metabolic interactions in the pathogenesis of diabetic neuropathy. Diabetologia 2001; 44:1973–1988.
36. Gregg EW, Beckles GL, Williamson DF, et al. Diabetes and physical disability among older U.S. adults. Diabetes Care 2000; 23:1272–1277.
37. Volpato S, Blaum C, Resnick H, et al. Comorbidities and impairments explaining the association between diabetes and lower extremity disability: The Women's Health and Aging Study. Diabetes Care 2002; 5:678–683.
38. Tudor-Locke C, Hatano Y, Pangrazi RP, et al. Revisiting "how many steps are enough?". Med Sci Sports Exerc 2008; 40(suppl 7):S537–S543.
39. van Schie CHM. Neuropathy: mobility and quality of life. Diabetes Metab Res Rev. 2008; 24(suppl 1):S45–S51.
40. Mueller MJ, Minor SD, Sahrmann SA, et al. Differences in the gait characteristics of patients with diabetes and peripheral neuropathy compared with age-matched controls. Phys Ther 1994; 74:299–308.
41. Courtemanche R, Teasdale N, Boucher P, et al. Gait problems in diabetic neuropathic patients. Arch Phys Med Rehabil 1996; 77:849–855.
42. Menz HB, Lord SR, St. George R, et al. Walking stability and sensorimotor function in older people with diabetic peripheral neuropathy. Arch Phys Med Rehabil 2004; 85:245–252.
43. Allet L, Armand S, De Bie RA, et al. Gait alterations of diabetic patients while walking on different surfaces. Gait Posture 2009; 29:488–493.
44. Richardson JK, Thies SB, Demott TK, et al. Gait analysis in a challenging environment differentiates between fallers and nonfallers among older patients with peripheral neuropathy. Arch Phys Med Rehabil 2005; 86:1539–1544.

45. van Deursen RW, Sanchez MM, Ulbrecht JS, et al. The role of muscle spindles in ankle movement perception in human subjects with diabetic neuropathy. Exp Brain Res 1998; 120:1–8.
46. van Schie CHM, Simoneau GG, Ulbrecht JS, et al. Postural instability in patients with diabetic sensory neuropathy. Diabetes Care 1994; 17:1411–1421.
47. Uccioli L, Giacomini PG, Pasqualetti P, et al. Contribution of central neuropathy to postural instability in IDDM patients with peripheral neuropathy. Diabetes Care 1997; 20:929–934.
48. Resnick H, Stansberry K, Harris TB, et al. Diabetes, peripheral neuropathy, and old age disability. Muscle Nerve 2002; 25:43–50.
49. Richardson JK, Ching C, Hurvitz EA. The relationship between electromyographically documented peripheral neuropathy and falls. J Am Geriatr Soc 1992; 40:1008–1012.
50. Vileikyte L, Peyrot M, Gonzalez JS, et al. Predictors of depressive symptoms in persons with diabetic peripheral neuropathy: A longitudinal study. Diabetologia 2009; 52:1265–1273.
51. Richardson JK, Sandman D, Vela S. A focused exercise regimen improves clinical measures of balance in patients with peripheral neuropathy. Arch Phys Med Rehabil 2001; 82:205–209.
52. Mueller MJ, Minor SD, Sahrmann SA, et al. Differences in the gait characteristics of patients with diabetes and peripheral neuropathy compared with age-matched controls. Phys Ther 1994; 74:299–308.
53. Kwon O-Y, Minor SD, Maluf KS, et al. Comparison of muscle activity during walking in subjects with and without diabetic neuropathy. Gait Posture 2003; 18:105–113.
54. Katoulis EC, Ebdon-Parry M, Lanshammar H, et al. Gait abnormalities in diabetic neuropathy. Diabetes Care 1997; 20:1904–1907.
55. Yavuzer G, Yetkin I, Toruner FB, et al. Gait deviations of patients with diabetes mellitus: Looking beyond peripheral neuropathy. Eura Medicophys 2006; 42:127–133.
56. Savelberg HH, Schaper NC, Willems PJ, et al. Redistribution of joint moments is associated with changed plantar pressure in diabetic polyneuropathy. BMC Musculoskelet Disord 2009; 10:16.
57. Andersen H, Poulsen PL, Mogensen CE, et al. Isokinetic muscle strength in long-term IDDM patients in relation to diabetic complications. Diabetes 1996; 45:440–445.
58. Andersen H, Nielsen S, Mogensen CE, et al. Muscle strength in type 2 diabetes. Diabetes 2004; 53:1543–1548.
59. van Schie CHM, Vermigli C, Carrington AL, et al. Muscle weakness and foot deformities in diabetes: Relationship to neuropathy and foot ulceration in Caucasian diabetic men. Diabetes Care 2004; 27:1668–1673.
60. Brash PD, Foster J, Vennart W, et al. Magnetic resonance imaging techniques demonstrate soft tissue damage in the diabetic foot. Diabet Med 1999; 16:55–61.
61. Bus SA, Yang QX, Wang JH, et al. Intrinsic muscle atrophy and toe deformity in the diabetic neuropathic foot: A magnetic resonance imaging study. Diabetes Care 2002; 25:1444–1450.
62. Andersen H, Gjerstad MD, Jakobsen J. Atrophy of foot muscles: A measure of diabetic neuropathy. Diabetes Care 2004; 27:2382–2385.
63. Andersen H, Gadeberg PC, Brock B, et al. Muscular atrophy in diabetic neuropathy: A stereological magnetic resonance imaging study. Diabetologia 1997; 40:1062–1069.
64. Andreassen CS, Jakobsen J, Andersen H. Muscle weakness: A progressive late complication in diabetic distal symmetric polyneuropathy. Diabetes 2006; 55:806–812.
65. Veves A, Murray HJ, Young MJ, et al. The risk of foot ulceration in diabetic patients with high foot pressure: A prospective study. Diabetologia 1992; 35:660–663.
66. Frykberg RG, Lavery LA, Pham H, et al. Role of neuropathy and high foot pressures in diabetic foot ulceration. Diabetes Care 1998; 21:1714–1719.

67. Pataky Z, Assal JP, Conne P, et al. Plantar pressure distribution in type 2 diabetic patients without peripheral neuropathy and peripheral vascular disease. Diabet Med 2005; 22:762–767.
68. Caselli A, Pham H, Giurini JM, et al. The forefoot-to-rear foot plantar pressure ratio is increased in severe diabetic neuropathy and can predict foot ulceration. Diabetes Care 2002; 25:1066–1071.
69. Höhne A, Stark C, Brüggemann GP. Plantar pressure distribution in gait is not affected by targeted reduced plantar cutaneous sensation. Clin Biomech 2009; 24:308–313.
70. Lavery LA, Armstrong DG, Wunderlich RP, et al. Predictive value of foot pressure assessment as part of a population-based diabetes disease management program. Diabetes Care 2003; 26:1069–1073.
71. Guldemond NA, Leffers P, Sanders AP, et al. Daily-life activities and in-shoe forefoot plantar pressure in patients with diabetes. Diabetes Res Clin Pract 2007; 77:203–209.
72. Armstrong DG, Lavery LA. Elevated peak plantar pressures in patients who have Charcot arthropathy. J Bone Joint Surg Am 1998; 80:365–369.
73. Bus SA. Foot structure and footwear prescription in diabetes mellitus. Diabetes Metab Res Rev 2008; 24(suppl 1):S90–S95.
74. Abouaesha F, van Schie CH, Armstrong DG, et al. Plantar soft-tissue thickness predicts high peak plantar pressure in the diabetic foot. J Am Podiatr Med Assoc 2004; 94:39–42.
75. Zimny S, Schatz H, Pfohl M. The role of limited joint mobility in diabetic patients with an at-risk foot. Diabetes Care 2004; 27:942–946.
76. Masson EA, Hay EM, Stockley I, et al. Abnormal foot pressures alone may not cause ulceration. Diabet Med 1989; 6:426–428.
77. Guldemond NA, Leffers P, Walenkamp GH, et al. Prediction of peak pressure from clinical and radiological measurements in patients with diabetes. BMC Endocr Disord 2008; 8:16.
78. Steinhoff M, Sander S, Seeliger S, et al. Modern aspects of cutaneous neurogenic inflammation. Arch Dermatol 2003; 139:1479–1488.
79. Shepherd AJ, Downing JE, Miyan JA. Without nerves, immunology remains incomplete—In vivo veritas. Immunology 2005; 116:145–163.
80. Schaper NC, Kitslaar PJEHM. Peripheral vascular disease in diabetes mellitus. In: DeFronzo RA, Ferannini E, Zimmet P, et al., eds. International Textbook of Diabetes Mellitus. Oxford, UK: John Wiley and Sons, 2004:1515–1527.
81. Daemen MJ, De Mey JG. Regional heterogeneity of arterial structural changes. Hypertension 1995; 25:464–473.
82. Edmonds ME, Morrison N, Laws JW, et al. Medial arterial calcification and diabetic neuropathy. Br Med J 1982; 284:928–930.
83. Goebel FD, Füessl HS. Mönckeberg's sclerosis after sympathetic denervation in diabetic and non-diabetic subjects. Diabetologia 1983; 24:347–350.
84. Shroff RC, Shanahan CM. The vascular biology of calcification. Semin Dial 2007; 20:103–109.
85. Jeffcoate W. Vascular calcification and osteolysis in diabetic neuropathy—Is RANK-L the missing link? Diabetologia 2004; 47:1488–1492.
86. Gilbey SG, Walters H, Edmonds ME, et al. Vascular calcification, autonomic neuropathy, and peripheral blood flow in patients with diabetic nephropathy. Diabet Med 1989; 6:37–42.
87. Everhart JE, Pettitt DJ, Knowler WC, et al. Medial arterial calcification and its association with mortality and complications of diabetes. Diabetologia 1988; 31: 16–23.
88. Criqui MH, Langer RD, Fronek A, et al. Mortality over a period of 10 years in patients with peripheral arterial disease. N Engl J Med 1992; 326:381–386.
89. Lehto S, Niskanen L, Suhonen M, et al. Medial artery calcification: A neglected harbinger of cardiovascular complications in non-insulin-dependent diabetes mellitus. Arterioscler Thromb Vasc Biol 1999; 16:978–983.

90. Costacou T, Huskey ND, Edmundowicz D, et al. Lower-extremity arterial calcification as a correlate of coronary artery calcification. Metabolism 2006; 55:1689–1696.
91. Meyer C, Milat F, McGrath BP, et al. Vascular dysfunction and autonomic neuropathy in type 2 diabetes. Diabet Med 2004; 21:746–751.
92. Yokoyama H, Yokota Y, Tada J, et al. Diabetic neuropathy is closely associated with arterial stiffening and thickness in type 2 diabetes. Diabet Med 2007; 24:1329–1335.
93. Sutton-Tyrrell K, Najjar SS, Boudreau RM, et al. Elevated aortic pulse wave velocity, a marker of arterial stiffness, predicts cardiovascular events in well-functioning older adults. Circulation 2005; 111:3384–3390.
94. Willum-Hansen T, Staessen JA, Torp-Pedersen C, et al. Prognostic value of aortic pulse wave velocity as index of arterial stiffness in the general population. Circulation 2006; 113:664–670.
95. Maser RE, Mitchell BD, Vinik AI, et al. The association between cardiovascular autonomic neuropathy and mortality in individuals with diabetes: A meta-analysis. Diabetes Care 2003; 26:1895–1901.
96. Dolan NC, Liu K, Criqui MH, et al. Peripheral artery disease, diabetes, and reduced lower extremity functioning. Diabetes Care 2002; 25:113–120.
97. Prompers L, Schaper N, Apelqvist J, et al. Prediction of outcome in individuals with diabetic foot ulcers: Focus on the differences between individuals with and without peripheral arterial disease: The EURODIALE Study. Diabetologia 2008; 51:747–755.
98. Williams DT, Harding KG, Price P. An evaluation of the efficacy of methods used in screening for lower-limb arterial disease in diabetes. Diabetes Care 2005; 28:2206–2210.
99. Purewal TS, Goss DE, Watkins PJ, et al. Lower limb venous pressure in diabetic neuropathy. Diabetes Care 1995; 18:377–381.
100. Lefrandt JD, Bosma E, Oomen PH, et al. Sympathetic mediated vasomotion and skin capillary permeability in diabetic patients with peripheral neuropathy. Diabetologia 2003; 46:40–47.
101. Nabuurs-Franssen MH, Houben AJ, Tooke JE, et al. The effect of polyneuropathy on foot microcirculation in type II diabetes. Diabetologia 2002; 45:1164–1171.
102. Lower RF, Kenzora JE. The diabetic neuropathic foot: A triple crush syndrome—Measurement of compartmental pressures of normal and diabetic feet. Orthopedics 1994; 17:241–248.
103. Greenman RL, Panasyuk S, Wang X, et al. Early changes in the skin microcirculation and muscle metabolism of the diabetic foot. Lancet 2005; 366:1711–1717.
104. Suzuki E, Kashiwagi A, Hidaka H, et al. 1H- and 31P-magnetic resonance spectroscopy and imaging as a new diagnostic tool to evaluate neuropathic foot ulcers in type II diabetic patients. Diabetologia 2000; 43:165–172.
105. Richards AM, Floyd DC, Terenghi G, et al. Cellular changes in denervated tissue during wound healing in a rat model. Br J Dermatol 1999; 140:1093–1099.
106. Smith PG, Liu M. Impaired cutaneous wound healing after sensory denervation in developing rats: Effects on cell proliferation and apoptosis. Cell Tissue Res 2002; 307:281–291.
107. Nabuurs-Franssen MH, Sleegers R, Huijberts MS, et al. Total contact casting of the diabetic foot in daily practice: A prospective follow-up study. Diabetes Care 2005; 28:243–247.
108. Flynn MD, Tooke JE. Diabetic neuropathy and the microcirculation. Diabet Med 1995; 12:298–301.
109. Pfutzner A, Forst T, Engelbach M, et al. The influence of isolated small nerve fibre dysfunction on microvascular control in patients with diabetes mellitus. Diabet Med 2001; 18:489–494.
110. Kramer HH, Schmelz M, Birklein F, et al. Electrically stimulated axon reflexes are diminished in diabetic small fiber neuropathies. Diabetes 2004; 53:769–774.
111. Krishnan ST, Rayman G. The LDI flare: A novel test of C-fiber function demonstrates early neuropathy in type 2 diabetes. Diabetes Care 2004; 27:2930–2935.

112. Lipsky BA, International consensus group on diagnosing and treating the infected diabetic foot. A report from the international consensus on diagnosing and treating the infected diabetic foot. Diabetes Metab Res Rev 2004; 20(suppl 1):S68–S77.
113. Beresford L, Orange O, Bell EB, et al. Nerve fibres are required to evoke a contact sensitivity response in mice. Immunology 2004; 111:118–125.
114. Dyck PJ, Kratz KM, Lehman KA, et al. The Rochester Diabetic Neuropathy Study: Design, criteria for types of neuropathy, selection bias, and reproducibility of neuropathic tests. Neurology 1991; 41:799–807.
115. Boulton AJ. The diabetic foot: Grand overview, epidemiology and pathogenesis. Diabetes Metab Res Rev 2008; 24(suppl 1):S3–S6.

6 Painful diabetic neuropathy

Lee C. Rogers and Rayaz A. Malik

Pain; The gift nobody wants

—Paul Wilson Brand

Diabetic polyneuropathy (DPN) is a devastating complication of diabetes that can lead to foot ulceration, Charcot foot, amputation, severe pain, and major psychological disorders. In 2000, it was estimated that 2.8% (171 million) of the world population had diabetes mellitus, and the WHO predicts that by the year 2030, this will rise to 4.4% (366 million). The greatest increases in diabetes prevalence will be seen in the Middle East, sub-Saharan Africa, and India (1). In the United States, recent reports estimate that 23.6 million people have diabetes (2). Roughly 50% of those with diabetes will develop DPN (3,4), and it is the leading cause of foot ulcers and nontraumatic limb amputation (5). In 2003, the annual cost of diabetic neuropathy was estimated to exceed $10.9 billion (6). The rise in diabetes and hence neuropathy prevalence with the high physical and financial costs demand greater attention and focused research in prevention and treatment of this debilitating complication.

PATHOPHYSIOLOGY

Four major pathways are considered to be key to the development of DPN: (1) increased polyol pathway activity, (2) nonenzymatic glycation of proteins resulting in advanced glycation end products, (3) activation of protein kinase C (PKC), and (4) increased hexosamine pathway flux (7). The common initiating factor for all the pathways is hyperglycemia with the generation of reactive oxygen species leading to oxidative stress that can itself be directly neurotoxic and that secondarily can cause neural ischemia from damage to the microvasculature (8). It has been shown that free radical defenses are reduced in the peripheral nerve as compared with the brain or liver, perhaps making the peripheral nerve more susceptible to damage from oxidative stress (9). It is also becoming evident that not only those with overt diabetes, and hence constant hyperglycemia, but also a percentage of patients with impaired glucose tolerance, and hence intermittent or moderate glucose perturbations, are at risk for neuropathy (10,11).

DPN is one of the three main diabetic microvascular complications of retinopathy, nephropathy, and neuropathy, which together constitute the "diabetic triopathy." Although microangiopathy has been considered a priori to underlie both retinopathy and nephropathy, much debate has revolved around the role of microangiopathy in neuropathy. However, Malik and colleagues (12) studied the extent of microangiopathy by employing electron microscopy in sural nerve biopsies from patients with varying degrees of neuropathy and age-matched controls, and they found decreased endoneurial capillary density that correlated directly with reduced myelinated fiber density. Also, increased capillary basement membrane area was associated with increasing neuropathic severity, which is consistent with the findings of Dyck and associates (13) who found basement membrane reduplication and pericyte degeneration in endoneurial capillaries. Basement membrane thickening is proposed to increase the distance and the density of the interstitial space through which oxygen must diffuse, thereby resulting in neural ischemia. And of course, endoneurial oxygen tension has been shown to be decreased in patients with DPN (14). Furthermore, the histologic pattern of nerve fiber loss in DPN supports the role of nerve ischemia (15). Although nerve fiber damage definitely occurs, there is current disagreement by neurobiologists whether axonal degeneration occurs primarily followed by demyelination or vice versa (16). Dyck and colleagues have studied this extensively and published reports supporting primary axonal loss with secondary demyelination and remyelination (13,17). However, studies in diabetic patients with early neuropathy do suggest demyelination before overt axonal degeneration (18).

DIAGNOSIS

A working clinical definition of DPN was first established in the San Antonio Consensus Conference (19) and was later simplified by Boulton et al. (20) as "the presence of symptoms and/or signs of peripheral nerve dysfunction in people with diabetes after exclusion of other causes." *After exclusion of other causes* is the crucial statement in the aforementioned definition. The Rochester Diabetic Neuropathy Study, the longest running longitudinal population-based study of patients with DPN, has shown that up to 10% of diabetic patients who present with neuropathy have an etiology other than diabetes as the cause of the neuropathy (21). A thorough differential diagnosis must enter clinicians' mind each time they examine a diabetic patient with suspected neuropathy. The reader is referred to detailed reviews published on the differential diagnosis of diabetic neuropathy (22,23). Some of the more prevalent clinical imitators of DPN are presented in Table 1.

The clinical features of DPN are that of a distal, symmetrical, length-dependent sensory loss beginning in the toes and progressing proximally with time. The longest axons are affected first; thus, hypoesthesia in the feet occurs before the hands. The classic descriptor of stocking-glove distribution is correct if you think of stockings as "knee-high" and not "ankle-high," since the anatomic length of the axons in the finger tips (cervical spine to finger tips) equals that of the axons to the skin just below the knee (lumbosacral spine to knee). The length-dependent process has been confirmed histopathologically by Dyck, who assessed multiple sections of nerves in 15 patients who died with DPN and compared them with 9 controls who died without peripheral neuropathies. He found the number and size of myelinated fibers normal to be slightly decreased in the lumbar roots of the diabetic patients, with a progressive increase in pathology in the sciatic nerve, which was greatest in the most distal nerves such as the sural nerve (15).

Patients may complain of "positive" symptoms of burning, lancinating pains, formication, allodynia, or pins and needles. However, most patients will have "negative" symptoms that can be elicited by the clinician only after careful questioning, such as numbness, dead/asleep feeling, loss of balance, or painless

Table 1 Differential Diagnosis in the Patient Presenting with Distal Symmetric Peripheral Neuropathy, Where Diabetic Neuropathy Is Being Considered

Diabetic neuropathy
HIV/highly active anti-retroviral therapy (HAART)
Alcoholism/malnutrition
Vasculitis
Primary vasculitis[a]: polyarteritis nodosa, Churg-Strauss syndrome
Wegnener granulomatosis
Secondary vasculitis: Sjorgren syndrome, sarcoidosis
Cryoglobulinemia
Renal failure
Idiopathic
Hereditary motor and sensory neuropathy (Charcot-Marie-Tooth disease)
Hepatitis
Hypothyrodism
Medications: chemotherapeutic drugs, statins, linezolid, quinolones
Monoclonal gammopathies
Amyloidosis
Vitamin B_{12} deficiency
Industrial agents
Lead poisoning
Neoplasms (paraneoplastic syndrome)
Nerve compression/entrapment[a]
Leprosy[a]
Lyme disease[a]
Lumbar radiculopathy[a]

[a] Generally not presenting as symmetric length-dependent pattern.

injury/ulcer. This fact makes "screening" for neuropathy imperative at every diabetic visit. There are two forms of inquiries for DPN: *screening* and *diagnosis*.

Diabetic peripheral neuropathy screening should be performed annually in those with diabetes and consists of simple clinical tests with high sensitivity but moderate to low specificity. Two screening tools are currently popular and sensitive for loss of protective sensation (LOPS) associated with DPN: the Semmes-Weinstein monofilament (SWM) and the biothesiometer (neurothesiometer, vibrometer). The monofilament was first developed by neurologist von Frey by using horse tail hairs of different diameters to test pressure sensation. The SWM is a nylon filament that exerts 10 g of force at the point it buckles. The SWM is also called a *5.07 monofilament* from the equation used to derive 10 g of buckling strength. Paul Wilson Brand, neuropathy researcher and orthopedic surgeon, popularized the use of the SWM in India during his mission work, while treating lepers with peripheral neuropathy. The sensitivity of the SWM has been reported to be 92%–95% (24,25). There is debate over how many points to test on the plantar surface of the foot. Common belief is that 10 points should be tested with 4 or more missed points considered to represent increased risk for ulceration. This may be true for lepromatous neuropathy in which a patchy nerve involvement is hallmark, but in DPN, a distal-to-proximal progression dictates that the distal-most points would be the most sensitive. In fact, in diabetic neuropathy, four distal sites showed the only discrimination between those with LOPS and those without LOPS (26). The correct usage of the SWM is dependent

Table 2 Laboratory Analysis for the Patient with Peripheral Neuropathy in Diabetes to Exclude the Most Common Other Causes

Laboratory test	Utility
CBC	Anemia (lead toxicity), eosinophilia (Churg-Strauss syndrome)
Basic metabolic panel (BMP)	Renal disease, uremia
AST/ALT	Liver dysfunction (suggest alcoholic neuropathy or hepatitis)
ESR and CRP	Vasculitis or other inflammatory diseases
TSH	Thyroid disease
Vitamin B_{12}	Pernicious anemia
Heavy metal screen, Lyme titer, hepatitis screen, serum cryoglobulins, paraneoplastic screen	Not needed routinely, use when suggested by history

Abbreviations: CBC, complete blood cell count; AST, aspartate aminotransferase; ALT, alanine aminotransferase; ESR, erythrocyte sedimentation rate; CRP, C-reactive protein; TSH, thyroid-stimulating hormone.

on the patient's response to a stimulus, thus it is considered a psychophysical test. Both psychological and physical pathways are needed to properly assess nerve function with the SWM, such that testing a patient with mental illness or degenerative brain disease or indeed lack of concentration will not produce a reliable result.

An accurate diagnosis should be established in any patient who has failed the screening, but this consists of more expensive, more invasive tests that have higher specificity. However, much of diagnosis is ruling out other causes for peripheral neuropathy since we have no highly specific test for DPN per se. A battery of tests for diagnosis of patients who failed the screening can be found in Table 2. In general, hereditary neuropathies are far more common than the other causes and probably make up the bulk of undiagnosed or "idiopathic" peripheral neuropathies. Hereditary motor and sensory neuropathies (HMSN) are a group of genetic peripheral neuropathies formerly known by the eponym *Charcot-Marie-Tooth diseases.* They are as prevalent as 1 in 2500 persons (27), are genetically heterogeneous, may be either autosomal dominant or autosomal recessive, and on occasion occur as point mutations in previously unaffected families (26,28). Their slow progression, distal-to-proximal involvement, and appearance later in life can lead to confusion with DPN. Expensive genetic testing exists for many forms of HMSN, but a complete family pedigree can generally reveal its presence. Fabry disease, an X-linked recessive disorder resulting in lipid accumulation in peripheral tissues secondary to a genetic defect in the enzyme α-galactosidase should be considered in all young men presenting with painful small-fiber neuropathy (29).

Lepromatous, syphilitic, and Lyme neuropathy all need to be considered as infectious causes. Hepatitis C viral infections may lead to an increase in circulating cryoglobulins (30), which can underlie a vasculitic neuropathy and may have a prevalence of up to 50% in those infected. There are several HIV-associated neuropathies; the most common is a distal sensory polyneuropathy due to axonal damage mediated by macrophage activation and proinflammatory cytokines initiating nerve damage (31).

Immune-mediated neuropathies are another underdiagnosed category of peripheral neuropathies. Monoclonal gammopathy is associated with peripheral neuropathy and an elevation of IgM, IgG, or IgA (in decreasing order of frequency) levels may be detected on laboratory analysis (32). Chronic renal insufficiency is a common complication of diabetes and may lead to uremia. An accumulation of uremic toxins may be responsible for a change in nerve function. The course of uremic neuropathy is that of a distal, symmetric, motor, and sensory polyneuropathy, which may be easily confused with DPN (33). Nerve function generally improves after the initiation of dialysis or renal transplantation (34).

Peripheral neuropathy may be the presenting symptom of a malignant process, classically a small cell lung cancer (35). The patient's smoking history should be noted and a chest radiograph ordered if necessary. Anti-Hu antibodies are associated with this type of paraneoplastic neuropathy. Although less common, peripheral neuropathies have also been reported in those with breast cancer (36).

Toxins responsible for peripheral neuropathies are drugs such as metronidazole, taxol, amiodarone, vinca alkaloids, cisplatin, linezolid, and ethanol. Alcoholic polyneuropathy previously thought to be nutritional from folate and thiamine deficiencies seen in chronic alcoholics is now believed to be a direct neurotoxic effect of alcohol (37). Alcoholic polyneuropathy is a distal axonopathy that affects both large and small fibers (38). When it presents as a painful peripheral neuropathy, it is difficult to distinguish from DPN (39). Patients should be questioned about their quantity and type of ethanol intake. Risk factors for the development of alcoholic neuropathy include type and duration of ethanol use and family history of alcoholism (37).

Any process deviating from the length-dependent nature of DPN should be referred to a neurologist with an interest in peripheral neuropathies. Sensory examination should confirm a stocking-glove, toes before fingers deficit. Motor examination should look for weakness of the interossei of the hands. The patient should be asked to walk on the heels and walk on the toes. Since the posterior muscles of the leg are larger and receive a more proximal innervation than do the anterior muscles, in a length-dependent process, it would be expected that the patient would first lose the ability to walk on the heels. If the opposite occurs (the Pierre Bourque sign), this is not consistent with DPN and may represent an intraspinal lesion (40).

Since neuropathy is a microvascular complication of diabetes and occurs temporally together with nephropathy and retinopathy, a diagnosis of DPN can be supported by a diagnosis of diabetic retinopathy or nephropathy (41). A urine screen for microalbumin should be ordered on all diabetic patients with neuropathy. Furthermore, the patient should be examined for retinopathy by using a dilated retinal examination. The presence of microabuminuria or retinopathy supports the diagnosis of DPN, and equally, the absence should indicate the search for other causes of neuropathy.

Electrophysiological tests can be used to confirm the presence of a neuropathy or to differentiate axonal from demyelinating neuropathies and may therefore be particularly useful in patients who may have chronic inflammatory demyelinating polyneuropathy. An electromyogram/nerve conduction velocity will show abnormalities in DPN before the patient may exhibit clinical signs and symptoms (42).

The nerve biopsy will show characteristic changes associated with DPN; however, it should be reserved for the patient who meets the following three criteria: (1) there is evidence for a disorder other than DPN, (2) the suspected disease is capable of causing diagnostically relevant changes in the nerve, and (3) identification of the neuropathy is likely to influence subsequent treatments (22). The technique of the sural nerve biopsy has been described by Bevilacqua et al. (43).

Two newer diagnostic techniques, skin biopsy and corneal confocal microscopy (CCM), currently available to researchers, may find clinical use in the near future. Skin biopsy is minimally invasive and requires considerable laboratory expertise to quantify intraepidermal nerve fiber density (IENFD) but correlates well with quantitative sensory tests and detects early small fiber neuropathy before electrophysiological abnormalities occur (44,45). Similarly, CCM also quantifies small nerve fiber damage and repair but in a noninvasive way by imaging corneal nerves that are quantified using image analysis. CCM has been shown to be as sensitive as IENFD assessment in skin biopsies, particularly in detecting early somatic neuropathy and may also have future value in staging DPN and assessing therapeutic efficacy following treatment (46–48).

TREATMENT

When discussing treatment, diabetic peripheral neuropathy can be clinically classified into two entities: hypoesthetic (painless) and nociceptive (painful). The physician should realize that the patient with nociceptive DPN will likely have some features of hypoesthetic DPN in addition.

Hypoesthetic Diabetic Peripheral Neuropathy

Hypoesthetic DPN is often falsely considered not as severe by both patient and physician since the patient does not present with any noticeable symptoms. However, hypoesthetic DPN is the single-most important risk factor for neuropathic ulceration and subsequent amputation (49,50). Therefore, the diagnosis of hypoesthetic DPN should alarm the physician of the possibility of limb loss, and the phrase "at-risk for foot ulceration" should be entered into the patient's problem list.

The primary treatment for hypoesthetic DPN is prevention of foot ulceration. This is accomplished by regular visits to the podiatrist or diabetic foot specialist and prescription of custom shoes, with "patient education." However, a recent randomized controlled trial (RCT) to determine the effect of a foot care education program in the secondary prevention of foot ulcers demonstrated that although the intervention was associated with improved foot care behavior, it was not associated with a reduction in reulceration at either 6 or 12 months (51). Nevertheless the patient's feet should be examined at each clinic visit. Calluses (52) and foot deformities such as hammertoes, bunions, or Charcot collapse should be identified as they are risk factors for ulceration (24). Footwear should be wide enough and deep enough to accommodate deformities. Onychomycosis with severely thickened toenails can be subject to increased pressure by the toe box of the shoe and cause subungual ulcers. Patients should wear shoes at all times, including while indoors, to prevent accidental injury. Prophylactic surgery to off-load high-pressure points can be performed in some patients (53).

No currently available pharmacologic agents have been shown to reverse hypoesthetic neuropathy to any clinically significant degree. Angiotensin-converting enzyme inhibitors (ACEIs) have been shown to improve diabetic nephropathy, and it was thought that this drug class might have some effect on

DPN since the development and progression of neuropathy, nephropathy, and retinopathy are closely related. ACEIs ameliorate vascular dysfunction and promote vasodilation by preventing the generation of the pressor agent angiotensin II and the breakdown of the vasodilator bradykinin (54). An RCT of 41 diabetic patients using trandalopril for 12 months showed modest improvement of electrophysiological measures of nerve function (55). ACEI may play an important role in preventing DPN (56).

Ruboxistaurin, a PKC-β inhibitor, was under investigation by the U.S. Food and Drug Administration for the slowing or prevention of diabetic sensory neuropathy. In a phase II, 12-month RCT, ruboxistaurin improved DPN as assessed by vibratory examination, objective measures of nerve function, and in the patients who experienced symptoms—an improvement in the Neuropathy Total Symptom Score-6 (57). However, two subsequent phase III trials proved to be negative, and ruboxistaurin has therefore been withdrawn from further study.

Published studies using monochromatic near-infrared photo energy (MIRE) claim reversal of sensory loss in diabetic patients with neuropathy. Of the published studies, three are RCTs involving a total of 103 patients (58,59). The studies used cutaneous pressure perception thresholds either with the SWM or other instrument and found a decrease in points missed after usage of the MIRE system. However, there were no objective measures of nerve function employed. Another study (60) was a retrospective cohort that may have included the same patients from a previous study (59). This study claimed a reduction in the incidence of ulceration at 1 year. Serious questions about this study's design are posed regarding low (57%) patient participation, no mention of footwear, and the absence of a true control group. More recently, Lavery and colleagues (61) found no benefit in using MIRE in a blinded RCT.

Painful Diabetic Peripheral Neuropathy

In painful DPN, few patients actually achieve 100% pain relief. Most studies consider 50% relief of pain a success and 70% relief as an exceptional result. The goal of treatment should be sufficient relief of pain to allow the patient to complete activities of daily living without significant side effects. This must be expressed to the patient prior to the initiation of therapy as unreasonable expectations can be a cause of treatment failure.

A PubMed review (in April 2008) of "diabetic neuropathy" with the limits "randomized controlled trial" returned 499 abstracts from 1974 to 2008. The abstracts were scanned and those that did not pertain to peripheral neuropathy were excluded. The pharmaceutical agents and number of studies for *painful diabetic peripheral neuropathy* included amitriptyline (15), gabapentin (11), duloxetine (10), oxcarbazepine/carbamazepine (7), pregabalin (6), lamotrigine (6), mexiletine (5), lidocaine (5), topical capsaicin (5), α-lipoic acid (4), tramadol (3), with oxycodone, aldose reductase inhibitors, imipramine, desipramine, valproate, topiramate, clonidine, venlafaxine, nitroglycerin spray, amantadine, pentoxifylline, ACE inhibitors, and neurotrophic peptides/factors being evaluated in two or less RCTs.

When evaluating the literature, it is difficult to assess the real efficacy of medications for painful symptoms of diabetic neuropathy due to the large placebo response experienced and the expected, incomplete relief of pain in those being treated for painful DPN. The most rigorous system of assessment of efficacy is

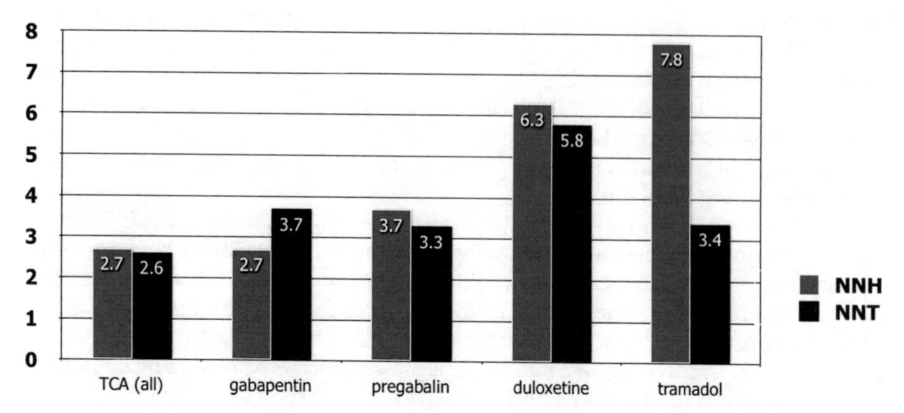

Figure 1 The number needed to treat (NNT) and number needed to harm (NNH) for common drugs used in painful diabetic neuropathy. The most desirable drug has a low NNT and a high NNH.

the number needed to treat (NNT) (62). The NNT for painful DPN is the number of patients needed to treat to get one patient with at least 50% pain relief. An NNT of 2.5 means that 2.5 patients need to receive treatment before you see one patient who will be show success (50% better) on therapy. Thus, the lower the NNT, the more efficacious the drug is. Where possible, we include the NNT for drugs discussed in this chapter. In addition, the safety profile can be measured by using the number needed to harm (NNH), which reflects the number of patients needed to treat until an adverse event occurs. Ideally a drug should have a low NNT (most efficacious) and high NNH (safest).

Four drugs or drug classes have been shown in several repeated placebo-controlled trial to be efficacious (Level A evidence). These are the tricyclic antidepressants (TCAs), gabapentinoids, tramadol, and duloxetine. Figure 1 shows the NNT and NNH for these agents, and each one will be discussed individually.

TCAs have been the mainstay of treatment for painful symptoms of DPN for 30 years. They inhibit serotonin (5-HT) and norepinephrine (nEpi) in the synapse and act principally by augmenting descending inhibitory pathways (63). Amitriptyline, imipramine, and desipramine are all effective versus placebo in treating nociceptive DPN. The TCAs—as a class—have an NNT of 2.6, with imipramine being the most efficacious drug with an NNT of 1.4. Amitriptyline has an NNT of 2.4. As a class, TCAs have many side effects that include sedation, dry mouth, constipation, and urinary retention. Rarely TCAs can cause malignant arrhythmias due to their quinidine-like effect on sodium channels (64) and should be avoided in patients with recent myocardial infarction or arrhythmia (65).

Duloxetine is a newer class of antidepressant called *selective serotonin norepinephrine reuptake inhibitor* (*SSNRI*). It is dosed at 60 to 120 mg daily and has an effect within 1 or 2 weeks, with a maximal effect in 6 weeks (Fig. 2). It has an NNT of 5.8 (66). Side effects include nausea, dizziness, somnolence, fatigue, and dry mouth. A 14% discontinuation rate from side effects is reported in the pivotal trials, which led to the FDA approval. As with the TCA group, it is precautioned in those with a recent myocardial infarction or dysrhythmia.

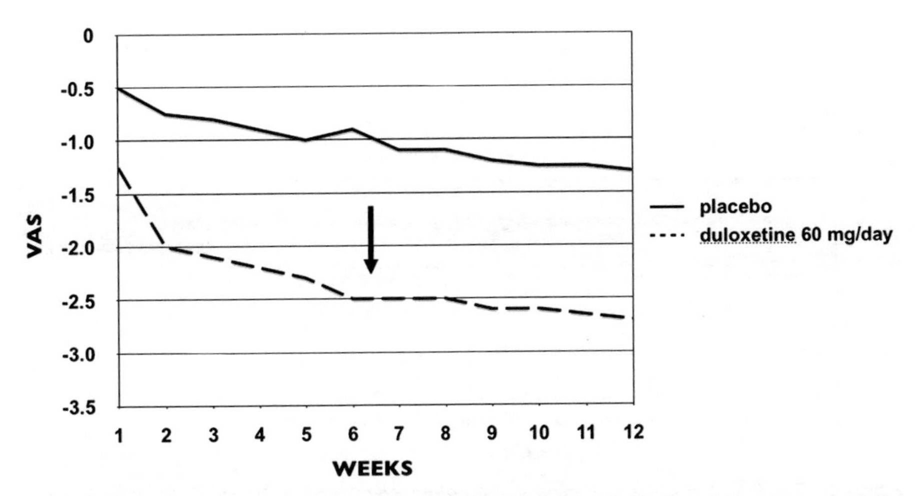

Figure 2 The maximal sustained pain relief experienced by duloxetine occurs near week 6, indicates the need for an adequate duration of treatment.

Gabapentin is a γ-amino butyric acid (GABA) analogue without direct action on GABA. It is thought to act by reducing calcium influx in the neurons of the central nervous system. When used in painful DPN, gabapentin should be rapidly titrated to doses above 1800 mg/day up to 3600 mg/day. Duration of an adequate trial should be 2 weeks at maximum-tolerated dose. Side effects include dizziness, somnolence, ataxia, and peripheral edema (67). The NNT for gabapentin is 3.8. Comparative studies between gabapentin and amitriptyline are limited, but one small randomized trial demonstrated no significant difference between the two groups for pain relief, with the mean dose of gabapentin given at 1600 mg/day and amitriptyline at 60 mg/day (68). Another smaller study compared gabapentin 2400 mg/day with amitriptyline 90 mg/day. Adverse events occurred much more frequently in the amitriptyline group, showing better tolerability of gabapentin (69).

Pregabalin is a newer gabapentinoid that selectively binds to the $\alpha_2\delta$ subunit of the neuronal voltage-gated calcium channel. There have been seven published RCTs with a total of 1510 patients. The NNT is 3.3. Study subjects can experience some pain relief within 1 week, but maximal effect is not experienced until week 8 (Fig. 3) (70). A recent meta-analysis attempted to establish the most efficacious dose (71). The authors found that 600 mg/day divided two or three times daily provided the most patients with both 30% and 50% pain relief (Fig. 4). In addition, as the dose escalated from 150 to 300 to 600 mg/day, so did the discontinuation rate secondary to adverse events. Even at the highest dose, the discontinuation rate was only 19%. The side effect profile is similar to gabapentin, with somnolence, ataxia, and peripheral edema being most common.

Tramadol is a centrally acting analgesic that binds to opioid receptors but with additional effect on norepinephrine and serotonin reuptake. Tramadol has an NNT of 3.4. One RCT evaluated its use in painful DPN at an average dose of 200 mg/day over 6 weeks (72). Tramadol significantly reduced pain and improved physical functioning but with a 14% discontinuation rate due to nausea, headache,

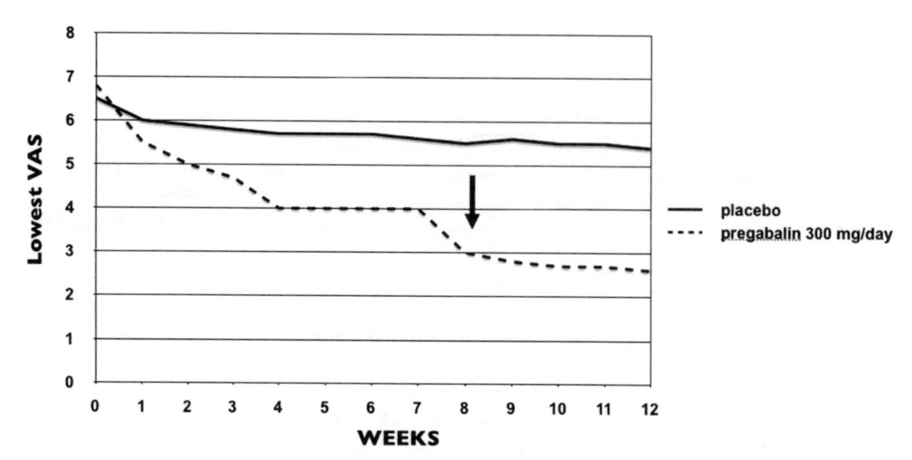

Figure 3 The maximal sustained pain relief experienced by pregabalin occurs at week 8, indicates the need for an adequate duration of treatment.

constipation, and somnolence. The NNH is 7.8. Tramadol lowers the seizure threshold and should be avoided in those at risk of seizures. One of the main benefits of tramadol is the low NNT and high NNH, making it fairly efficacious and one of the safer options for treatment. However, long-term use may result in opiate tolerance and requires caution.

Other pharmacological options include opiates and nonsteroidal anti-inflammatory drugs (NSAIDs). Extended release of oxycodone relieved neuropathic pain in two trials at a dose of 20 to 80 mg/day (73,74). The side effects, risk of tolerance, and addiction potential, all prohibit long-term usage. Opiates

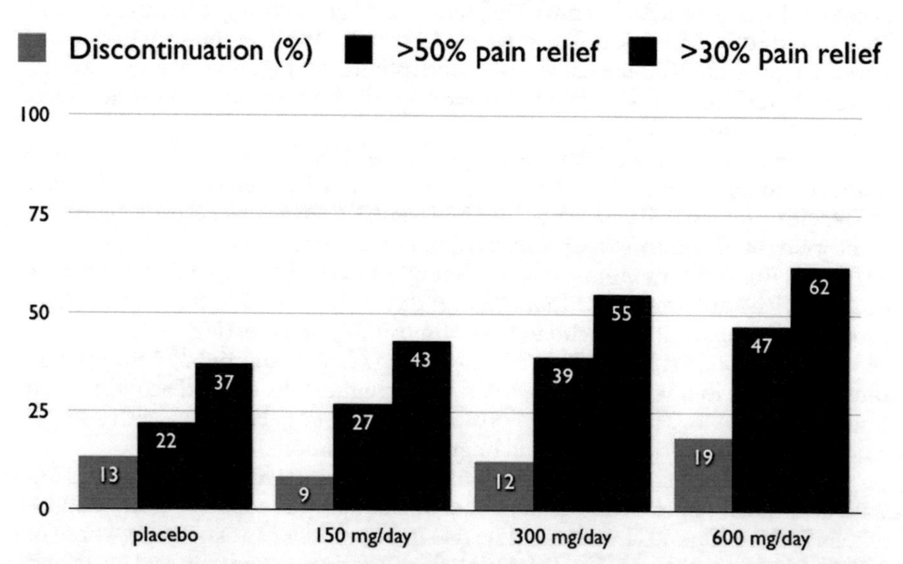

Figure 4 A comparison of varying doses of pregabalin with placebo and the effect on 30% pain relief, 50% pain relief, and discontinuation rates.

might be best suited for early combination therapy with antidepressants or anticonvulsants if DPN pain is intolerable. NSAIDs have been used in painful DPN (75,76) but have the risk of gastrointestinal, renal, and cardiac toxicities. In those with diabetes, where renal function might be impaired and who may be at risk for coronary artery disease, the use of NSAIDs is generally not recommended.

A recently published trial of benfotiamine (vitamin B_1) for painful DPN had an RCT design with 165 subjects (77). There was minimal benefit from the use of this supplement for the main study outcome, the Neuropathy Symptom Score (NSS). While the NSS may be a good diagnostic questionnaire for DPN, it has poor reproducibility and is not the best tool for longitudinal studies of DPN (78,79). The other measures in the study failed to reach statistical significance.

Surgical decompression of peripheral nerves for both painful neuropathy and to restore sensation has been advocated. However, we are critical of this method since it does not address the underlying pathophysiology of DPN, uses nonstandard and unaccepted methods to "prove" its effect, and many of the studies require the use of a proprietary device (Pressure-Specific Sensory Device) to show significance. The American Academy of Neurology (80) and the American Diabetes Association (81) have published position statements cautioning against using this unsubstantiated modality for DPN. In addition, a recent Cochrane review found that the use of decompressive surgery for diabetic symmetric distal neuropathy is unproven (82).

SUMMARY

Peripheral neuropathy occurs commonly in those with diabetes and approximately 30% will experience painful symptoms. The painful symptoms can be particularly troublesome and difficult to treat. Drug treatments for DPN have many adverse effects, and a balance must be achieved between effects and side effects. Evidence-based medicine should be employed to choose an efficacious and safe therapy. Many patients who suffer from painful DPN will become painless after a period of years. It is recommended to take a "drug holiday" during treatment to determine whether the therapy directed at pain is still required.

There have been no effective treatments (medical, physical, or surgical) that have been unequivocally proven to reverse sensory neuropathy due to diabetes. The focus should be to prevent sensory loss perhaps by tight control of not only blood glucose but also the other traditional cardiovascular risk factors such as blood pressure and lipids (83). Once sensory neuropathy is present, careful attention should be placed on regular foot screening and diabetic ulcer prevention to reduce the worst sequel of DPN, the lower extremity amputation.

REFERENCES

1. Wild S, Roglic G, Green A, et al. Global prevalence of diabetes: Estimates for the year 2000 and projections for 2030. Diabetes Care 2004; 27(5):1047–1053.
2. Centers for Disease Control and Prevention. National Diabetes Fact Sheet. In: National Estimates on Diabetes. Department of Health and Human Services circular, 2007.
3. de Neeling JN, Beks PJ, Bertelsmann FW, et al. Peripheral somatic nerve function in relation to glucose tolerance in an elderly Caucasian population: The Hoorn study. Diabet Med 1996; 13(11):960–966.

4. Adler AI, Boyko EJ, Ahroni JH, et al. Risk factors for diabetic peripheral sensory neuropathy: Results of the Seattle Prospective Diabetic Foot Study. Diabetes Care 1997; 20(7):1162–1167.
5. Thomas PK. Diabetic peripheral neuropathies: Their cost to patient and society and the value of knowledge of risk factors for development of interventions. Eur Neurol 1999; 41(suppl 1):35–43.
6. Gordois A, Scuffham P, Shearer A, et al. The health care costs of diabetic peripheral neuropathy in the US. Diabetes Care 2003; 26(6):1790–1795.
7. Feldman EL, Vincent AM. The prevalence, impact, and multifactoral pathogenesis of diabetic peripheral neuropathy. Adv Stud Med 2004; 4:S642–S649.
8. Sima AA. New insights into the metabolic and molecular basis for diabetic neuropathy. Cell Mol Life Sci 2003; 60(11):2445–2464.
9. Low PA. Oxidative stress: An integrative view. In: Gries FA, Cameron NE, Low PA, Ziegler D, eds. Textbook of Diabetic Neuropathy. New York, NY: Thieme, 2003: 123–128.
10. Sumner CJ, Sheth S, Griffin JW, et al. The spectrum of neuropathy in diabetes and impaired glucose tolerance. Neurology 2003; 60(1):108–111.
11. Smith AG, Ramachandran P, Tripp S, et al. Epidermal nerve innervation in impaired glucose tolerance and diabetes-associated neuropathy. Neurology 2001; 57(9): 1701–1704.
12. Malik RA, Veves A, Masson EA, et al. Endoneurial capillary abnormalities in mild human diabetic neuropathy. J Neurol Neurosurg Psychiatry 1992; 55(7): 557–561.
13. Dyck PJ, Giannini C, Lais A. Pathologic alterations of nerves. In: Dyck PJ, Thomas PK, Griffin JW, eds. Peripheral Neuropathy. 3rd ed. Philadelphia, PA: WB Saunders, 1998:514–595.
14. Newrick PG, Wilson AJ, Jakubowski J, et al. Sural nerve oxygen tension in diabetes. Br Med J (Clin Res Ed) 1986; 293(6554):1053–1054.
15. Dyck PJ, Karnes JL, O'Brien P, et al. The spatial distribution of fiber loss in diabetic polyneuropathy suggests ischemia. Ann Neurol 1986; 19(5):440–449.
16. Boulton AJ, Malik RA. Diabetic neuropathy. Med Clin North Am 1998; 82(4):909–929.
17. Dyck PJ, Lais A, Karnes JL, et al. Fiber loss is primary and multifocal in sural nerves in diabetic polyneuropathy. Ann Neurol 1986; 19(5):425–439.
18. Malik RA, Tesfaye S, Newrick PG, et al. Sural nerve pathology in diabetic patients with minimal but progressive neuropathy. Diabetologia 2005; 48(3):578–585.
19. American Diabetes Association. Joint report and recommendations of the San Antonio Conference on diabetic neuropathy. Diabetes Care 1998; 11:582–597.
20. Boulton AJ, Gries FA, Jervell JA. Guidelines for the diagnosis and outpatient management of diabetic peripheral neuropathy. Diabet Med 1998; 15(6):508–514.
21. Dyck PJ. Severity and staging of diabetic polyneuropathy. In: Gries FA, Cameron NE, Low PA, Ziegler D, eds. Textbook of Diabetic Neuropathy. New York, NY: Thieme, 2003:170–175.
22. Grant IA. Differential diagnosis of diabetic neuropathies. In: Dyck PJ, Thomas PK, eds. Diabetic Neuropathy. 2nd ed. Philadelphia, PA: WB Saunders, 1999: 415–444.
23. Thomas PK. Classification, differential diagnosis, and staging of diabetic neuropathy. Diabetes 1997; 46:S54–S57.
24. Armstrong DG, Lavery LA, Vela SA, et al. Choosing a practical screening instrument to identify patients at risk for diabetic foot ulceration. Arch Intern Med 1998; 158: 289–292.
25. Vileikyte L, Hutchings G, Hollis S, et al. The tactile circumferential discriminator: A new, simple screening device to identify diabetic patients at risk of foot ulceration [see comments]. Diabetes Care 1997; 20(4):623–626.
26. Smieja M, Hunt DL, Edelman D, et al. Clinical examination for the detection of protective sensation in the feet of diabetic patients: International Cooperative Group for Clinical Examination Research. J Gen Intern Med 1999; 14(7):418–424.

27. Reilly MM, Hanna MG. Genetic neuromuscular disease. J Neurol Neurosurg Psychiatry 2002; 73(suppl 2):II12–II21.
28. Berciano J, Combarros O. Hereditary neuropathies. Curr Opin Neurol 2003; 16(5): 613–622.
29. Brady RO. Fabry disease. In: Dyck PJ, Thomas PK, Griffin JW, eds. Peripheral Neuropathy. Philadelphia, PA: WB Saunders, 1993:1169–1178.
30. Poynard T, Yuen MF, Ratziu V, et al. Viral hepatitis C. Lancet 2003; 362(9401): 2095–2100.
31. Pardo CA, McArthur JC, Griffin JW. HIV neuropathy: Insights in the pathology of HIV peripheral nerve disease. J Peripher Nerv Syst 2001; 6(1):21–27.
32. Magy L, Chassande B, Maisonobe T, et al. Polyneuropathy associated with IgG/IgA monoclonal gammopathy: A clinical and electrophysiological study of 15 cases. Eur J Neurol 2003; 10(6):677–685.
33. Asbury AK. Uremic neuropathy. In: Dyck PJ, Thomas PK, eds. Peripheral neuropathy. Philadelphia, PA: WB Saunders, 1975:982.
34. Asbury AK. Neuropathies with renal failure, hepatic disorders, chronic respiratory insufficiency, and critical illness. In: Dyck PJ, Thomas PK, Griffin JW, eds. Peripheral neuropathy. Philadelphia, PA: WB Saunders, 1993:1251–1265.
35. Ansari J, Nagabhushan N, Syed R, et al. Small cell lung cancer associated with anti-Hu paraneoplastic sensory neuropathy and peripheral nerve microvasculitis: Case report and literature review. Clin Oncol (R Coll Radiol) 2004; 16(1):71–76.
36. Altaha R, Abraham J. Paraneoplastic neurologic syndrome associated with occult breast cancer: A case report and review of literature. Breast J 2003; 9(5):417–419.
37. Ammendola A, Tata MR, Aurilio C, et al. Peripheral neuropathy in chronic alcoholism: A retrospective cross-sectional study in 76 subjects. Alcohol Alcohol 2001; 36(3): 271–275.
38. Vittadini G, Buonocore M, Colli G, et al. Alcoholic polyneuropathy: A clinical and epidemiological study. Alcohol Alcohol 2001; 36(5):393–400.
39. Koike H, Mori K, Misu K, et al. Painful alcoholic polyneuropathy with predominant small-fiber loss and normal thiamine status. Neurology 2001; 56(12):1727–1732.
40. Bourque PR, Dyck PJ. Selective calf weakness suggests intraspinal pathology, not peripheral neuropathy. Arch Neurol 1990; 47(1):79–80.
41. Dyck PJ. Detection, characterization, and staging of polyneuropathy: Assessed in diabetics. Muscle Nerve 1988; 11:21–32.
42. Braune HJ. Early detection of diabetic neuropathy: A neurophysiological study on 100 patients. Electromyogr Clin Neurophysiol 1997; 37(7):399–407.
43. Bevilacqua NJ, Rogers LC, Malik RA, et al. Technique of the sural nerve biopsy. J Foot Ankle Surg 2007; 46(2):139–142.
44. Herrmann DN, Ferguson ML, Pannoni V, et al. Plantar nerve AP and skin biopsy in sensory neuropathies with normal routine conduction studies. Neurology 2004; 63(5):879–885.
45. Periquet MI, Novak V, Collins MP, et al. Painful sensory neuropathy: Prospective evaluation using skin biopsy. Neurology 1999; 53(8):1641–1647.
46. Malik RA, Kallinikos P, Abbott CA, et al. Corneal confocal microscopy: A non-invasive surrogate of nerve fibre damage and repair in diabetic patients. Diabetologia 2003; 46(5):683–688.
47. Quattrini C, Tavakoli M, Jeziorska M, et al. Surrogate markers of small fiber damage in human diabetic neuropathy. Diabetes 2007; 56(8):2148–2154.
48. Mehra S, Tavakoli M, Kallinikos PA, et al. Corneal confocal microscopy detects early nerve regeneration after pancreas transplantation in patients with type 1 diabetes. Diabetes Care 2007; 30(10):2608–2612.
49. Pecoraro RE, Reiber GE, Burgess EM. Pathways to diabetic limb amputation: Basis for prevention. Diabetes Care 1990; 13:513–521.
50. Reiber GE, Vileikyte L, Boyko EJ, et al. Causal pathways for incident lower-extremity ulcers in patients with diabetes from two settings. Diabetes Care 1999;22(1): 157–162.

51. Lincoln NB, Radford KA, Game FL, et al. Education for secondary prevention of foot ulcers in people with diabetes: A randomised controlled trial. Diabetologia 2008; 51(11):1954–1961.
52. Murray HJ, Young MJ, Hollis S, et al. The association between callus formation, high pressures and neuropathy in diabetic foot ulceration. Diabetic Med 1996; 13(11): 979–982.
53. Armstrong DG, Frykberg RG. Classification of diabetic foot surgery: Toward a rational definition. Diabet Med 2003; 20(4):329–331.
54. Curzen NC, Timmis A. Endothelial dysfunction in chronic heart failure. In: Coats A, Cleland JG, eds. Controversies in the Management of Heart Failure. Edinburgh, England: Churchill-Livingstone, 1997:25–40.
55. Malik RA, Williamson S, Abbott C, et al. Effect of angiotensin-converting-enzyme (ACE) inhibitor trandolapril on human diabetic neuropathy: Randomised double-blind controlled trial [see comments]. Lancet 1998; 352(9145):1978–1981.
56. Malik RA. Can diabetic neuropathy be prevented by angiotensin-converting enzyme inhibitors? Ann Med 2000; 32(1):1–5.
57. Wheeler GD. Ruboxistaurin (Eli Lilly). IDrugs. 2003; 6:159–163.
58. Prendergast JJ, Miranda G, Sanchez M. Improvement of sensory impairment in patients with peripheral neuropathy. Endocr Pract 2004; 10(1):24–30.
59. Kochman AB, Carnegie DH, Burke TJ. Symptomatic reversal of peripheral neuropathy in patients with diabetes. J Am Podiatr Med Assoc 2002; 92(3):125–130.
60. Powell MW, Carnegie DE, Burke TJ. Reversal of diabetic peripheral neuropathy and new wound incidence: The role of MIRE. Adv Skin Wound Care 2004; 17(6): 295–300.
61. Lavery LA, Murdoch DP, Williams J, et al. Does anodyne light therapy improve peripheral neuropathy in diabetes? A double-blind, sham-controlled, randomized trial to evaluate monochromatic infrared photoenergy. Diabetes Care 2008; 31(2): 316–321.
62. Sinclair JC, Cook RJ, Guyatt GH, et al. When should an effective treatment be used? Derivation of the threshold number needed to treat and the minimum event rate for treatment. J Clin Epidemiol 2001; 54(3):253–262.
63. Barbano R, Hart-Gouleau S, Pennella-Vaughan J, et al. Pharmacotherapy of painful diabetic neuropathy. Curr Pain Headache Rep 2003; 7(3):169–177.
64. Semenchuk MR, Sherman S, Davis B. Double-blind, randomized trial of bupropion SR for the treatment of neuropathic pain. Neurology 2001; 57(9):1583–1588.
65. Sindrup SH, Jensen TS. Pharmacologic treatment of pain in polyneuropathy. Neurology 2000; 55(7):915–920.
66. Sultan A, Gaskell H, Derry S, et al. Duloxetine for painful diabetic neuropathy and fibromyalgia pain: Systematic review of randomised trials. BMC Neurol 2008; 8:29.
67. Vinik A. Use of antiepileptic drugs in the treatment of chronic painful diabetic neuropathy. J Clin Endocrinol Metab 2005; 90(8):4936–4945.
68. Morello CM, Leckband SG, Stoner CP, et al. Randomized double-blind study comparing the efficacy of gabapentin with amitriptyline on diabetic peripheral neuropathy pain. Arch Intern Med 1999; 159(16):1931–1937.
69. Dallocchio C, Buffa C, Mazzarello P, et al. Gabapentin vs. amitriptyline in painful diabetic neuropathy: An open-label pilot study. J Pain Symptom Manage 2000; 20(4): 280–285.
70. Freynhagen R, Strojek K, Griesing T, et al. Efficacy of pregabalin in neuropathic pain evaluated in a 12-week, randomised, double-blind, multicentre, placebo-controlled trial of flexible- and fixed-dose regimens. Pain 2005; 115(3):254–263.
71. Freeman R, Durso-Decruz E, Emir B. Efficacy, safety, and tolerability of pregabalin treatment for painful diabetic peripheral neuropathy: Findings from seven randomized, controlled trials across a range of doses. Diabetes Care 2008; 31(7): 1448–1454.
72. Harati Y, Gooch C, Swenson M, et al. Double-blind randomized trial of tramadol for the treatment of the pain of diabetic neuropathy. Neurology 1998; 50(6):1842–1846.

73. Gimbel JS, Richards P, Portenoy RK. Controlled-release oxycodone for pain in diabetic neuropathy: A randomized controlled trial. Neurology 2003; 60(6):927–934.
74. Watson CP, Moulin D, Watt-Watson J, et al. Controlled-release oxycodone relieves neuropathic pain: A randomized controlled trial in painful diabetic neuropathy. Pain 2003; 105(1/2):71–78.
75. Cohen KL, Harris S. Efficacy and safety of nonsteroidal anti-inflammatory drugs in the therapy of diabetic neuropathy. Arch Intern Med 1987; 147(8):1442–1444.
76. Kellogg AP, Cheng HT, Pop-Busui R. Cyclooxygenase-2 pathway as a potential therapeutic target in diabetic peripheral neuropathy. Curr Drug Targets 2008; 9(1):68–76.
77. Stracke H, Gaus W, Achenbach U, et al. Benfotiamine in diabetic polyneuropathy (BENDIP): Results of a randomised, double blind, placebo-controlled clinical study. Exp Clin Endocrinol Diabetes 2008; 116(10):600–605.
78. Veves A. Diagnosis of diabetic neuropathy. In: Veves A, ed. Clinical Management of Diabetic Neuropathy. Humana Press, Inc. Totowa, New Jersey, 1998:61–75.
79. Dyck PJ, Kratz KM, Lehman KA, et al. The Rochester Diabetic Neuropathy Study: Design, criteria for types of neuropathy, selection bias, and reproducibility of neuropathic tests. Neurology 1991; 41(6):799–807.
80. Chaudhry V, Stevens JC, Kincaid J, et al. Practice Advisory: Utility of surgical decompression for treatment of diabetic neuropathy: Report of the Therapeutics and Technology Assessment Subcommittee of the American Academy of Neurology. Neurology 2006; 66(12):1805–1808.
81. Cornblath DR, Vinik A, Feldman E, et al. Surgical decompression for diabetic sensorimotor polyneuropathy. Diabetes Care 2007; 30(2):421–422.
82. Chaudhry V, Russell J, Belzberg A. Decompressive surgery of lower limbs for symmetrical diabetic peripheral neuropathy. Cochrane Database Syst Rev 2008; (3):CD006152.
83. Tesfaye S, Chaturvedi N, Eaton SE, et al. Vascular risk factors and diabetic neuropathy. N Engl J Med 2005; 352(4):341–350.

7 Advanced therapies to treat diabetic foot ulcers

Lawrence A. Lavery and George T. Liu

Historically, outcomes of diabetic foot ulcers (DFUs) have been poor. In a meta-analysis of control groups from randomized clinical trials (RCTs) for DFUs, only 24.2% of wounds that received "standard therapy" healed in 12 weeks (1). However, outcomes may be even worse in clinical practice because the exclusion and inclusion criteria used in RCTs exclude the least desirable and most challenging patients. RCTs that evaluate treatments for DFUs exclude high-risk patients such as those with poor glycated hemoglobin, peripheral arterial disease (PAD), and large, deep, or infected wounds. Most industry-sponsored studies do not reflect the majority of patients who are treated in clinical practice. For instance, Carter et al. (2) used a large electronic medical records database from wound clinics and found that more than half of patients would have been excluded from 15 of 17 RCTs. Most RCTs use less than optimal techniques for "off-loading" the ulcer, such as shoes and healing sandals. In fact, most descriptive cohort studies of total contact casts and RCTs that study off-loading devices have a healing rate that is twice that of "advanced therapies" such as bioengineered tissue, growth factors and negative pressure wound therapy (NWPT) (3,4).

Advanced therapies are often much more expensive than standard therapies; therefore, they must improve healing rates and healing time to be cost-effective. One way to do this is to stratify the wounds into categories and identify which wounds are most likely to fail standard therapy. There are several classifications systems that have attempted to do this.

CLINICAL EXAMINATION AND CLASSIFICATION

Examination and classification of DFUs is an essential aspect of wound assessment. Wound duration, depth, size, perfusion, and underlying infections are associated with wound healing and amputation risk (5–7). Most wound classification systems use some or all of these factors in their systems to score wound severity and help predict clinical outcomes. The two most-cited ulcer classifications are the Wagner and University of Texas (UT) ulcer classifications.

Wagner Ulcer Classification

Meggitt (8) first described his DFU classification in 1976. The same system was subsequently popularized by Wagner and bears his name (9). The Meggitt-Wagner ulcer classification is a six-tiered system that inconsistently includes components of depth, infection, and gangrene. The first tier is level 0. It is described as intact skin. Ulcer classification 1 is a superficial ulceration, and classification 2 is based on depth that penetrates to tendon, bone, or joint. None of the first

Table 1 University of Texas Ulcer Classification

	0	1	2	3
A	Preulcerative lesion	Full thickness ulcer not involving tendon, capsule, or bone	Penetrates to tendon or capsule	Penetrates to bone
B	Infection	Infection	Infection	Infection
C	PAD	PAD	PAD	PAD
D	PAD and infection	PAD and infection	PAD and infection	PAD and infection

Abbreviation: PAD, peripheral arterial occlusive disease.

three tiers of the Meggitt-Wagner classification include any criteria for infection or PAD. Classification 3 is an ulcer that penetrates to deep structures with abscess or osteitis. Level 4 is described as forefoot gangrene, and level 5 is gangrene of the whole foot. The last two tiers are the only ones that suggest the presence of PAD, although gangrene can be caused by embolism, frostbite, or sepsis in addition to PAD.

The University of Texas DFU Classification

The UT ulcer classification uses a 4 × 4 matrix to classify ulcer depth (ulcer grade) and the presence of infection and PAD (ulcer stage) (Table 1) (10). The four criteria for recording wound depth are similar to the Meggitt-Wagner classification. Grade 0 is designated as pre- or postulcerative skin that is intact. Grade 1 is for full thickness ulcerations, and Grade 2 is for ulcers that penetrate to tendon or capsule. Grade 3 ulcers are those that probe to bone. The y-axis of the ulcer classification matrix describes the ulcer stage and includes scores for the presence of infection and PAD. Stage A is designated as no signs of either infection or PAD. Stage B is infection with no PAD, and Stage C is PAD with no infection. Stager D includes both PAD and infection. One of the advantages of the UT ulcer classification system is that it includes two of the most common comorbidities related to wound failure and amputation to be included in every wound assessment.

Armstrong et al. conducted a retrospective cohort study of 360 consecutive patients with DFUs to validate the UT Ulcer Classification system (6). The study indicated that as wound depth increases and as wound stage progresses from A to D, the frequency and level of lower extremity amputation increases. For instance, ulcers that penetrated to bone were 11 times more likely to result in a midfoot or higher level of amputation. In a subsequent study, Oyibo et al. (11) compared the Wagner and UT ulcer classification using a similar study design with 194 DFUs. He found that healing times were not different for each grade of the UT classification ($P = 0.07$) or the Wagner classification ($P = 0.1$). However, a stepwise increase in the time to heal was identified with each stage of the UT system, and the ulcer stage predicted healing. Gul et al. (12) compared healing time and amputations in a cohort of 200 patients with DFUs and found that the median time to heal ulcerations increased as the UT stage and grade increased and as the Wagner grade increased. As the UT ulcer grade or depth of the ulceration increased, the risk of amputation increased as well. Both Gul et al. and Oyibo et al. concluded that including the stage and grade in the ulcer classification improved its ability to predict outcomes (11,12).

WOUND HEALING TRAJECTORIES

Another way to maximize the use of advanced therapies is to identify wounds that are unlikey to heal more quickly. This has been done by identifying wound healing rates that predict complete healing. Several studies have suggested that evaluation of the velocity of wound healing or the percentage change in wound area can help predict wound healing potential. Regular wound evaluation and measurement gives the clinician objective data to reassess both the patient and the effectiveness of the wound care plan. Perhaps the clinical value of assessing wound trajectories will be to identify wounds that are likely to fail standard therapy and use this information as a mechanism to institute more expensive, advanced therapies earlier during treatment.

Studies by Sheehan et al. (13) and Lavery et al. (14) evaluated surrogate endpoints to predict wound healing in DFUs and open amputation wounds. Sheehan et al. (13) reported that DFUs that did not have a median percentage wound area reduction of at least 54% in 28 days were significantly less likely to heal in 12 weeks. Likewise, Lavery et al. did a post hoc analysis of data from a RCT of NWPT in open foot amputation wounds and reported similar results. However, in addition to evaluating percentage wound area reduction at 4 weeks, they looked at 1-week percentage wound area reduction. Patients who did not have at least a 15% wound area reduction at 1 week and a 60% wound area reduction at 4 weeks were significantly less likely to heal over a 16-week evaluation period compared with patients who met or exceeded those benchmarks (14). In addition, the initial size and depth of the wound, history of wound healing, infection, PAD, glycated hemoglobin, renal disease, and nutrition could impact the risk of healing, infection, amputation, and death. The time to initiate expensive "advanced therapies" such as hyperbaric medicine, bioengineered tissue, electrical stimulation, and NWPT is unclear. By identifying high-risk populations such as patients with chronic kidney disease (CKD) or patients with wounds that do not progress on the basis of a change in wound area, we could target "advanced" therapies earlier in the course of treatment when they might have a better clinical and economic impact.

WOUND DEBRIDEMENT

The rational for debridement is to remove nonviable tissue, reduce wound bioburden, decrease the risk of infection, and convert chronic to acute wounds. There are many recommendations for the type and the level of debridement that should be provided to DFUs. Some authors suggest that surgical debridement should be used to remove tissue from the wound edges and bed (15–17). Others advocate topical, chemical debridement agents or larval therapy for regular debridement. Unfortunately there is very little prospective evidence to guide decision making or product selection.

There is little evidence to support the effectiveness of debridement to improve DFU healing. Much of wound care in this respect is driven by convention rather than clinical evidence. Some physicians believe that wounds should be surgically debrided every week or two. Others rely on nonsurgical debridement and use chemical or larval debridement. And they look for specific changes in the wound bed to trigger the need to continue or stop debridement. Because the local signs of changes in wounds are subjective, they are difficult to define and standardize even among clinicians in the same clinic. There is a need for clinicians to perform more objective wound measurement and understand when, how, and to what extent a wound should be debrided.

There are only a few studies that have reported the benefit of wound debridement in DFUs. All three studies we identified performed post hoc analysis using data from RCTs and assessed if wounds were debrided or the extent of debridement and attempted to identify an association with wound healing. Steed and colleagues' data included 118 patients from a multicenter RCT of topical platelet-derived growth factor. Surgical debridement of DFUs was performed at the discretion of the treating physician over the 20-week study period. The average percentage of visits where debridement was performed was 47% for patients assigned to the growth factor treatment group and 48% for patients assigned to the control group. A significantly higher rate of healing was identified at centers that had more-frequent debridement independent of the treatment group. And a lower rate of healing was observed in those centers that performed less-frequent debridement (17).

Cardinal et al. (18) performed a similar study, using data from large RCTs, and evaluated the frequency of debridement. He evaluated data from a venous stasis ulcer study ($N = 366$) and a DFU study ($N = 310$). In both studies, there was a higher proportion of wounds that healed at centers that debrided wounds more frequently (18). However, the frequency of debridement per subject was not statistically correlated to higher rates of wound closure ($P = 0.069$).

Saap and Falanga (16) evaluated the predictive value of a wound debridement using a wound debridement scoring system (Debridement Performance Index) to identify healing over a 12-week study period. They evaluated 143 wounds using the Apligraf RCT pivotal study data. The DPI attempts to evaluate and score (1) if wound debridement was needed and (2) the level of debridement. The system evaluates there areas (callus, undermining edge, and necrotic tissue) and scores each from 0 to 1 based on whether debridement was needed but not done (0), needed and done (1), or not needed and not done (2). Scores could range from 0 to 6, with the highest score identifying the best debridement care. On the basis of Saap's evaluation, patients who had appropriate wound debridement based on the Debridement Performance Index scores (scored 3–6) were 2.4 times more likely to heal (16).

Larval Debridement

While larval therapy seems to have growing acceptance and use, there are still only a few clinical studies in DFUs. There are three retrospective cohort studies (*level B*) and one prospective study (*level A*) that describe the benefit of maggot debridement in DFU (15,19–21). Wound debridement and bacterial load is improved with larval therapy but the proportion of wounds that heal and clinical infections are not significantly different than wounds treated with conventional debridement. Paul et al. (19) compared *Lucillia cuprina* larval therapy ($n = 29$) to conventional therapy ($n = 30$) in patients with DFUs. There was no difference in the proportion of wounds that healed with maggot debridement (48.3%) compared with conventional debridement (60.0%) (19) (*level B*). Likewise, Armstrong evaluated 60 subjects with UT Ulcer classification C or D ulcers over a 6-month period. There was no difference in the proportion of wounds that healed in larval debridement and conventional debridement (57% vs. 33%) or in wounds that developed infection (80% vs. 60%). However, among patients who healed, time to healing was shorter (15) (*level B*).

Sherman (20) compared a cohort of 18 patients with 20 wounds and their response to conventional and maggot wound debridement. After 5 weeks of treatment, wounds that had conventional therapy had an average of 33% of the wound surface covered with necrotic tissue. Wounds treated with maggots were completely debrided in 4 weeks. Sherman (20) also reported work on the benefit of larval therapy for wound debridement. In a descriptive cohort of 10 patients with 13 ulcers treated with *Lucillia sericata* treated for 3 days a week, all wounds were completely debrided in an average of 1.9 weeks. The average weekly wound area reduction was 16%. In addition, the bacterial load was reduced after the first application (20). Larval therapy has also been shown to eliminate methicillin-resistant *Staphylococcus aureus* colonization in DFUs (22).

The use of larval debridement is limited because of patient acceptance, the need for frequent clinic visits to have the dressings changed and new maggots added to the wound bed, and patient tolerance because of pain during maggot treatment.

Electrical Stimulation

There are several applications of electrical stimulation described in the medical literature for wound healing, including pulsed electromagnetic fields, high-voltage galvanic electrical stimulation, and transcutaneous electrical stimulation. Electrical stimulation and pulsed electromagnetic field therapy have been shown to increase local perfusion (23) and stimulate the release of growth factors (24). Electrical stimulation to improve wound healing has a relatively large number of randomized clinical studies and cohort studies to support its effectiveness (*level A*). There are more randomized clinical studies that report the effectiveness of electrical stimulation in wound healing than any other wound therapy. The studies reported in Table 2 provide some examples of the clinical applications and outcomes. The RCTs in this area evaluate a variety of wounds. All of the studies have positive results; however, most of the studies are small studies of short duration, and they evaluate the percentage change in wound area reduction rather than complete wound healing as the primary outcome in most studies. These studies evaluate pressure ulcers, arterial ulcers, venous ulcerations, and DFUs. In addition, the type of electrical stimulation, the duration of the electrical stimulation therapy per day, the type of waveform, and polarity at the wound are variable.

Peters et al. evaluated DFUs among patients with diabetes, and Lundeberg et al. studied venous leg ulcers in persons with diabetes (25,26) (*level A*). Peters et al. conducted a double-blinded sham-controlled RCT of 40 patients with UT Ulcer classification 1A and 2A ulcers. Patients in the active treatment arm received a subsensory level of electrical stimulation given at home and the control group used a sham electrical stimulation device. Both groups used the device at home at night while they slept 7 days a week. Patients in both groups were given DH Pressure Relief Walking boots to off-load the ulcer site. Over a 12-week evaluation period, 65% of patients with active electrical stimulation units healed compared with 35% of sham patients ($P = 0.058$). However, after adjusting for compliance, there was a significant trend in healing with electrical stimulation (26). Peter and colleagues' study was unique because it was a home, self-administered application, and they were able to download data from the electrical stimulation device

Table 2 Electrical Stimulation Studies

Study	Stimulation	Study type	Wound type	Treatment group	N	Initial wound size	% Healed or % change
Griffin (27) 1991	HVPC	Single-blind RCT	Decubitis Grades II–IV	HVPC	8	2.34 cm^2	80% WAR
				Sham	9	2.72 cm^2	52% WAR
Feedar (28) 1991	PDC	Double-blind RCT	Mixed	PDC	26	14.7 cm^2	14% per week WAR
				Sham	24	16.9 cm^2	8.5% per week WAR
Sarma (29) 1997	PC	Double-blind RCT	Leprosy Foot ulcer	PEMF	18	2843 cu mm	86% WAR
				Sham	15	2428 cu mm	40% WAR
Houghton (30) 2003	HVPC	Double-blind RCT	Mixed Leg	HVPC	14	6.4 cm^2	44% WAR
				Sham	13	5.5 cm^2	16% WAR
Stiller (31) 1992	PEMF	Double-blind RCT	Venous stasis	PEMF	18	7.3 cm^2	47.1 WAR
				Sham	13	7.7 cm^2	48.7 increase
Carley (32) 1985	Low-intensity direct current	RCT	Mixed	HVPC	15	4.7cm^2	89% WAR
				Wet-dry	15	3.9 cm^2	45% WAR
Peters (26) 2001	HVPC	Double-blind RCT	DFU	HVPC	20	1.4 cm^2	65% healed
				Sham	20	1.3 cm^2	35% healed
Lundeberg (25) 1992	TENS	Double-blind RCT	Diabetic Venous stasis	TENS	32	24.2 cm^2	31% healed
				Sham	32	22.0 cm^2	12.5% healed
Wood (33) 1993	PDC	Double-blind RCT	Decubitis Stage II/III	PDC	43	2.61 cm^2	56% healed
				Sham	31	1.91 cm^2	3% healed

Abbreviations: HVPC, high-voltage pulsed current; PDC, pulsed direct current; PC, pulsed current; PEMF, pulsed electromagnetic field; TENS, transcutaneous electrical nerve stimulation; WAR, wound area reduction.

to identify the number of hours electrical stimulation was self-applied each week. In other studies, the application of electrical stimulation was usually performed in a clinic or a hospital setting, so compliance was not an issue. Peters et al. (26) found that compliant patients had better clinical outcomes. Patients who used the electrical stimulation device at least 3 days a week were more likely to heal than those who used it 0 to 2 days a week.

Lundeberg and colleagues' study included 64 patients with diabetes and venous stasis ulcerations. Patients who were assigned to the active electrical stimulation group received alternating constant current at 80 Hz for 20 minutes twice a day for 12 weeks. The wound area reduction and proportion of wounds that healed were significantly greater in the active treatment group (61% wound area reduction, 31% healed) compared with sham treatment (41% wound area reduction, 12.5% healed, $P < 0.05$) (25).

Negative Pressure Wound Therapy

Topical subatmospheric therapy has been one of the most studied wound therapies in the medical literature over the past decade. Most of the published work involves animal studies and retrospective cohort studies. Laboratory studies have demonstrated that NPWT increases local perfusion (34), increases granulation tissue formation (35), reduces bacterial load in wounds, and reduces matrix metalloproteinases in the wound bed (36).

There are several RCTs in patients with DFUs or open surgical wounds conducted using NPWT. Armstrong and Lavery (37) reported the results of a RCT that compared NPWT to standard wound care in patients with diabetes who had open amputation wounds over a 16-week evaluation period *(level A)*. There were 77 patients randomized to NPWT and 85 to the control arm. During the 16-week evaluation period, a significantly higher proportion of wounds healed (56%) compared with the control group (39%). The median treatment duration in the NPWT group was 59 days and 106 days in the standard therapy group ($P < 0.001$). There were fewer additional amputations in the NPWT group ($n = 2$) compared with that in the control group ($n = 9$, $P = 0.06$).

Blume et al. (39) reported a subsequent RCT that evaluated DFUs *(level A)*. The study used a similar design and randomized 342 patients with diabetes and neuropathic foot ulcers to receive NPWT or moist wound therapy for a 16-week treatment period. A higher proportion of wounds healed in the NPWT group (43.2%) than in the control arm (28.9%, $P = 0.007$). In addition, there were significantly fewer amputations in the NPWT (4.1% vs. 10.2%, $P = 0.035$) and a significant increase in granulation tissue.

One of the difficulties evaluating NPWT for diabetic foot wounds is selecting a clinical outcome that matches the objectives of therapy. NPWT is not a modality that is usually used throughout the wound treatment cycle, especially when treating DFUs. NWPT is used to stimulate and prepare the wound bed. Often in DFUs, wounds are too small to continue therapy. Advances in NPWT devices and application techniques have expanded the use of this technology. Many NPWT devices are small, light-weight, and battery-operated, so patients can wear them on their waist and perform activities of daily living without being tethered to their bed. In addition, bridging techniques to extend the foam interface from wounds on the sole of the foot to the top of the foot allow the connections to be off weight-bearing surfaces. Patients can walk without the NPWT injuring the bottom of the foot. Armstrong et al. (39) performed a gait laboratory study for pressures before and after application of NPWT for plantar foot wounds and showed that there was not a significant change in pressures when a bridging technique was used.

NWPT is one of the innovations that has changed wound care. There are several new products that are available. Most of the publications in the area of NPWT use the same device, so most of the new products have little evidence that specifically describe their "take-off" on NPWT. It is still unclear whether newer approaches are the same, worse, or better than the initial VAC product (KCI San Antonio, Texas).

HYPERBARIC MEDICINE

Systemic hyperbaric oxygen therapy for DFUs has been available for many years. Even though it is widely available in the United States, there are only a handful of small RCTs. There is evidence from RCTs that hyperbaric oxygen therapy increases the proportion of DFUs that heal and that hyperbaric oxygen (HBO) reduces lower extremity amputations (Table 3). The prospective studies for wound healing are small and probably inadequately powered to study different severities of DFUs.

Abidia et al. (40) randomized 18 patients with Wagner 1–2 ulcers for 6 weeks. Patients in the HBO group had more ulcers that healed and a significantly greater median reduction in wound area compared with the sham group. In the HBO group, five patients healed (55.6%), and only one patient healed in the sham arm (11.1%, $P = 0.04$). The median wound area reduction was 100% with HBO and 52% in the sham group ($P = 0.27$). There was one major amputation in each group (40) *(level A)*.

Kessler et al. (41) randomized 28 patients with Wagner 1–3 wounds. After 4 weeks, there was no difference in the reduction of ulcer size between the two treatment groups (HBO 61.9 ± 23.3 vs. control 55.1 ± 21.5). There was no difference in wound healing. Two patients healed in the HBO group, and none of the patients in the control arm healed ($P = 0.33$) (41) *(level A)*.

Table 3 Hyperbaric Oxygen Therapy and Diabetic Foot Ulcers

Author	RCT	HBO controls (*n*)	Primary outcome	Average number dives	atm	Dive duration (min)	% Outcome in HBO group
Faglia (42)	Yes	35–33	Major amputation	38	2.5	90	8.3 vs. 32.3
Doctor (43)	Yes	15–15	Major amputation	4	3	45	13.3 vs. 46.7
Baroni (48)	No	18–10	DFU healing	34	2.5–2.8	90	88.9 vs. 10
Kessler (41)	Yes	14–14	DFU healing	28	2.5	90	14.3 vs. 0
Abidia (40)	Yes	9–9	DFU healing	30	2.4	90	55.6 vs. 11.1

Faglia and coworkers (42) randomized 36 subjects to receive HBO and 34 to receive standard therapy. The HBO group received 38 ± 8 treatments on average at pressures ranging from 2.2 to 2.5 atm. There were three major amputations in the HBO group (8.3%) and 11 in the control arm (32.3%, $P < 0.05$). The authors reported significantly fewer major amputations (below-the-knee or above-the-knee) for the HBO group but only among patients with Wagner grade IV ulcers. There were no statistical differences in minor amputations between the HBO and control groups and no intergroup difference in major amputations among patients with Wagner grade II or III wounds (42) *(level A)*.

Doctor and coworkers (43) reported the results of a prospective, randomized, controlled study of 30 patients randomized to hyperbaric therapy or a control group. The duration of hyperbaric therapy was only four sessions at a pressure of 3 atm for 45 minutes per session. Despite the short treatment period, the authors reported fewer major amputations in the HBO group (13.3%) compared with the control group (46.7%, $P < 0.05$) *(level A)*.

BIOENGINEERED TISSUE

There are a variety of cellular and acellular wound scaffold products that are used for DFUs, such as Graftjacket (Wright Medical, Arlington, TN), Oasis (Healthpoint, Fort Worth, Texas), Apligraf (Organogenesis, Canton, MA), and Dermagraft (Advanced Biohealing, La Jolla, CA). Several products have double-blinded RCTs that demonstrate that these products improve DFU healing. The bioactive products are suggested to increase local growth factors. The acellular products may provide a scaffold for wound regeneration.

Graftjacket and Oasis are acellular wound matrix products. Graftjacket is a cryopreserved product from human skin, and Oasis is dry packaged porcine small intestine mucosa. Brigido et al. (44) conducted a single center RCT to evaluate a single application of Graftjacket compared with standard therapy over a 16-week evaluation period. There was a higher proportion of wounds that healed with Graftjacket (85.7%) compared with patients who received standard therapy (28.6%, $P = 0.001$) *(level A)*.

Niezgoda et al. (45) compared Oasis to Regranex gel, platelet-derived growth factor, in a 12-week study of DFUs. They randomized 73 patients to receive Oasis ($n = 37$) or Regranex gel ($n = 36$). There was a trend that indicated the Oasis application healed a higher proportion of DFUs (49%) compared with topical platelet-derived growth factor (28%, $P = 0.055$) (45) *(level A)*.

There are two commercially available bioengineered active wound products in the United States, Dermagraft and Apligraf. Both have level A evidence that they heal a higher proportion of DFUs compared with standard therapy. Dermagraft is cryopreserved human dermal fibroblast product seeded on a bioabsorbable polyglactin scaffold. Dermagraft is derived from newborn foreskin. Apligraf is a bilayered epidermal-dermal product. The upper layer consists of human keratinocytes, and the lower dermal layer combines bovine collagen and human fibroblasts.

A multicenter RCT randomized 245 patients with DFUs. Patients in both treatment groups had wound debridement ad lib and off-loading with extra-depth shoes and custom insoles or healing sandals. Patients assigned to the Dermagraft group had up to 8 weekly applications of Dermagraft. More patients healed after 12 weeks in the Dermagraft group (30%) compared with those in controls (18%, $P = 0.023$). In addition, the Dermagraft group healed ulcers faster than controls. The median percentage wound closure was 78% in the control group and 91% in the Dermagraft group ($P = 0.044$). The Dermagraft group also had few complications such as soft tissue or bone infections (Dermagraft 19% vs. control 32%, $P = 0.007$) (46) *(level A)*.

There were similar results reported from an Apligraf pivotal trial. Veves et al. (47) reported the results of a multicenter RCT in which 112 patients were randomized to receive up to 5 weekly applications of Apligraf, and 96 were randomized to receive saline moistened gauze. Off-loading was provided with a custom sandal. A significantly higher proportion of wounds healed in the Apligraf group (56%) compared with those in the control group (38%, $P = 0.004$). The time to wound healing in the treatment group was less than that for controls. The median time to complete epithelialization was 65 days with Apligraf and 90 days with saline-moistened gauze (47) *(level A)*.

CONCLUSION

Wound healings is a complex process that is difficult to study in animals and in humans. There are many challenges and opportunities in wound healing in patients with diabetes. A decade or two ago, most of the content of this chapter would have been based on expert opinion. Our understanding of debridement, off-loading, and evolving technologies has improved over the last decade, but in many ways, it is still at its infancy. Most of the studies in DFUs that are not phase 3 clinical trials are small. And studies that are sponsored by industry, selectively exclude the type of wounds and patients who are most often seen in clinical practice. So, it is still a challenge to generalize many published studies to the bedside.

REFERENCES

1. Margolis DJ, Kantor J, Berlin JA. Healing of diabetic neuropathic foot ulcers receiving standard treatment: A meta-analysis. Diabetes Care 1999; 22:692–695.
2. Carter MJ, Fife CE, Walker D, et al. Estimating the applicability of wound care randomized controlled trials to general wound care populations by estimating the percentage of individuals excluded from a typical wound care population in such trials. Adv Skin Wound Care 2009; 22:316–324.
3. Mueller MJ, Diamond JE, Sinacore DR, et al. Total contact casting in treatment of diabetic plantar ulcers: Controlled clinical trial. Diabetes Care 1989; 12:384–388.
4. Armstrong DG, Nguyen HC, Lavery LA, et al. Off-loading the diabetic foot wound: A randomized clinical trial. Diabetes Care 2001; 24:1019–1022.
5. Ince P, Game FL, Jeffcoate WJ. Rate of healing of neuropathic ulcers of the foot in diabetes and its relationship to ulcer duration and ulcer area. Diabetes Care 2007; 30:660–663.
6. Armstrong DG, Lavery LA, Harkless LB. Validation of a diabetic wound classification system: The contribution of depth, infection, and ischemia to risk of amputation. Diabetes Care 1998; 21:855–859.
7. Margolis DJ, Allen-Taylor L, Hoffstad O, et al. Diabetic neuropathic foot ulcers: The association of wound size, wound duration, and wound grade on healing. Diabetes Care 2002; 25:1835–1839.
8. Meggitt B. Surgical management of the diabetic foot. Br J Hosp Med 1976; 16:227–232.
9. Wagner FW Jr. The dysvascular foot: A system for diagnosis and treatment. Foot Ankle 1981; 2:64–122.

10. Lavery LA, Armstrong DG, Harkless LB. Classification of diabetic foot wounds. J Foot Ankle Surg 1996; 35:528–531.
11. Oyibo SO, Jude EB, Tarawneh I, et al. The effects of ulcer size and site, patient's age, sex and type and duration of diabetes on the outcome of diabetic foot ulcers. Diabet Med 2001; 18:133–138.
12. Gul A, Basit A, Ali SM, et al. Role of wound classification in predicting the outcome of diabetic foot ulcer. J Pak Med Assoc 2006; 56:444–447.
13. Sheehan P, Jones P, Caselli A, et al. Percent change in wound area of diabetic foot ulcers over a 4-week period is a robust predictor of complete healing in a 12-week prospective trial. Diabetes Care 2003; 26:1879–1882.
14. Lavery LA, Boulton AJ, Niezgoda JA, et al. A comparison of diabetic foot ulcer outcomes using negative pressure wound therapy versus historical standard of care. Int Wound J 2007; 4:103–113.
15. Armstrong DG, Salas P, Short B, et al. Maggot therapy in "lower-extremity hospice" wound care: Fewer amputations and more antibiotic-free days. J Am Podiatr Med Assoc 2005; 95:254–257.
16. Saap LJ, Falanga V. Debridement performance index and its correlation with complete closure of diabetic foot ulcers. Wound Repair Regen 2002; 10:354–359.
17. Steed DL, Donohoe D, Webster MW, et al. Effect of extensive debridement and treatment on the healing of diabetic foot ulcers: Diabetic Ulcer Study Group. J Am Coll Surg 1996; 183:61–64.
18. Cardinal M, Eisenbud DE, Armstrong DG, et al. Serial surgical debridement: A retrospective study on clinical outcomes in chronic lower extremity wounds. Wound Repair Regen 2009; 17:306–311.
19. Paul AG, Ahmad NW, Lee HL, et al. Maggot debridement therapy with *Lucilia cuprina*: A comparison with conventional debridement in diabetic foot ulcers. Int Wound J 2009; 6:39–46.
20. Sherman RA. Maggot therapy for treating diabetic foot ulcers unresponsive to conventional therapy. Diabetes Care 2003; 26:446–451.
21. Tantawi TI, Gohar YM, Kotb MM, et al. Clinical and microbiological efficacy of MDT in the treatment of diabetic foot ulcers. J Wound Care 2007; 16:379–383.
22. Bowling FL, Salgami EV, Boulton AJ. Larval therapy: A novel treatment in eliminating methicillin-resistant *Staphylococcus aureus* from diabetic foot ulcers. Diabetes Care 2007; 30:370–371.
23. Smith TL, Wong-Gibbons D, Maultsby J. Microcirculatory effects of pulsed electromagnetic fields. J Orthop Res 2004; 22:80–84.
24. Aaron RK, Boyan BD, Ciombor DM, et al. Stimulation of growth factor synthesis by electric and electromagnetic fields. Clin Orthop Relat Res 2004; (419):30–37.
25. Lundeberg TC, Eriksson SV, Malm M. Electrical nerve stimulation improves healing of diabetic ulcers. Ann Plast Surg 1992; 29:328–331.
26. Peters EJ, Lavery LA, Armstrong DG, et al. Electric stimulation as an adjunct to heal diabetic foot ulcers: A randomized clinical trial. Arch Phys Med Rehabil 2001; 82: 721–725.
27. Griffin JW, Tooms RE, Mendius RA, et al. Efficacy of high voltage pulsed current for healing of pressure ulcers in patients with spinal cord injury. Phys Ther 1991; 71:433–442, discussion 442–444.
28. Feedar JA, Kloth LC, Gentzkow GD. Chronic dermal ulcer healing enhanced with monophasic pulsed electrical stimulation. Phys Ther 1991; 71:639–649.
29. Sarma GR, Subrahmanyam S, Deenabandhu A, et al. Exposure to pulsed magnetic fields in the treatment of plantar ulcers in leprosy patients—A pilot, randomized, double-blind, controlled clinical trial. Indian J Lepr 1997; 69:241–250.
30. Houghton PE, Kincaid CB, Lovell M, et al. Effect of electrical stimulation on chronic leg ulcer size and appearance. Phys Ther 2003; 83:17–28.
31. Stiller MJ, Pak GH, Shupack JL, et al. A portable pulsed electromagnetic field (PEMF) device to enhance healing of recalcitrant venous ulcers: A double-blind, placebo-controlled clinical trial. Br J Dermatol 1992; 127:147–154.

32. Carley PJ, Wainapel SF. Electrotherapy for acceleration of wound healing: Low intensity direct current. Arch Phys Med Rehabil 1985; 66:443–446.
33. Wood JM, Evans PE III, Schallreuter KU, et al. A multicenter study on the use of pulsed low-intensity direct current for healing chronic stage II and stage III decubitus ulcers. Arch Dermatol 1993; 129:999–1009.
34. Morykwas MJ, Argenta LC, Shelton-Brown EI, et al. Vacuum-assisted closure: A new method for wound control and treatment: Animal studies and basic foundation. Ann Plast Surg 1997; 38:553–562.
35. Morykwas MJ, Faler BJ, Pearce DJ, et al. Effects of varying levels of subatmospheric pressure on the rate of granulation tissue formation in experimental wounds in swine. Ann Plast Surg 2001; 47:547–551.
36. Shi B, Chen SZ, Zhang P, et al. [Effects of vacuum-assisted closure (VAC) on the expressions of MMP-1, 2, 13 in human granulation wound]. Zhonghua Zheng Xing Wai Ke Za Zhi 2003; 19:279–281.
37. Armstrong DG, Lavery LA. Negative pressure wound therapy after partial diabetic foot amputation: A multicentre, randomised controlled trial. Lancet 2005; 366: 1704–1710.
38. Blume PA, Walters J, Payne W, et al. Comparison of negative pressure wound therapy using vacuum-assisted closure with advanced moist wound therapy in the treatment of diabetic foot ulcers: A multicenter randomized controlled trial. Diabetes Care 2008; 31:631–636.
39. Armstrong DG, Kunze K, Martin BR, et al. Plantar pressure changes using a novel negative pressure wound therapy technique. J Am Podiatr Med Assoc 2004; 94: 456–460.
40. Abidia A, Laden G, Kuhan G, et al. The role of hyperbaric oxygen therapy in ischaemic diabetic lower extremity ulcers: A double-blind randomised-controlled trial. Eur J Vasc Endovasc Surg 2003; 25:513–518.
41. Kessler L, Bilbault P, Ortega F, et al. Hyperbaric oxygenation accelerates the healing rate of nonischemic chronic diabetic foot ulcers: A prospective randomized study. Diabetes Care 2003; 26:2378–2382.
42. Faglia E, Favales F, Aldeghi A, et al. Adjunctive systemic hyperbaric oxygen therapy in treatment of severe prevalently ischemic diabetic foot ulcer: A randomized study. Diabetes Care 1996; 19:1338–1343.
43. Doctor N, Pandya S, Supe A. Hyperbaric oxygen therapy in diabetic foot. J Postgrad Med 1992; 38:112–114.
44. Brigido SA, Boc SF, Lopez RC. Effective management of major lower extremity wounds using an acellular regenerative tissue matrix: A pilot study. Orthopedics 2004; 27: s145–s149.
45. Niezgoda JA, Van Gils CC, Frykberg RG, et al. Randomized clinical trial comparing OASIS Wound Matrix to Regranex Gel for diabetic ulcers. Adv Skin Wound Care 2005; 18:258–266.
46. Marston WA, Hanft J, Norwood P, et al. The efficacy and safety of Dermagraft in improving the healing of chronic diabetic foot ulcers: Results of a prospective randomized trial. Diabetes Care 2003; 26:1701–1705.
47. Veves A, Falanga V, Armstrong DG, et al. Graftskin, a human skin equivalent, is effective in the management of noninfected neuropathic diabetic foot ulcers: A prospective randomized multicenter clinical trial. Diabetes Care 2001; 24:290–295.
48. Baroni G, Porro T, Faglia E, et al. Hyperbaric oxygen in diabetic gangrene treatment. Diabetes Care 1987; 10(1):81–86.

8 The infected diabetic foot

Edgar J. G. Peters

INTRODUCTION AND EPIDEMIOLOGY

Infections of the foot are common in patients with diabetes mellitus. It is estimated that 4% of patients with diabetes get a foot infection or ulcer in their lifetime (1). A foot infection is often the pivotal event leading to an amputation (2–5). A study by Eneroth and coworkers in Sweden showed that approximately 50% of 223 patients with an infection received an amputation, 10% of which were proximal (6). Most patients with a foot infection also have a foot wound. A foot ulcer can serve as a *porte d'entrée* for pathogens. Furthermore, infections in the presence of ischemia can lead to necrosis and thus to further failure of the integument. In most risk classifications, patients with foot infections are considered to have a high risk for amputation. Given the crucial role infections play in the cascade towards amputation, it makes sense to treat them aggressively.

The cost of treatment of a diabetic foot infection (corrected for inflation in June 2010, calculated from Swedish Kronor) is $23.493 without amputation and up to $45.227 with amputation. Of these costs, 95% is related to the duration of healing and surgical procedures, 51% to bandages and topical treatment, and only 4% to antibiotics (7–9).

Definitions

Diabetic foot: infection, ulceration, or destruction of deep tissues of the foot associated with neuropathy and/or peripheral arterial disease in the lower extremity of people with diabetes (7).

Infection: a pathologic state caused by invasion and multiplication of microorganisms in tissues, accompanied by tissue destruction and/or a host inflammatory response (2,3,7).

Superficial infection: an infection of the skin not extending to any structure below the dermis (2,10).

Deep infection: an infection deeper than the skin, with evidence of abscess, septic arthritis, osteomyelitis, septic tenosynovitis, or necrotizing fasciitis (10).

Contamination: external introduction of nonresident bacteria into host tissue. The number and virulence of the organisms and the robustness of the host's immune system determine the next steps (7). It can also mean contamination of a culture sample after obtaining it from the patient.

Colonization: new bacteria introduced into and ulcer, replicate, and establish a physiological state of coexistence without overt tissue damage or host response (7).

Osteitis: infection of bone without the involvement of bone marrow.

Osteomyelitis: infection of bone, with involvement of bone marrow.
Septic arthritis: infection of a joint.
Acute osteomyelitis: osteomyelitis without necrosis (11).
Chronic osteomyelitis: osteomyelitis with necrosis. Necrosis can be present early in the natural course of the disease (11).

PATHOPHYSIOLOGY OF INFECTIONS IN DIABETES MELLITUS

It has long been thought that people with diabetes are more prone to diabetes, but data to support this theory were scarce. In a review in 1980, Wheat wrote that it seemed that infections are more common in patients with diabetes, but that only bacteriuria seemed more prevalent in patients with diabetes (12). In a more recent publication, however, a group from Toronto, Canada, has retrospectively studied insurance claims of a cohort of more than 500,000 subjects with diabetes matched with a cohort of subjects without diabetes (13). Almost 50% of patients with diabetes were admitted or had a physician claim for an infection compared with 38% in the cohort of patients without diabetes (risk ratio of 1.2). The relative risk for hospitalization was 2.2; the risk ratio for hospitalization for infection was 2.0. In addition, the risk ratio for osteomyelitis was 4, sepsis 2, and death due to any infection 1.84. Furthermore, subjects with diabetes had an 80% increased risk for cellulitis. Another 12-month cohort study in 7417 patients with diabetes, conducted as part of the Second Dutch National Survey of General Practice, also showed that patients with diabetes had a higher incidence of pneumonia, urinary tract infection, and skin infections (14). These data clearly demonstrate the higher risk of infection associated with diabetes. Other landmark studies have linked better survival on an intensive care unit with better glucose control (15,16).

What happens on a physiological level, however, has not been fully uncovered. There have been numerous in vitro studies to the effect of hyperglycemia and other metabolic disturbances on the immune system. The influence of diabetes seems to be multifactorial and has an effect on different parts of the immune system.

The early innate immune response comprises, amongst other things, the local vasoactive cytokines, the complement system, and proinflammatory cytokines. The local vasoactive cytokines such as bradykinin lead to vasodilatation through a nitric oxide (NO) response. In hyperglycemia, however, the dysregulation of the endothelial nitric oxide synthase (eNOS)/NO system can lead to vasoconstriction instead, which in turn can lead to hypoxia and inhibition of phagocytes to reach an inflammatory state (17,18). In a study in 1991, complement activation was seen more often in patients with type 2 diabetes who used insulin (19). Other, more recent studies have shown that elevated glucose concentrations can inhibit complement-mediated immune activities. Complement receptor-3 and Fcγ receptor–mediated phagocytosis is decreased in normal human neutrophils by activation of protein kinases C α and β (20,21). The proinflammatory cytokines such as tumor necrosis factor-α, interleukin (IL) 1β, IL-6 and IL-18 levels are elevated in hyperglycemia. The higher levels of these cytokines can lead to more insulin resistance through a couple of pathways such as reduced mRNA expression of glucose transporter, increased lipolysis, and activation of stress hormones through the pituitary-adrenal axis. The increased insulin resistance can lead to a vicious circle of more hyperglycemia, further elevated proinflammatory cytokine levels, and insulin resistance (22).

Phagocytes or polymorphonuclear (PMN) cells are at the basis of the cellular innate immune system and destroy microorganisms by a wide variety of functions. Patients with diabetes have an impaired function of phagocytes in chemotaxis, adherence, phagocytosis, and intracellular killing (23). Insulin treatment normalizes these functions probably through metabolic control. In one study, however, these improvements were also seen in healthy subjects during euglycemic insulin clamp, suggesting a more direct effect of insulin (24). Advanced glycation end products lead to impaired PMN transendothelial migration (25). There have been some studies to the effect of diabetes in chemotaxis of PMN cells. In some studies, hyperglycemia has shown a decrease in phagocyte chemotaxis, which could be improved by insulin therapy (26,27). Other studies have shown that PMN chemotaxis is reduced in diabetes independent of metabolic control (23,28). Monocytes as well have been reported to function less in patients with diabetes (29).

Superoxide, a key antimicrobial agent in phagocytes, is produced by the activity of NADPH oxidase. High glucose concentrations have been shown to impair the production of superoxide formation (23,30). The way this occurs is through inhibition of glucose-6-phosphate dehydrogenase (G6PD), which catalyzes the formation of NADPH (30). NADPH is a part of the polyol pathway. Its increased utilization may be at the expense of reduced levels of superoxide production (31,32). The activity of myeloperoxidase—an enzyme that also has a function in the production of superoxides—however, seems unaffected by hyperglycemia (31). Improving leukocyte function has been a field of interest, given the loss of function of the innate cellular immunity in diabetes. There are some conflicting data on the effectiveness of agents that might improve leukocyte function such as granulocyte colony-stimulating factor (G-CSF) in diabetic foot infections (32,33). In a meta-analysis of five randomized controlled trials (RCTs) in 2005, G-CSF did not seem to have an effect on cure of infection or healing of ulcers. Patients who received G-CSF, however, did need significantly less surgery (13% vs. 35%) and underwent fewer amputations (7% vs. 18%) (34).

The influence of diabetes on the adaptive immune system with T cells and immunoglobulins is less well-characterized. There seems to be an impaired T-lymphocyte function. Some specific defects in the cellular adaptive immune system have been identified in vaccination studies in both poorly controlled and adequately controlled patients with type 1 diabetes (35–37). Another study, however, in patients with good metabolic control in type 1 and 2 diabetes showed a normal immune response suggesting normal T-memory cell and CD4-positive lymphocyte function (38). This suggests that better metabolic control helps optimize the adaptive immune system *(level D)*.

Glycation of IgG is correlated to the level of glycated hemoglobin (HbA1c). It seems that the antigen-binding fragment (Fab) of IgG is glycated, leading to an inhibition of molecular recognition between antibody and antigen (39). That being said, the protection after vaccination against influenza, pneumococcal disease, and hepatitis B has been proven adequate in clinical studies (40–43). Therefore, the clinical relevance of the findings from in vitro studies to glycation of immunoglobulins is low.

RISK FACTORS FOR INFECTION

Risk factors for diabetic foot infection were a specific study subject in only two studies. One was a prospective, multicenter study that compared 150 patients with 199 episodes of diabetic foot infection (20% of which were complicated by osteomyelitis), with 97 diabetic controls who did not develop a foot infection (44). Factors that were significantly associated (by multivariate analysis) with developing a foot infection included having a wound that extended to bone [based on a positive probe to bone test; odds ratio (OR) of 6.7], a foot ulcer with a duration of more than 30 days (OR 4.7), a history of recurrent foot ulcers (OR 2.4), a wound of traumatic etiology (OR 2.4), and the presence of peripheral vascular disease defined as absent peripheral arterial pulsation or an ankle-brachial index (ABI) less than 0.9 (OR 1.9). Only one infection occurred in a patient without a previous or concomitant foot ulcer.

The second study was a retrospective review of 112 patients with a severe diabetic foot infection, possibly requiring an amputation (45). By multivariate analysis, factors associated with developing an infection were a previous amputation (OR 19.9); peripheral vascular disease, defined as any missing pedal pulsation or an ABI less than 0.8 (OR 5.5); or loss of protective sensation (OR 3.4). Psychological and economical factors did not contribute significantly to infection (45).

Several other studies examined the association between a specific medical condition and various diabetic foot complications, including infections. These types of studies lack a control group of patients without foot infection and are therefore subject to selection bias. Some studies have suggested an association between renal failure and diabetic foot infections. One retrospective Czech study (for which we could only obtain the abstract) of 64 patients with renal and pancreatic transplantation reported that 30% of patients developed a foot infection during a follow-up period ranging from 6 months to 7 years (46). In an Indian study of 192 patients with diabetes, 17 had undergone renal transplantation. Of all patients with a renal transplantation, 8.8% presented with a foot infection. No numbers were given regarding the risk of infection for patients with a renal transplant (47). In another study, among 60 patients with end-stage renal disease, there were more infections (15% vs. 4%) and amputations (11% vs. 4%) than among 72 patients with diabetes but without end-stage renal disease (48). Finally, a report from Sri Lanka found that, compared with patients who wore shoes, those who walked barefoot for more than 10 hours per day had more web space and nail infections (14% vs. 40%, respectively, $P < 0.01$) (49).

CLINICAL SIGNS AND SYMPTOMS

The diagnosis of infection is made based on clinical parameters. Given the subjective nature of clinical signs and symptoms, it is hard to define strict criteria for infection. There is, however, consensus on the use of the classic signs and symptoms of inflammation, such as redness, warmth, swelling, pain, and loss of function (Table 1).Other signs indicative of infection are purulent discharge, fetid odor, necrosis, and lack of wound healing. Systemic signs such as fever, malaise, leukocytosis, and elevated erythrocyte sedimentation rate (ESR) and C-reactive protein level are not always present, not even in severe infections. If these are present, however, the infection is regarded severe (6,53–55). Microbiological data by themselves are not easy to interpret without clinical data. Use of outcomes of

Table 1 IWGDF (PEDIS) and IDSA Classifications on Diabetic Foot Infection (1–4). In All Cases, Other Causes of an Inflammatory Response of the Skin Should be Excluded (e.g. Trauma, Gout, Acute Charcot Neuro-Osteoarthropathy, Fracture, Thrombosis, Venous Stasis)

Clinical manifestation of infection	IWGDF (PEDIS) grade	IDSA infection severity
No symptoms or signs of infection	1	Uninfected
Infection involving the skin and the subcutaneous tissue only (without involvement of deeper tissues and without systemic signs as described below). At least 2 of the following items are present: • Local swelling or induration • Erythema > 0.5 to 2 cm around the ulcer • Local tenderness or pain • Local warmth • Purulent discharge (thick, opaque to white or sanguineous secretion)	2	Mild
Erythema > 2 cm plus one of the items described above (swelling, tenderness, warmth, discharge), *or* Infection involving structures deeper than skin and subcutaneous tissues as abscess, osteomyelitis, septic arthritis, fasciitis. No systemic inflammatory response signs, as described below	3	Moderate
Any foot infection with the following signs of a systemic inflammatory response syndrome (SIRS). This response is manifested by two or more of the following conditions: • Temperature >38°C or <36°C • Heart rate > 90 beats/min • Respiratory rate > 20 breaths/min or $PaCO_2$ < 32 mm Hg • White blood cell count >12,000 or <4,000 mm^3 or 10% immature (band) forms	4	Severe

Source: From Refs. 7, 50–52.

cultures or Gram stains in defining infection can be misleading as all wounds are colonized with bacteria.

In patients with diabetes, the signs and symptoms are usually less present (56). On top of this, the infected diabetic foot is often not adequately evaluated by hospital staff. In one 4-year study in a teaching hospital in the United States, only 14% of patients received what was considered to be the minimally acceptable level of evaluation (53). There are several reasons for the absence of clinical signs in infection. In diabetes, pain may be mitigated because of neuropathy. Therefore, an absence of pain does not exclude a severe infection. The signs can also be less visible, partly because of decreased influx of blood in case of peripheral arterial disease. The influx can be less due to autonomous neuropathy and diminished skin blood flow. Second, the influx can also be impaired because of peripheral arterial disease. A final issue is improper functioning of leukocytes, as discussed in "Pathophysiology of Infections in Diabetes Mellitus" section.

CLASSIFICATION

Assessing the severity is considered useful in determining appropriate empirical therapy. There are several classification schemes available to assess infection severity. Most of these are subsections of ulcer classifications. There is no consensus on which classification to use, predominantly because these classifications often have different purposes. A clinical classification should be simple and descriptive and all patients should fit into it. A classification for research purposes, on the other hand, should be selective and exclusive to allow comparison of different study populations (50). Examples of classifications are the Meggit-Wagner, PEDIS, SAD/SAD, and the University of Texas (UT) classifications. All are originally ulcer classifications but have a separate section to assess infection severity. Other schemes were specifically developed as wound scores. Examples of these are the ulcer severity index, the Diabetic Ulcer Severity Score (DUSS), and the diabetic foot infection (DFI). All classifications and scores are discussed in the following sections.

Meggit-Wagner

One of the oldest and most widespread is the Meggit-Wagner classification, first described by Meggit but popularized by Wagner (57,58), this classification consists of five grades of ulcers, ranging from superficial ulcer, deep ulcer, infection, localized gangrene to widespread gangrene. The classification exclusively assesses ulcer depth without comorbidities as ischemia unless it comes in such a severe form as gangrene. It is unsuitable for grading of infection severity in individual cases, since it has only one grade for infection.

PEDIS and IDSA

The PEDIS ulcer classification—which stands for perfusion, extent (size), depth (tissue loss), infection, sensation (neuropathy)—was originally developed by the International Working Group on the Diabetic Foot (IWGDF) for research purposes (7,50,51). It can, however, be used for clinical practice as well. It offers a semiquantitative gradation of ulcer severity. The infection part of the classification is practically the same as the one by the Infectious Disease Society of America (IOSA) (52). Both are shown in Table 1. There are slight differences between the two classifications. The IDSA classification describes a moderate infection as a mild infection with more extensive cellulitis, lymphangitic streaks and deep infection, and gangrene. The IWGDF defines it as more extensive cellulitis plus one other sign of inflammation or a deep infection. Furthermore, severe foot infection in the IDSA classification is defined as an infection with systemic toxicity or metabolic disturbance, whereas in the PEDIS classification, this is more strictly defined as a patient with sepsis: a foot infection and two or more criteria of the systemic inflammatory response syndrome (SIRS). In clinical practice, however, these classifications are unlikely to differ. A major advantage of both classifications is that the analogy with other infections makes it easier for clinicians with less experience with diabetic foot management to use these classifications. Another advantage is that the system has been validated by being applied to a prospective studies of diabetic patients (59–61); it predicts the need for hospitalization and for limb amputation (59). It was originally set up to include all types of foot ulcers, which led to a relatively complicated system. As a consequence, the schemes were hard to remember and thus not easy to apply in clinical practice. In a recent study, the system was used for a comparative audit between 14 European diabetic foot centers but not for prospective research (60). In another recent study, it was used to study the effectiveness of procalcitonin and C-reactive protein (61).

SAD/SAD and SINBAD

The S(AD)/SAD system was originally devised to facilitate classification of different ulcers into groups to select populations for prospective research (62–64). The name is an acronym for the five key points: (Size), Area, Depth, Sepsis (infection), Arteriopathy, and Denervation (neuropathy). Each point has four grades, thus creating a semiquantitative scale. The authors claim good agreement between observers. Significant contributors correlated with the outcome of ulcers were area, depth, and arteriopathy (63). Infection (sepsis) was not related to outcome in that particular study. Infection was graded as none, surface, cellulitis, and osteomyelitis. More exact criteria were not given. Like the PEDIS classification, this system is somewhat complicated, making it hard to apply into clinical practice. The SINBAD classification is a simplified version of the S(AD)/SAD system that keeps the same five key points but decreases the number of grades to two (65). Presence of any type of infection versus no infection predicted unfavorable outcome in a multicenter trial; but with only one variable, the SINBAD can not be used to classify infection in clinical practice.

University of Texas Classification

Investigators at the UT (at San Antonio) have promoted an ulcer classification based on four grades (related to the depth of the wound) and four stages (related to the presence or absence of infection or ischemia) (64,66,67). When combined, the stages and grades form a matrix. The different grades are based on the depth and range, from superficial to subcutaneous, tendon, and bone. The stages are: no infection or ischemia, ischemia, infection, and a combination of infection and ischemia. The main difference between the UT and the S(AD)/SAD systems is that the UT does not include loss of protective sensation. The idea of the authors was that virtually all patients with ulcers would have neuropathy; thus, it does not add anything to the classification. The classification successfully predicted the substantially higher likelihood of complications in patients with a higher stage and grade groups. A subanalysis in the infectious ulcer groups also showed a significantly higher percentage of amputations in the deeper wounds than in the superficial ulcers (67). Another study demonstrated a positive correlation between the Meggit-Wagner and the UT classifications (66). A more recent study conducted in Tanzania with 326 persons with diabetes compared the UT, S(AD)SAD, and PEDIS classifications (68). Regrettably, there was inadequate follow-up for 104 of the cases. The authors noted a correlation between infection and adverse outcome in both the S(AD)SAD system and the PEDIS system. Results from Tanzania may not be entirely applicable for more developed countries of course; and even in Western countries, practices vary considerably. For example, surgical resection of infected bone more common in the United States than in the United Kingdom (69).

Ulcer Severity Index

Knighton and coworkers devised and prospectively evaluated a wound severity index based on 20 clinical parameters that generated scores ranging from 0 to

97 (70). A total of 58% of the subjects studied had diabetes. An infection score could be determined by combining the scores for erythema, edema, and purulence, whereas exposed bone was counted in a separate score. The published report gave no data on the association of infection with outcome. The index was specifically developed for a study investigating growth factors for treating diabetic foot ulcers. Because of its complexity, it is an awkward tool to use for clinical practice.

Diabetic Ulcer Severity Score and MAID (71,72)

The authors of the DUSS scoring system evaluated the tool in a study of 1000 patients (71). Similar to the Ulcer Severity Index, the score is based on specific wound characteristics associated with stages of wound repair. Four parameters were included in the score: palpable pedal pulses, probing to bone results, ulcer location, and presence of multiple ulcers. Patients with a low score were more likely to heal and less likely to undergo a lower extremity amputation during a 1-year follow-up period. In fact, an increase in the score by 1 point reduced the chance of healing by 35%. The same group of authors published data in 2009 on 2019 subjects with another wound score with four parameters: the MAID (72). The acronym stands for *m*ultiple ulcers, wound *a*rea larger than 4 cm^2, nonpalpable pedal pulses (*I*), and ulcer *d*uration of more than 130 days. Neither infection nor probing to bone is part of the MAID wound score. The authors found no significant correlation between soft tissue infection and wound healing, although there was a trend toward more infection in the higher-risk groups.

DFI Wound Score

This 10-item scoring system was developed for use in studies of the outcome of various antimicrobial treatments of diabetic foot infections (Table 2) (73). The authors employed a preliminary version of this score in two studies of antibiotic therapy for diabetic foot infections (74,75) and then used a modified version in a large prospective study of the effectiveness of two antibiotics (76,77). The score consists of a semiquantitative assessment of the presence of signs of inflammation, combined with measurements of wound size and depth. Explicit definitions are available to score wound parameters. An evaluation of the wound score for 371 patients demonstrated that it significantly correlated with the clinical response and that scores demonstrated good internal consistency. Surprisingly, excluding scores for wound discharge (purulent and nonpurulent), leaving an 8-item score, provided better measurement statistics (73). The DFI Wound Score appears to be a useful tool for predicting clinical outcomes in treatment trials and clinical practice, but its complexity would likely require clinicians to use a scoring sheet.

Clinical Use of the Classifications and Wound Scores

The Meggit-Wagner and SINBAD classifications are not useful to describe infection because they provide only a dichotomous description of infection without further definitions of infection. The UT classification uses a dichotomous description for infection as well, but infection is better defined in stages and there is evidence that the system adequately predicts outcome (*level C*). The PEDIS, IDSA, and S(AD)/SAD classifications provide a semiquantitative 4-point scale to describe infection and may better predict the outcome of a diabetic foot infection. The Ulcer Severity Index is complex, and there are no data available on the predictive qualities for infection (*level D*). The DUSS and DFI systems are less complex

Table 2 Items Comprising the Diabetic Foot Infection Wound Score Wound Parameters and Wound Measurements and the Method for Scoring Each (73)

Item	Assessment	Preassigned scoring
Wound parameters	Absent	0
Purulent discharge	Present	3
Other signs & symptoms of inflammation[a]	Absent	0
Nonpurulent discharge[a]	Mild	1
Erythema[a]		
Induration[a]	Moderate	2
Tenderness[a]		
Pain[a]		
Local warmth[a]	Severe	3
Range of Wound Parameter (10-Item) Subtotal		0–21
Range of Wound Parameter (8-Item) Subtotal		0–15
Wound Measurements		
Size (cm^2)	<1	0
	1–2	1
	>2–5	3
	>5–10	6
	>10–30	8
	>30	10
Depth (mm)	<5	0
	5–9	3
	10–20	7
	>20	10
Undermining (mm)	<2	3
	2–5	5
	>5	8
Range of Wound Measurement Subtotal		3–28
Range of Total 10-Item DFI Wound Score		3–49
Range of Total 8-Item DFI Wound Score		3–43

NOTE: DEFINITION OF TERMS

Wound Measurements

– Size (cm^2): The ulcer area as traced with a fine-tipped felt pen on a sterile clear plastic film applied over the wound. Scored as shown (0 to 10) based on size of ulcer (0 to >30 cm^2)

– Depth (mm): Measured in the deepest apparent part of the wound by using a sterile cotton-tipped wooden swab held at 90° to the wound and marked with a pen held parallel to the surface of the intact skin.

– Undermining (mm): Measurement of any tunneling, subepithelial tissue loss, or shearing, as measured using a sterile cotton-tipped wooden swab. Scored as shown (3–8) based on the measured amount (<2 to >5 mm)

Wound Parameters

– Purulent drainage: A viscous, yellowish-white, or greenish fluid formed in infected tissue.

– Nonpurulent drainage: A serous, sanguineous, or sero-sanguineous collection of fluid in the tissue surrounding the wound. Graded: absent, none present; mild: scant drainage noted on dressing (<0.5 cm diameter) not requiring additional dressings; moderate: > scant but < copious drainage on dressing (>2 cm diameter) requiring additional dressing changes; and severe: copious drainage on dressing (>2 cm diameter) requiring additional dressing changes.

– Erythema: Congestive or exudative redness surrounding the wound caused by engorgement of the capillaries in the lower layers of the skin. Graded: none: absent; mild: pink, barely perceptible; moderate: pale red with defined edges; and severe/extreme: red to dark red.

– Induration: Inflammatory hardening or thickening of tissues, sometimes called *brawny edema*. Graded: none: absent; mild: localized to the site of infection; moderate: limited extension from the site of infection; and severe: extending from the site of infection to involve a substantial portion of the affected lower extremity.

– Tenderness (sign): Palpation of the site of infection elicits a report of tenderness by the patient; measured on a 0 (no tenderness)-to-10 (the worst imaginable tenderness) scale. Graded: none: absent; mild: score of ≤5; moderate: score of 6–8; and severe: score of ≥9.

– Pain (symptom): Subjective reporting of discomfort or the perception of pain at the site of the infection as reported by the patient; measured on a 0 (no pain)-to-10 (the worst imaginable pain) scale. Graded: none: absent; mild: score of ≤5; moderate: score of 6–8; and severe: score of ≥9.

– Local warmth (sign): Increase in skin temperature relative to the uninfected contralateral foot. Graded: none: temperature of the two sides the same; mild: temperature slightly, but perceptibly, warmer; moderate: temperature clearly warmer (perceived as 1°F–2°F); and severe: marked difference in temperature (perceived as >2°F)

[a] Each assessed as mild, moderate, or severe and placed in one of the preassigned categories.

and are wound scores that have been successfully tested in large clinical trials *(level B)*. There is no evidence that one classification or wound score is better than any other *(level D)*.

Microbiology

Microbiological data are not easy—if not impossible—to interpret without clinical data. Use of outcomes of cultures or Gram stains in defining infection can be misleading as all wounds are colonized with bacteria. There is a substantial chance that the identified organisms might be nothing more than colonization, and treating a colonized wound without clinical infection has not been proven to be effective in healing of ulcers (78–80) *(level B)*.

Microbiology is useful to select the most appropriate antibiotic for the infection. In case an infection is present, results from cultures or Gram stains are effective in determining the causative organism(s). Care needs to be given to proper sampling technique. Vital tissues, in general, do not have colonizing organisms. A sample from deep and vital tissue through noncolonized surroundings, or of pus, can therefore lessen the chance of a false-positive culture due to contamination or colonization. It is essential that the wound be sampled after proper debridement of necrotic tissue. For the same reason, superficial cultures obtained with cotton swabs are less suitable than tissue biopsies. In one study, superficial swab cultures in a cohort of patients with distal foot ulcers without previous treatment matched results of biopsy in only 22.5% of patients (81,82).

The most probable organisms causing infections in previously untreated wounds are aerobic Gram-positive cocci, predominantly *Staphylococcus aureus* and β-hemolytic streptococci (7,83–86). In developing countries, the contribution of *S. aureus* species in diabetic foot infections seems less than in Western countries (approximately 30% vs. 75%) (87,88). Deep and moderate to severe infections are predominantly due to mixed flora of gram-positive cocci and gram-negative rods. Besides the organisms found in superficial mild infected wound, enterococci, different enterobacteriaceae (*Escherichia coli*, *Proteus*, *Klebsiella*), nonfermentative Gram-negative rods (*Pseudomonas*), and anaerobes (*Peptostreptococcus*, *Bacteroides*) can cause infections (86,89–94). Of special note is that severe and direct limb-threatening infections can harbor *P. aeruginosa*, especially in case of deep puncture wound and in patients who wear tennis shoes (56,86,95). Anaerobes can be expected in case of gangrene or severe ischemia (96). The different expected microorganisms in selected cases are summarized in Table 3.

The mixed infections usually occur in chronic and complex wounds. Often, but not always, these wounds have been unsuccessfully treated with antibiotics, leading to selection of less usual and drug-resistant flora (97–99). Studies to the outcome of ulcers infected with resistant organisms such as methicillin-resistant *S. aureus* (MRSA) or vancomycin-resistant enterococcus (VRE) have produced conflicting data. In one study, patients with ulcers harboring multidrug-resistant organisms, including 25% patients with osteomyelitis, did not seem to do worse than patients without resistant bacteria (97,100). Other studies, however, suggested that patients with MRSA did seem to have a worse outcome (87,101). A potential confounder in these studies might be that patients colonized with MRSA might have been subjected to earlier unsuccessful treatments or hospitalizations that led to the colonization with resistant organisms. Another point that makes generalization of these statements difficult is that most specimens were

Table 3 Expected Microorganisms Related to the Severity of Infection and Subsequent Empirical Antibiotic Regimen *(level D)*

Severity of infection	Usual pathogens	Potential antimicrobial regimens
Nonsevere (oral for entire course)		
No complicating features	Gram-positive cocci	Semisynthetic penicillin or first-generation cephalosporin
Recent antibiotic therapy	Gram-positive cocci ± Gram-negative rods	Fluoroquinolone, β-lactamase–resistant β-lactam
Drug allergies		Clindamycin, fluoroquinolone, trimethoprim/sulfamethoxazole
Severe (intravenous until stable, then switch to oral equivalent)		
No complicating features	Gram-positive cocci[a] ± Gram-negative rods	β-lactamase–resistant β-lactam, second-/third-generation cephalosporin
Recent antibiotic/ necrosis	Gram-positive cocci + Gram-negative rods/anaerobes	Third-/fourth-generation cephalosporin, fluoroquinolone+clindamycin
Life-threatening (prolonged intravenous)		
MRSA unlikely	Gram-positive cocci + Gram-negative rods + anaerobes	Carbapenem, clindamycin + aminoglycoside
MRSA likely		Glycopeptide or linezolid + 3/4 generation cephalosporin or fluoroquinolone + metronidazole

Abbreviation: MRSA, methicillin-resistant *Staphylococci aureus*.
[a] A high local prevalence of methicillin resistance among staphylococci may require using vancomycin or other appropriate antistaphylococcal agents active against these organisms.
Source: From Ref. 7.

cultured from superficial swabs instead of tissue biopsies. This might also explain why most of the patients who did well in spite of multidrug-resistant organisms healed without antimicrobial drugs specifically targeted at these bacteria (74) *(level C)*. These considerations kept aside, the contribution of MRSA in diabetic foot infections is rising, as shown by several reports (85,98–100). Especially in the United States, these bacteria, not only hospital-associated pathogens but also community-acquired MRSA, can cause severe soft tissue infections (102). Besides MRSA, extended-spectrum β-lactamase (ESBL)–producing *Enterobacteriaceae* are an emerging global problem in diabetic foot infections (87). Identified risk factors for resistant bacteria in foot infections include previous antibiotic therapy and long duration of previous antibiotic therapy, frequency of hospitalization for the same ulcer, duration of hospital stay, and osteomyelitis (97,103).

TREATMENT

General Measurements

Treatment of a diabetic foot infection consists of a combination of different strategies. Antibiotics alone will not heal a severe infection but should be combined with appropriate debridement, proper off-loading, and often surgical procedures as discussed in other chapters. Surgical management will encompass cleansing, removal of callus, and necrotectomy and drainage in severe cases. Edema should be treated with elevation or compression of the limb and, in selected cases, with diuretics. Furthermore, vascular interventions to optimize supply of nutrients and immune cells are crucial in case of ischemia. These essential elements of therapy are discussed in other chapters in this book. This chapter will focus on the antibiotic treatment of diabetic foot infection.

Topical Treatment

Several studies have been conducted to understand the effectiveness of topical antimicrobial treatment in patients with infected diabetic foot ulcers. Most of these studies looked at topical agents (e.g., silver dressings, mafenide acetate, povidone-iodine solutions, hypochlorite, peroxide, zinc oxide) as adjuncts to systemic antibiotic treatment. No single agent has been proven superior (104–106) *(level D)*. Most agents, however, also seem to have nonantimicrobial effects on the process of wound healing itself (107). Despite its widespread use, two recent systematic reviews could not identify any data on the effectiveness of topical silver (104,108) *(level D)*.

Effectiveness of Adjunctive Therapy

Revascularization to enable debridement and minor surgery is often propagated (7,109). A restoration of vascular supply could help to treat the infection and might prevent necrosis. Wound healing after debridement of necrotic and infected tissue might also benefit from revascularization. However, probably because of the face value, studies to improved outcome in revascularization in foot infections or to the timing of revascularization are not available *(level D)*. No studies could be found on the effectiveness of vacuum-assisted closure (VAC) therapy on diabetic foot infections (104,110) *(level D)*.

Larvae

In a systematic review published in 2008, two studies were identified regarding the effect of larvae in diabetic foot ulcers (104). In one of these studies, in patients with vascular disease, application of larvae seemed to decrease the use of antibiotics and the need for amputations, suggesting a potential antibacterial effect as well as an effect on ulcer healing (111) *(level B)*. Other nonclinical studies have suggested that larvae have a direct antimicrobial effect and an effect on biofilm formation (112,113).

Hyperbaric Oxygen Treatment

Regarding anaerobic bacteria, hyperbaric oxygen treatment might be an option. There is much debate on the usefulness of the modality (114,115). In a Cochrane review analysis in 2004, it was concluded that hyperbaric oxygen therapy reduces the risk for major amputation related to diabetic foot ulcers (116) *(level B)*. The review identified five trials. The authors concluded that there was limited evidence based on three trials that hyperbaric oxygen decreases amputation in patients with diabetic foot ulcers (117–119) *(level B)*. Another more recent systematic review found the same reviews and came to the same conclusion (104). Both reviews raised questions on how to select patients to optimize allocation of this expensive treatment modality. There are no direct data regarding the effect of hyperbaric oxygen to diabetic foot infections.

Antibiotic Treatment

Assessing the severity is useful in determining appropriate empirical antibiotic therapy (120). The classifications mentioned earlier can be used to assess the severity. After the results of cultures become available, the empirical therapy can be adapted to tailor the therapy. Suggested empirical therapies are summarized in Table 3 (7). Most of these recommendations are expert opinion *(level D)*. In 2008, a meta-analysis was published on factors associated with treatment failure. The authors found 18 RCTs in a systematic review, of which 11 were exclusively conducted in patients with diabetes (120). Factors associated with treatment failure in a total studied number of 1715 subjects were the use of antibiotic another than a carbapenem and the presence of MRSA and streptococci. It has to be emphasized that the reported studies were likely to suffer from bias and that the outcomes of these studies are dependent on local antibiotic resistance. Another systematic review in 2006 identified 23 trials with 19 unique comparisons between interventions (121). In both those systematic reviews and one study published in 1999, no single antibiotic regimen was proven superior over the other (120–122). The conclusion of the reviews is that there are not many trials conducted and that the methodological quality of the available studies is poor. Sample sizes in most studies were insufficient to identify differences between antibiotic regimes. There was variability in definitions and outcomes used. On the basis of available data, there is no strong evidence for recommendations of particular antimicrobial agent for prevention of amputation, resolution of infection, or healing of ulcer *(level D)*.

One literature review has described studies regarding serum and tissue levels of antibiotics (122). In one study by Seabrook and coworkers, in 26 patients who received intravenous antibiotics in diabetic foot infections, antibiotic levels in viable tissues of gentamicin and clindamycin adjacent to the surgical site were low (123). Concentrations of β-lactam and biotics in tissue were generally higher than in serum. In contrast, two other studies suggested that, with the exception of ceftazidime, β-lactams only achieved low tissue levels (124,125). In these studies however, four patients were studied. In contrast with Seabrook et al., three other studies on small samples have suggested that clindamycin and quinolones do have good penetration in bone, biofilm, and necrotic tissue (126–128). Important is that the oral absorption is high enough to make oral therapy possible, even in case of gastropathy due to autonomic neuropathy (129). An important caveat with those studies is that a direct relationship between antibiotic level and clinical outcome still needs to be proven.

In case of drug resistance, some newer drugs have shown efficacy. These drugs include linezolid orally or intravenously for Gram-positive and anaerobic organisms (74,130–132); once-daily parenteral daptomycin for gram-positive organisms (133); quinupristin/dalfopristin parenterally for Gram-positive organisms; dalbavancin once-weekly parenterally for Gram-positive organisms (134,135); once-daily parenteral telavancin for Gram-positive organisms including glycopeptide-resistant strains (136); tigecycline twice-daily parenterally for Gram-positive and Gram-negative bacteria including anaerobes, VRE, and ESBL-producers but not *Pseudomonas* (137); ceftobiprole parenterally twice-daily for Gram-positive organisms (138,139); moxifloxacin parenterally or orally once-daily, broad-spectrum but not for multidrug-resistant organisms (140); and ertapenem parenterally once-daily for Gram-positive and Gram-negative organisms but not for *Pseudomonas* (77).

Uninfected Wounds

Some argue for using systemic antibiotic treatment in uninfected ulcers, believing that high levels of surface colonization may inhibit healing or that overt signs of infection are obscured in diabetes (78,141). In one small nonrandomized study, published only as an abstract, patients with uninfected wound who were prescribed antibiotics received few amputations (80). However, larger trials to treatment of a colonized wound without clinical infection (PEDIS grade 1) have not proven antibiotics to be effective in healing of ulcers or as prophylaxis against infections (142–144). In fact, prescription of antibiotics is discouraged in present guidelines because of the unproven efficacy and the fact that the antibiotics are costly and can cause adverse effects and antimicrobial resistance (7,52) *(level C)*. The adverse effects can range from mild such as upset stomach to fatal reactions or bacteriological complication such as *Clostridium difficile*–associated disease. On a population level, prescribing antibiotics to patients needs to be weighed against the spread of antibiotic resistance. More studies are needed regarding the efficacy of treating uninfected wounds with antibiotics.

Mild Infections

Mild infections (PEDIS grade 2) that have not been treated previously are usually caused by streptococci and staphylococci. Outpatient treatment is considered to be safe in mild infection provided that the social and cognitive circumstances allow this (74) *(level D)*. Although Gram-negative rods are sometimes cultured, these are usually thought to colonize and not infect the wound. Data from a study regarding the effectiveness of linezolid with only Gram-positive coverage performed even better than amoxicillin/clavunate acid, which has a broader coverage, including Gram-negative rods and anaerobes (7). In areas where MRSA is unlikely, a semisynthetic penicillin with staphylococcal activity such as flucloxacillin or oxacillin, or a first-generation cephalosporin such as cephalexin, for 2 weeks is appropriate *(level D)*. An alternative is clindamycin (145,146). In contrast to areas with a low prevalence of MRSA, wound cultures are advisable in case of endemic MRSA to prevent prescription of inadequate antibiotics (122,147,148) *(level D)*.

Moderate Infections

Patients with a moderate infection (PEDIS grade 3) who need antibiotic therapy require broad-spectrum coverage for Gram-positive cocci and Gram-negative rods *(level D)*. The latter two are often present in wounds with necrosis and in patients who have been previously treated with antibiotics. Anaerobes are not encountered frequently in mild to moderate infections (7,122,149) *(level C)*. In presence of necrosis or severe ischemia, however, they can play a role.

Options for empirical therapy are combinations of a fluoroquinolone (e.g., ciprofloxacin or levofloxacin) with clindamycin or a β-lactam antibiotic with anti–β-lactamase activity (e.g., amoxicillin-clavulanate or piperacillin/tazobactam) (150) *(level D)*. In case of (expected) colonization with multidrug-resistant organisms, a carbapenem might also be an option (151) *(level D)*. Hospitalization is usually necessary for surgical or diagnostic procedures or intravenous administration of antibiotics. Although hospitalization is usually the case, it is not obligatory with these types of infections. It has to be kept in mind, however, that inappropriate treatment can lead to more proximal amputations in 10% of cases (2,122,150). After the result of cultures, Gram stains, or clinical response are available, the empirical antibiotic treatment should be switched to the most adequate regime. The duration of therapy depends on infection severity, clinical response, the need for surgical intervention such as vascular reconstruction or debridement, and the presence of osteomyelitis (94) *(level D)*.

Severe Infections

The antibiotic treatment for PEDIS grade 4 ulcers is essentially the same as that for moderate infections. The main difference is that patients are systemically ill, and resistant bacteria are more likely to play a role in the disease process. Anaerobic organisms seem to play a larger role in these severe infections (7,122) *(level D)*. It is not clear whether they cause the more serious nature of the infection or are merely bystanders. The antibiotics commonly prescribed in these categories of patients are broad-spectrum and intravenously administered, mainly because the consequences for treating an infection with an antibiotic without effectiveness against a causing organism are grave (148,149,152) *(level D)*.

Switch to Oral Antibiotics

Initial treatment in moderate and severe infections is often intravenously, as the pathogen load is high, the margins for error are small, and adequate serum levels need to be attained. After the first phase of treatment is over, a switch to oral antibiotics is often possible. Oral treatment is cheaper, safer, and easier for patients and medical staff. As mentioned under the section "Antibiotic Treatment," the oral availability and effectiveness of certain antibiotics is excellent (129,153). In one study in osteomyelitis, long-term oral antibiotic treatment seemed an effective alternative to prolonged intravenous treatment and surgery (120) *(level D)*. No studies are available to the most optimal timing of switch to oral antibiotics *(level D)*.

OSTEOMYELITIS

A separate entity within diabetic foot infections is osteomyelitis. Osteomyelitis is the infection of bone, with the involvement of bone marrow (7). In the diabetic foot, infections of bone are usually due to contiguous spread, usually from a chronic ulcer. In other cases of osteomyelitis, for instance, in tuberculosis or in children, spread is usually hematogenous. It is a common condition; up to 15% of patients with an ulcer eventually develop osteomyelitis (154). Approximately 20% of cases of foot infection in persons with diabetes involve bone (155). The diagnosis of osteomyelitis has serious consequences. The treatment typically involves prolonged antibiotic treatment combined with (repeated) surgical procedures *(level D)*. Infection of bone greatly increases the likelihood that the patient will require a lower extremity amputation (44,156).

Microbiology of Osteomyelitis and Biofilm Formation

Osteomyelitis in the foot of a patient with diabetes generally occurs by contiguous spread. Therefore, the causative microorganisms are similar to those isolated from complicated soft tissue infections mentioned earlier. The most commonly isolated microbe is *S. aureus*, whereas in case of chronically infected wounds, the infection is often polymicrobial (82,87,157–159). Bone infection can be particularly persistent. Reasons for this phenomenon include impaired immune and inflammatory responses, reduced leukocyte count, and biofilm formation. All these circumstances are especially present in the case of necrotic bone or a sequestrum (160–163). A biofilm typically consists of colonies of bacteria in a matrix of hydrated polysaccharides, protein, and other molecules (164,165). In contrast to bacteria in a free-living, planktonic phase, bacteria in a biofilm have a slower metabolism and a lower replication rate. Antimicrobials are less effective in this milieu. Slower penetration of antibiotics in the extracellular matrix of the biofilm and the expression and exchange of biofilm-specific resistance genes also play a role (166–168).

Diagnosis of Osteomyelitis

The clinical presentation of osteomyelitis in the diabetic foot can vary, depending on the site involved, the extent of infected and dead bone, any associated abscess and soft tissue involvement, the causative organism(s), and the presence of limb ischemia. The diagnosis of osteomyelitis is difficult but is essential to ensure appropriate treatment. Especially early infection can be missed because it takes several weeks for the infection to show on radiographs. Furthermore, the symptoms and results of imaging studies are hard to distinguish from those by neuro-osteo (Charcot) arthropathy. Recent reviews have been published that sum up the available evidence for current tests (110,169,170).

Symptoms

In general, a nonhealing ulcer with an underlying bony prominence despite adequate off-loading, especially in the presence of poor vascular supply, should raise the suspicion of underlying osteomyelitis. However, no studies regarding the diagnostic value of medical history are available.

Signs on Physical Examination

Several studies have focused on physical examination to diagnose diabetic foot osteomyelitis. The accuracy of a physician's clinical judgment without formal rules or weighing of findings for the presence of osteomyelitis is high, with a likelihood ratio (LR) of 5.5 and a 95% confidence interval (CI) of 1.8–17. A physician's clinical judgment, or "gestalt," that osteomyelitis is not present in a patient has a reported negative LR of 0.54 (CI, 0.30–0.97) (155,171,172). Of the different diagnostic modalities, temperature has a reported sensitivity of only 19% (173). Presence of bone exposure on the other hand, suggests osteomyelitis with a LR of 9.2 but with a large 95% CI of 0.57–146 (155). In the same study, an ulcer area larger than 2 cm^2 increased the likelihood of osteomyelitis with an LR of 7.2 (CI, 1.1–49), whereas an ulcer smaller than 2 cm^2 decreased the likelihood (LR, 0.48; CI, 0.31–0.76) (155). Presence of local signs of inflammation did not alter the pretest possibility of osteomyelitis (155).

A sterile probe is used to palpate bone in the base of an ulcer or sinus tract. The test is positive if a rock-hard gritty structure can be found at the bottom. A negative probe to bone test in experienced physicians can practically rule out osteomyelitis, both in outpatient and inpatient settings, with a reported negative predictive value of up to 98%, a positive LR of 4.3–9.4 and a negative LR ranging

Table 4 Features of Osteomyelitis on Plain Radiography (155,180–182)

Periosteal reaction or elevation
Loss of cortex with bony erosion
Focal loss of trabecular pattern or marrow radiolucency
New bone formation
Bone sclerosis with or without erosion
Sequestration
Devitalized bone with radiodense appearance that has become separated from normal bone
Involucrum
A layer of new bone growth outside existing bone resulting from the stripping off of the periosteum and new bone growing from the periosteum
Cloaca
Opening in involucrum or cortex through which sequestra or granulation tissue may be discharged
The bony changes are often accompanied by soft tissue swelling

from 0.14 to 0.68 (174–176). A negative probe to bone test could practically rule out osteomyelitis in outpatient setting with a negative LR of 0.14 (176).

Laboratory Studies

An elevated ESR of more than 70 mm/hr increases the likelihood of diabetic foot osteomyelitis (155,177,178). The pooled likelihood of osteomyelitis with an ESR > 70 mm/hr is 11 (CI, 1.6–79). An ESR < 70 mm/hr is less specific, with a pooled negative likelihood of 0.34 that osteomyelitis is absent (169,177,179). An elevated leukocyte count is not predictive of osteomyelitis with a sensitivity of 14% to 54% (173). A positive microbiology swab of an ulcer surface does not predict whether patients have underlying osteomyelitis or not with a positive and negative LR of 1.0 (178).

Radiological Studies—Plain Radiography

Characteristic features on radiographs of the foot are summed up in Table 4 (155,180–182). Most centers use two- or three-way views. Several studies have assessed the accuracy of plain radiography in osteomyelitis (155,171,172,180,182–194). Nine of these had a prospective setup (155,171,180,182–184,187,188,194). The reported sensitivity of plain radiography varied greatly, ranging from 28% to 75%. The timing of the examination is of course of great influence in this matter, as older lesions are more likely to show up on the radiograph. In the review by Dinh et al. (170), four studies were used to calculate the sensitivity and specificity. The pooled sensitivity of these four studies was reported to be 0.54, the pooled specificity 0.68, with a diagnostic OR of 2.84 and a Q statistic of 0.60 (155,180,182,194). In the review by Butalia (169), the summary positive likelihood of seven studies was found to be 2.3 (CI, 1.6–3.3) for plain radiographs. The negative likelihood was 0.63 (CI, 0.5–0.8) (155,180,182,186,190,191,193). The results indicate that radiographic results appear to be only marginally predictive if positive. A negative result was even less predictive of the absence of osteomyelitis. It has to be emphasized that no studies were identified in these two reviews that used sequentially obtained radiographs of the foot. It is felt that *changes* in

Table 5 Features of Osteomyelitis on MRI (155,171,180,195–197)

Low focal signal intensity on T-1 weighted images
High focal signal on T2-weighted images
Short tau inversion recovery sequences in bone marrow
Less specific or secondary changes:
Cortical disruption
Adjacent cutaneous ulcer
Soft tissue mass
Sinus tract
Adjacent soft tissue inflammation or edema

radiological appearance are far more likely to predict the presence of osteomyelitis than does a single radiograph.

Radiological Studies—Magnetic Resonance Imaging

Magnetic resonance imaging (MRI) is considered a valuable attribute to diagnose osteomyelitis (52). The features on MRI are summed up in Table 5. Two meta-analyses were recently published on the use of MRI in the diabetic foot (170,198). Dinh and coworkers (170) identified four trials, all of which had a prospective setup (180,182,195,199). Two used a consecutive recruitment method (180,182). Only one study was conducted for less than 10 years (195). The prevalence of osteomyelitis in the four studies ranged from 44% to 86%. The pooled sensitivity was 0.90 (CI, 0.82–0.95). The diagnostic OR was excellent with a value of 24.4. Kapoor et al. (198) found 16 trials in their meta-analysis (171,172,180,182,188,192,195,196,200–207). Nine of these had a prospective setup, and 11 studies exclusively included subjects with diabetes. The prevalence of standard defined osteomyelitis was 50% (range, 32%–89%). The pooled sensitivity in the meta-analysis by Kapoor et al. was 77% to 100%, the specificity 40% to 100%, with a diagnostic OR of 42 (CI, 15–120). The summary positive LR was 3.8 (CI, 0.2.5–5.8), the summary negative LR was 0.14 (CI, 0.08–0.26) in subjects with diabetes. Studies that were performed recently had a lower diagnostic OR (OR, 25; CI, 6–117) than older studies. This might be due to better design of the studies. The subgroups of patients with other diagnoses (e.g., Charcot arthropathy) was too low to analyze any differences.

Radiological Studies—Nuclear Medicine

Three recent meta-analysis have been identified that reviewed nuclear medicine techniques (170,198,208). In their meta-analysis, Capriotti and coworkers reviewed 57 papers, including 7 reviews on the clinical value of several nuclear medicine techniques (208). Several types of nuclear imaging scans are available. Bone scans are usually performed with ^{99m}Tc-methylene diphosphate. Osteomyelitis is diagnosed by increased blood pool activity and abnormally increased intensity localized to the bone (170). Capriotti et al. found in a total of 719 lesions that three-phase bone scans were sensitive (90%) but not specific (46%) (208). The calculated summary negative predictive value from 643 lesions was 71%; the positive predictive value was 65%. Dinh and coworkers (170) found six studies that qualified their search criteria (155,180,182,194,209,210). Dinh et al. found a pooled sensitivity of 80% and specificity of 28% in 185 subjects. The pooled diagnostic OR was 2.1, indicating poor discriminating ability. The Q statistic was 0.6, indicating moderate accuracy for the diagnosis of osteomyelitis (170). Seven studies were found by Kapoor et al. (198) that compared MRI with triple-phase bone scan (171,182,188,192,202,206,207). MRI performance was markedly superior with a diagnostic OR of 150 (CI, 55–411), compared with bone scan with a diagnostic OR of 3.5 (CI, 1.0–13) (198). Especially in the forefoot, healthy bone is also likely to have an increased uptake of the radiopharmacon (208). Although a positive bone scan is not specific for osteomyelitis, a negative bone scan can be used to rule out osteomyelitis or Charcot neuro-osteoarthropathy *(level C)*.

Radiolabeled white blood cells are generally not taken up in healthy bone and are therefore more specific for osteomyelitis (and Charcot osteoarthropathy) (208). The used radiopharmacons to label leukocytes are ^{99m}Tc and ^{111}In. The summary positive predictive values were reported to be 90% and 72%, respectively; the negative predictive values were 81% and 83%, respectively (208). The better predictive value of the ^{99m}Tc label is attributed to superior physical characteristics leading to better spatial resolution (208). Dinh and coworkers (170) identified six studies to ^{111}In–radiolabeled leukocytes. They found a pooled sensitivity of 74% and a specificity of 68% (155,180,182,194,209,210). The pooled diagnostic OR was 10, indicating a moderately good discriminating characteristics. The Q statistic of 0.59 indicated a low to moderate accuracy of ^{111}In–labeled leukocytes for the diagnosis of osteomyelitis (170). Kapoor et al. (198) found three studies that compared MRI with ^{99m}Tc (207)– or ^{111}In (188,192)–labeled leukocyte scan. Calculated from these studies, MRI outperformed leukocyte scanning with diagnostic ORs of 120 (CI, 62–234) and 3.4 (CI, 0.2–62), respectively (198) *(level B)*. Combination of labeled leukocytes with bone scan (dual tracer technique) does not improve diagnostic accuracy (189).

Other available nuclear medicine techniques include ^{99m}Tc–/^{111}In–labeled human immunoglobulin G (HIG) and anti-granulocyte antigen monoclonal antibodies and their fragments (208). ^{99m}Tc–/^{111}In–HIG uptake is related to vascular permeability and is not specific to inflamed tissue. Therefore, these tests are not as specific as radiolabeled leukocytes (193,211). The pooled positive and negative predictive values calculated from 97 lesions are 72% and 88%, respectively (208).

Radiological Studies—Other Techniques

Two studies using computed tomography (CT) and positron emission tomography (PET) scans for the diagnosis of osteomyelitis have been published (170). A histopathological examination was not included in these studies (212,213). However, there seems to be place for CT scan when MRI is not available or possible *(level D)*.

Bone Biopsy

The gold standard for diagnosis is the combination of microbiological culture and histological examination of bone (110,214). The culture will also identify the responsible pathogens and their antibiotic sensitivities. A bone specimen may be obtained either percutaneously (through uninfected skin) or as part of an operative procedure. Use of the proper technique is critically important. A false-positive result can occur when the biopsy is taken through an area of contamination or bacterial colonization, such as an ulcer. False-negative results can occur when the area of infection is missed while biopsying (110). It should be emphasized that bone cultures are important to guide appropriate therapy. In a French study, cultures of swabs were identical to bone culture in only 17% of patients. Furthermore, swabs will often overstate the number of pathogens involved (81,215). Fine-needle aspiration of bone has been suggested as an alternative to bone biopsy, but it gives the same result as bone biopsy in only 32% of cases (215). Where possible, antibiotics should be discontinued (for at least 48 hours and preferably longer) before the biopsy, to maximize the yield from cultures (216,217) *(level D)*. So far, the exact minimal duration to stop antibiotics before obtaining a culture specimen is not known.

Diagnostic Strategies

In 2007, the International Working Group on the Diabetic Foot reached an international consensus between representatives on the diagnosis and treatment of diabetic foot osteomyelitis (7,110,214) *(level D)*. It consists of four categories ranging from unlikely, possible, probable, to definite osteomyelitis. The patient falls into one of the categories, depending on the result of a combination of criteria. The criteria are made from symptoms and several tests from physical examination, simple bedside tests, laboratory tests, and imaging. In time, the diagnosis can become more or less likely depending on changing signs and symptoms, but this is not taken into account in the scheme. The scheme is so far the only agreed set of criteria for the diagnosis of osteomyelitis. The gold standard consists of a combination of a positive culture of a bone specimen and histopathological examination that shows bone death, acute or chronic inflammation, and reparative responses (110). Other criteria that lead to a definite diagnosis are detached bone fragments from an ulcer and an intraosseous abcess on MRI. Combinations of other positive tests can also lead to a definite, probable, or possible diagnosis of osteomyelitis (Table 6) (7,110). An important sign that should raise the suspicion of an underlying osteomyelitis is a nonhealing ulcer despite adequate vascular supply and off-loading. A positive probe to bone test can make the diagnosis more or less likely (174–176).

Treatment of Osteomyelitis

In the recent past, several (systematic) reviews have been published on the treatment of osteomyelitis of the foot of patients with diabetes. These include a review by a group from the International Working Group on the Diabetic Foot (7,110,214) and reviews of antibiotic treatment by Byren (218), Lazzarini (219), and, somewhat longer ago, Stengel et al. (220).

Role of Surgery

In their systematic review in 2008, Berendt et al. studied the value of surgery in the treatment of diabetic foot osteomyelitis (7,110). They concluded that there is little evidence to help choose between primarily medical and primarily surgical treatments in the management of diabetic foot osteomyelitis *(level D)*. They found no controlled studies on this subject but identified several observational studies (110). One study reported that amputation and death were less common in patients receiving early surgical intervention (221). The study was performed in 112 patients with a relatively high proportion of deep severe infections. Ha

Table 6 Scheme for the Diagnosis of Osteomyelitis (110)

Category	Post-test probability of osteomyelitis	Management advice	Criteria	Comments
Definite ('beyond reasonable doubt')	>90%	Treat for osteomyelitis	Bone sample with positive culture AND positive histology OR	Sample must be obtained at surgery or through uninvolved skin
			Purulence in bone found at surgery OR	Definite purulence identified by experienced surgeon
			Atraumatically detached bone fragment removed from ulcer by podiatrist/surgeon OR	Definite bone fragment identified by experienced surgeon/podiatrist
			Intraosseous abscess found on MRI OR	
			Any two probable criteria OR one probable and two possible criteria OR, any four possible criteria below	
Probable ('more likely than not');	51–90%	Consider treating, but further investigation may be needed	Visible cancellous bone in ulcer OR	
			MRI showing bone oedema with other signs of osteomyelitis OR	Sinus tract: sequestrum, heel or metatarsal head involved; doaca
			Bone sample with positive culture but negative or absent histology OR	
			Bone sample with positive histology but negative or absent culture OR	
			Any two possible criteria below	

Possible (but on balance, less rather than more likely)	10–50%	Treatment may be justifiable but further investigation usually advised	Plain X-rays show cortical destruction OR MRI shows bone oedema OR Cloaca, OR Probe to bone positive OR Visible cortical bone OR ESR >70 mm/h with no other plausible explanation OR Non-healing wound despite adequate offloading and perfusion for >6 weeks OR ulcer of >2 weeks duration with clinical evidence of infection
Unlikely	<10%	Usually no need for further investigation or treatment	No signs or symptoms of inflammation AND normal X-rays AND ulcer present for <2 weeks or absent AND any ulcer present is superficial OR Normal MRI OR Normal bone scan

Van and coworkers studied 32 patients treated with conservative orthopedic surgery (222). They compared the results with a historical control group that was treated only with antibiotics. The healing rate and days till healing were 78% and 181 days, respectively, for patients in the surgically treated group and 57% and 462 days, respectively, for the group treated only with antibiotics. Pittet and coworkers studied 50 patients with suspected osteomyelitis of deep foot infection. They found a healing rate of 70% in patients treated without surgery and reserved surgery for early failure of conservative therapy (223). Simpson et al. found in 50 patients that surgical resection was associated with significantly less relapse of chronic osteomyelitis (224). In a noncontrolled study of 237 patients, Henke and coworkers found that patients treated with surgery had a nonsignificantly different outcome in proximal amputations (80% vs. 81%) compared with patients treated only with antibiotics (225). Noncontrolled studies of outcomes of nonsurgical treatment have reported rates of healing comparable with those following surgery (153,226,227) *(level C–D)*. There are some advantages to surgical therapy such as shorter duration of treatment and less likely development of bacterial resistance against antibiotics (222) *(level D)*. Disadvantages are the higher likelihood of further foot complications, such as ulcers and amputations, after surgery (228–232). These additional complications are possibly due to changed biomechanical properties of the foot.

Choice of the Type of Surgical Therapy

In their systematic review, Berendt and coworkers could not identify a beneficial effect of certain types of surgical interventions (110) *(level D)*. A wide range of surgical interventions has been described. The most properly described ones include debridement to bleeding bone marrow with epidermal sheet grafting, two-stage debridement with secondary closure, and limb amputation (233–236).

Reviews on Antimicrobial Therapy

Stengel and coworkers found 22 controlled trials in their literature review (220). The review included both patients with and without diabetes. The authors made no distinction between studies regarding arthritis-, osteomyelitis-, and prosthesis-related joint infections. By excluding comparative studies, they ignored most trials on osteomyelitis. In their systematic review in 2005, Lazzarini and coworkers found 93 studies, of which 17 comparative studies pertained to the treatment of osteomyelitis in patients with and without diabetes (219). They found that many studies do not have a long period of follow-up. This period is necessary because the IDSA definition of a favorable outcome for osteomyelitis is a disease-free period of more than 1 year (11). Also, neither the duration of osteomyelitis is often defined nor is the distinction between acute and chronic osteomyelitis. Few studies specified the sensitivity of the causative organisms. Most studied infections were monobacterial, although some were polymicrobial. Information about surgical procedures or removal of surgical hardware (if present) was not provided in most studies. This is important, since surgery might have an impact on outcome.

Empirical Antibiotic Treatment

No systemic review has identified studies that demonstrate the superiority of any one antibiotic over another (110,219) *(level D)*. Both therapy against staphylococci and streptococci and broad-spectrum antibiotics against Gram-positive cocci, Gram-negative rods, and anaerobes seem to be equally effective (110,219) *(level D)*. No studies are available to answer if antibiotic therapy in osteomyelitis should be selected on the basis of the sensitivity of all present pathogens present or on the basis of most likely pathogens (usually Gram-positive cocci).

Oral Versus Parenteral Treatment

Oral treatment has the advantage over parenteral therapy that it is cheaper and it leads to less hospital admission days. Besides, it is easier to administer oral therapy, especially in remote and rural areas. There is evidence that oral therapy for osteomyelitis can be as effective as parenteral therapy *(level C)*. Fluoroquinolones and clindamycin with their high bioavailability and relatively high bone levels seem to be particularly suitable for this (219). Embil and coworkers published a retrospective study in 93 cases of patients with osteomyelitis treated with oral antibiotics and limited office debridement (153). Eighty-one percent of cases were put in remission after a mean of 40 weeks of culture-driven antibiotics. One article was published that compared oral and parenteral formulations of linezolid and aminopenicillin/β-lactamase inhibitor in 357 patients with diabetic foot infections, of whom 77 had osteomyelitis (74). The cure rates for oral and parenteral therapy were 77% and 83%, respectively, for linezolid and 68% and 72%, respectively, for aminopenicillin/β-lactamase inhibitor (differences not statistically significant).

Aminoglycoside-Impregnated Beads

Gentamicin-containing beads, usually made of polymethylmethacrylate (PMMA), are used in some clinics for treatment of chronic osteomyelitis *(level D)*. The theoretical advantage of this technique is that a high local dose of aminoglycosides can be given without systemic toxicity. There have been studies pertaining to the effectiveness of these beads in chronic osteomyelitis (not necessarily diabetic foot osteomyelitis) (237–240). Of these studies, one is an FDA-initiated, controlled trial of 190 patients treated with intravenous antibiotics, 49 with gentamicin PMMA beads, and 145 with a combination of beads and intravenous antibiotics (239). The patients in the combination group were significantly more likely to experience a relapse of infection compared with patients who were treated only with intravenous antibiotics (43% vs. 24%, respectively). The other uncontrolled studies reported healing rates of 89% to 92% (237,238,240).

Duration of Treatment

The optimal duration of antimicrobial therapy could not be identified in systematic reviews (110,219) *(level D)*. In most studies, patients were treated for 6 weeks. In a minority of (7 of 93) studies, patients were treated for 6 months (219). The optimal duration of treatment with antibiotics seems to vary with the amount of debridement. Treatment durations of 2 weeks have been reported following aggressive surgical debridement (44). A treatment duration on the other side of the spectrum was 40 weeks with limited debridement (153). No studies were found that identified a favorable outcome with longer treatment. The common presumption that osteomyelitis needs to be treated for 4 to 6 weeks seems to stem from animal studies where bacteria could be cultured from infected bone even after 2 weeks of appropriate treatment (241) *(level D)*.

Adjunctive Therapy for Osteomyelitis

There are no studies that suggest that the use of larvae, G-CSF, or VAC are helpful in treating diabetic foot osteomyelitis (110,242) *(level D)*.

REFERENCES

1. Verhoeven S, van Ballegooie E, Casparie AF. Impact of late complications in type 2 diabetes in a Dutch population. Diabet Med 1991; 8(5):435–438.
2. Eneroth M, Larsson J, Apelqvist J. Deep foot infections in patients with diabetes and foot ulcer: An entity with different characteristics, treatments, and prognosis. J Diabetes Complications 1999; 13(5–6):254–263.
3. Adler AI, Boyko EJ, Ahroni JH, et al. Lower extremity amputation in diabetes: The independent effects of peripheral vascular disease, sensory neuropathy, and foot ulcers. Diabetes Care 1999; 22(7):1029–1035.
4. Nather A, Bee CS, Huak CY, et al. Epidemiology of diabetic foot problems and predictive factors for limb loss. J Diabetes Complications 2008;22(2):77–82.
5. Pecoraro RE, Reiber GE, Burgess EM. Pathways to amputation: Basis for prevention. Diabetes Care 1990; 13(5):513–21.
6. Eneroth M, Apelqvist J, Stenstrom A. Clinical characteristics and outcome in 223 diabetic patients with deep foot infections. Foot Ankle Int 1997; 18(11):716–722.
7. International Working Group on the Diabetic Foot. International consensus on the diabetic foot and supplements [DVD]. In: Apelqvist J, Bakker K, Van Houtum WH, et al., eds. Amsterdam, The Netherlands: International Diabetes Federation, 2007.
8. Tennvall GR, Apelqvist J, Eneroth M. Costs of deep foot infections in patients with diabetes mellitus. Pharmacoeconomics 2000; 18(3):225–238.
9. Washington, DC: US Census Bureau, http://www.bls.gov/data/inflation_calculator.htm; http://www.xe.com/ucc. Accessed June 2, 2010.
10. Berendt AR, Lipsky BA. Infection in the diabetic foot. In: Armstrong DG, Lavery LA, eds. Clinical Care of the Diabetic Foot. Alexandria, VA: American Diabetes Association, 2005:90–98.
11. Mader JT, Shirtliff M, Calhoun JH. Staging and staging application in osteomyelitis. Clin Infect Dis 1997; 25(6):1303–1309.
12. Wheat LJ. Infection and diabetes mellitus. Diabetes Care 1980; 3(1):187–197.
13. Shah BR, Hux JE. Quantifying the risk of infectious diseases for people with diabetes. Diabetes Care 2003; 26(2):510–513.
14. Muller LM, Gorter KJ, Hak E, et al. Increased risk of common infections in patients with type 1 and type 2 diabetes mellitus. Clin Infect Dis 2005; 41(3):281–288.
15. van den Berghe G., Wouters P, Weekers F, et al. Intensive insulin therapy in the critically ill patients. N Engl J Med 2001; 345(19):1359–1367.
16. van den Berghe G, Wilmer A, Hermans G, et al. Intensive insulin therapy in the medical ICU. N Engl J Med 2006; 354(5):449–461.
17. Santilli F, Cipollone F, Mezzetti A, et al. The role of nitric oxide in the development of diabetic angiopathy. Horm Metab Res 2004; 36(5):319–335.
18. Kim SH, Park KW, Kim YS, et al. Effects of acute hyperglycemia on endothelium-dependent vasodilation in patients with diabetes mellitus or impaired glucose metabolism. Endothelium 2003; 10(2):65–70.
19. Bergamaschini L, Gardinali M, Poli M, et al. Complement activation in diabetes mellitus. J Clin Lab Immunol 1991; 35(3):121–127.
20. Saiepour D, Sehlin J, Oldenborg PA. Hyperglycemia-induced protein kinase C activation inhibits phagocytosis of C3b- and immunoglobulin G-opsonized yeast particles in normal human neutrophils. Exp Diabesity Res 2003; 4(2):125–132.
21. Saiepour D, Sehlin J, Oldenborg PA. Insulin inhibits phagocytosis in normal human neutrophils via PKCalpha/beta-dependent priming of F-actin assembly. Inflamm Res 2006; 55(3):85–91.
22. Turina M, Fry DE, Polk HC Jr. Acute hyperglycemia and the innate immune system: Clinical, cellular, and molecular aspects. Crit Care Med 2005; 33(7):1624–1633.

23. Delamaire M, Maugendre D, Moreno M, et al. Impaired leucocyte functions in diabetic patients. Diabet Med 1997; 14(1):29–34.
24. Walrand S, Guillet C, Boirie Y, et al. In vivo evidences that insulin regulates human polymorphonuclear neutrophil functions. J Leukoc Biol 2004; 76(6):1104–1110.
25. Collison KS, Parhar RS, Saleh SS, et al. RAGE-mediated neutrophil dysfunction is evoked by advanced glycation end products (AGEs). J Leukoc Biol 2002; 71(3):433–444.
26. Geerlings SE, Hoepelman AI. Immune dysfunction in patients with diabetes mellitus (DM). FEMS Immunol Med Microbiol 1999; 26(3–4):259–265.
27. Cavalot F, Anfossi G, Russo I, et al. Insulin, at physiological concentrations, enhances the polymorphonuclear leukocyte chemotactic properties. Horm Metab Res 1992; 24(5):225–228.
28. Mowat A, Baum J. Chemotaxis of polymorphonuclear leukocytes from patients with diabetes mellitus. N Engl J Med 1971; 284(12):621–627.
29. Hill HR, Augustine NH, Rallison ML, et al. Defective monocyte chemotactic responses in diabetes mellitus. J Clin Immunol 1983; 3(1):70–77.
30. Perner A, Nielsen SE, Rask-Madsen J. High glucose impairs superoxide production from isolated blood neutrophils. Intensive Care Med 2003; 29(4):642–645.
31. Sato N, Kashima K, Shimizu H, et al. Hypertonic glucose inhibits the production of oxygen-derived free radicals by rat neutrophils. Life Sci 1993; 52(18):1481–1486.
32. Gough A, Clapperton M, Rolando N, et al. Randomised placebo-controlled trial of granulocyte-colony stimulating factor in diabetic foot infection. Lancet 1997; 350(9081):855–859.
33. Yonem A, Cakir B, Guler S, et al. Effects of granulocyte-colony stimulating factor in the treatment of diabetic foot infection. Diabetes Obes Metab 2001; 3(5):332–337.
34. Cruciani M, Lipsky BA, Mengoli C, et al. Are granulocyte colony-stimulating factors beneficial in treating diabetic foot infections? A meta-analysis. Diabetes Care 2005; 28(2):454–460.
35. MacCuish AC, Urbaniak SJ, Campbell CJ, et al. Phytohemagglutinin transformation and circulating lymphocyte subpopulations in insulin-dependent diabetic patients. Diabetes 1974; 23(8):708–712.
36. Eibl N, Spatz M, Fischer GF, et al. Impaired primary immune response in type-1 diabetes: Results from a controlled vaccination study. Clin Immunol 2002; 103(3, pt 1):249–259.
37. Spatz M, Eibl N, Hink S, et al. Impaired primary immune response in type-1 diabetes. Functional impairment at the level of APCs and T-cells. Cell Immunol 2003; 221(1):15–26.
38. Pozzilli P, Pagani S, Arduini P, et al. In vivo determination of cell mediated immune response in diabetic patients using a multiple intradermal antigen dispenser. Diabetes Res 1987; 6(1):5–8.
39. Lapolla A, Tonani R, Fedele D, et al. Non-enzymatic glycation of IgG: An in vivo study. Horm Metab Res 2002; 34(5):260–264.
40. Diepersloot RJ, Bouter KP, van BR, et al. Cytotoxic T-cell response to influenza A subunit vaccine in patients with type 1 diabetes mellitus. Neth J Med 1989; 35 (1–2):68–75.
41. el-Madhun AS, Cox RJ, Seime A, et al. Systemic and local immune responses after parenteral influenza vaccination in juvenile diabetic patients and healthy controls: Results from a pilot study. Vaccine 1998; 16(2–3):156–160.
42. Lederman MM, Schiffman G, Rodman HM. Pneumococcal immunization in adult diabetics. Diabetes 1981; 30(2):119–121.
43. Marseglia G, Alibrandi A, d'Annunzio G, et al. Long term persistence of anti-HBs protective levels in young patients with type 1 diabetes after recombinant hepatitis B vaccine. Vaccine 2000; 19(7–8):680–683.
44. Lavery LA, Armstrong DG, Wunderlich RP, et al. Risk factors for foot infections in individuals with diabetes. Diabetes Care 2006; 29(6):1288–1293.

45. Peters EJ, Lavery LA, Armstrong DG. Diabetic lower extremity infection: Influence of physical, psychological, and social factors. J Diabetes Complications 2005; 19(2):107–112.
46. Bartos V, Jirkovska A, Koznarova R. [Risk factors for diabetic foot in recipients of renal and pancreatic transplants]. Cas Lek Cesk 1997; 136(17):527–529.
47. George RK, Verma AK, Agarwal A, et al. An audit of foot infections in patients with diabetes mellitus following renal transplantation. Int J Low Extrem Wounds 2004; 3(3):157–160.
48. Hill MN, Feldman HI, Hilton SC, et al. Risk of foot complications in long-term diabetic patients with and without ESRD: A preliminary study. ANNA J 1996; 23(4):381–386.
49. Jayasinghe SA, Atukorala I, Gunethilleke B, et al. Is walking barefoot a risk factor for diabetic foot disease in developing countries? Rural Remote Health 2007; 7(2):692.
50. Schaper NC. Diabetic foot ulcer classification system for research purposes: A progress report on criteria for including patients in research studies. Diabetes Metab Res Rev 2004; 20(suppl 1):90–95.
51. International Working Group on the Diabetic Foot. International Consensus on the Diabetic Foot and Supplements [DVD]. In: Apelqvist J, Bakker K, Van Houtum WH et al., eds. Amsterdam, The Netherlands: International Diabetes Federation, 2003.
52. Lipsky BA, Berendt AR, Deery HG, et al. Diagnosis and treatment of diabetic foot infections. Clin Infect Dis 2004; 39(7):885–910.
53. Edelson GW, Armstrong DG, Lavery LA, et al. The acutely infected diabetic foot is not adequately evaluated in an inpatient setting. Arch Intern Med 1996; 156(20):2373–2376.
54. Armstrong DG, Perales TA, Murff RT, et al. Value of white blood cell count with differential in the acute diabetic foot infection. J Am Podiatr Med Assoc 1996; 86(5):224–227.
55. Lavery LA, Armstrong DG, Quebedeaux TL, et al. Puncture wounds: The frequency of normal laboratory values in the face of severe foot infections of the foot in diabetic and non-diabetic adults. Am J Med 1996; 101:521–525.
56. Lavery LA, Walker SC, Harkless LB, et al. Infected puncture wounds in diabetic and nondiabetic adults. Diabetes Care 1995; 18(12):1588–1591.
57. Meggitt B. Surgical management of the diabetic foot. Br J Hosp Med 1976; 16:227–332.
58. Wagner FW. The dysvascular foot: A system for diagnosis and treatment. Foot Ankle 1981; 2:64–122.
59. Lavery LA, Armstrong DG, Murdoch DP, et al. Validation of the Infectious Diseases Society of America's Diabetic Foot Infection Classification system. Clin Infect Dis 2007; 44(4):562–565.
60. Prompers L, Huijberts M, Apelqvist J, et al. High prevalence of ischaemia, infection and serious comorbidity in patients with diabetic foot disease in Europe: Baseline results from the EURODIALE study. Diabetologia 2007; 50(1):18–25.
61. Jeandrot A, Richard JL, Combescure C, et al. Serum procalcitonin and C-reactive protein concentrations to distinguish mildly infected from non-infected diabetic foot ulcers: A pilot study. Diabetologia 2008; 51(2):347–352.
62. Macfarlane RM, Jeffcoate WJ. Classification of diabetic foot ulcers: The S(AD) SAD system. Diabetic Foot 1999; 2(4):123–131.
63. Treece KA, Macfarlane RM, Pound N, et al. Validation of a system of foot ulcer classification in diabetes mellitus. Diabet Med 2004; 21(9):987–991.
64. Jeffcoate WJ, Chipchase SY, Ince P, et al. Assessing the outcome of the management of diabetic foot ulcers using ulcer-related and person-related measures. Diabetes Care 2006; 29(8):1784–1787.
65. Ince P, Abbas ZG, Lutale JK, et al. Use of the SINBAD classification system and score in comparing outcome of foot ulcer management on three continents. Diabetes Care 2008; 31(5):964–967.
66. Oyibo SO, Jude EB, Tarawneh I, et al. A comparison of two diabetic foot ulcer classification systems: The Wagner and the University of Texas wound classification systems. Diabetes Care 2001; 24(1):84–88.

67. Armstrong DG, Lavery LA, Harkless LB. Validation of a diabetic wound classification system: The contribution of depth, infection, and ischemia to risk of amputation. Diabetes Care 1998; 21(5):855–859.
68. Abbas ZG, Lutale JK, Game FL, et al. Comparison of four systems of classification of diabetic foot ulcers in Tanzania. Diabet Med 2008; 25(2):134–137.
69. Jeffcoate WJ, Lipsky BA. Controversies in diagnosing and managing osteomyelitis of the foot in diabetes. Clin Infect Dis 2004; 39(suppl 2):S115–S122.
70. Knighton DR, Ciresi KF, Fiegel VD, et al. Classification and treatment of chronic nonhealing wounds: Successful treatment with autologous platelet-derived wound healing factors (PDWHF). Ann Surg 1986; 204(3):322–330.
71. Beckert S, Witte M, Wicke C, et al. A new wound-based severity score for diabetic foot ulcers: A prospective analysis of 1,000 patients. Diabetes Care 2006; 29(5):988–992.
72. Beckert S, Pietsch AM, Kuper M, et al. M. A.I.D.: A prognostic score estimating probability of healing in chronic lower extremity wounds. Ann Surg 2009; 249(4):677–681.
73. Lipsky BA, Polis AB, Lantz KC, et al. The value of a wound score for diabetic foot infections in predicting treatment outcome: A prospective analysis from the SIDESTEP trial. Wound Repair Regen 2009; 17(5):671–677.
74. Lipsky BA, Itani K, Norden C. Treating foot infections in diabetic patients: A randomized, multicenter, open-label trial of linezolid versus ampicillin-sulbactam/amoxicillin-clavulanate. Clin Infect Dis 2004; 38(1):17–24.
75. Ge Y, MacDonald D, Henry MM, et al. In vitro susceptibility to pexiganan of bacteria isolated from infected diabetic foot ulcers. Diagn Microbiol Infect Dis 1999; 35(1):45–53.
76. Lipsky BA, Armstrong DG, Baker NR, Macdonald IA. Does a diabetic foot infection (DFI) wound score correlate with the clinical response to antibiotic treatment? Data from the SIDESTEP study. Diabetologia 2005; 48(suppl 1):A354.
77. Lipsky BA, Armstrong DG, Citron DM, et al. Ertapenem versus piperacillin/tazobactam for diabetic foot infections (SIDESTEP): Prospective, randomised, controlled, double-blinded, multicentre trial. Lancet 2005; 366(9498):1695–1703.
78. Berendt AR, Lipsky BA. Should antibiotics be used in the treatment of the diabetic foot? Diabetic Foot 2003; 6:18–28.
79. Chantelau E, Tanudjaja T, Altenhofer F, et al. Antibiotic treatment for uncomplicated neuropathic forefoot ulcers in diabetes: A controlled trial. Diabet Med 1996; 13(2):156–159.
80. Foster AVM, Bates M, Doxford M, et al. Should oral antibiotics be given to "clean" foot ulcers with no cellulitis? In: Abstracts of the 3rd International Symposium of the Diabetic Foot. Noordwijkerhout, The Netherlands: International Working Group on the Diabetic Foot, 1999:Abstract O13.
81. Senneville E, Melliez H, Beltrand E, et al. Culture of percutaneous bone biopsy specimens for diagnosis of diabetic foot osteomyelitis: Concordance with ulcer swab cultures. Clin Infect Dis 2006; 42(1):57–62.
82. Embil JM, Trepman E. Microbiological evaluation of diabetic foot osteomyelitis. Clin Infect Dis 2006; 42(1):63–65.
83. Urbancic-Rovan V, Gubina M. Bacteria in superficial diabetic foot ulcers. Diabet Med 2000; 17(11):814–815.
84. Lipsky BA, Pecoraro RE, Wheat LJ. The diabetic foot: Soft tissue and bone infection. Infect Dis Clin North Am 1990; 4(3):409–432.
85. Goldstein EJ, Citron DM, Nesbit CA. Diabetic foot infections: Bacteriology and activity of 10 oral antimicrobial agents against bacteria isolated from consecutive cases. Diabetes Care 1996; 19(6):638–641.
86. Ge Y, MacDonald D, Hait H, et al. Microbiological profile of infected diabetic foot ulcers. Diabet Med 2002; 19(12):1032–1034.
87. Gadepalli R, Dhawan B, Sreenivas V, et al. A clinico-microbiological study of diabetic foot ulcers in an Indian tertiary care hospital. Diabetes Care 2006; 29(8):1727–1732.

88. Abdulrazak A, Bitar ZI, Al-Shamali AA, et al. Bacteriological study of diabetic foot infections. J Diabetes Complications 2005; 19(3):138–141.
89. Jones EW, Edwards R, Finch R, et al. A microbiological study of diabetic foot lesions. Diabet Med 1985; 2(3):213–215.
90. Sapico FL, Witte JL, Canawati HN, et al. The infected foot of the diabetic patient: Quantitative microbiology and analysis of clinical features. Rev Infect Dis 1984; 6(suppl 1):S171–S176.
91. Hunt JA. Foot infections in diabetes are rarely due to a single microorganism. Diabet Med 1992; 9(8):749–752.
92. Louie A, Baltch AL, Smith RP. Gram-negative bacterial surveillance in diabetic patients. Infect Med 1993; 10(2):33–34–39.
93. Candel Gonzalez FJ, Alramadan M, Matesanz M, et al. Infections in diabetic foot ulcers. Eur J Intern Med 2003; 14(5):341–343.
94. Wheat LJ, Allen SD, Henry M, et al. Diabetic foot infections: Bacteriologic analysis. Arch Intern Med 1986; 146(10):1935–1940.
95. Pathare NA, Bal A, Talvalkar GV, et al. Diabetic foot infections: A study of microorganisms associated with the different Wagner grades. Indian J Pathol Microbiol 1998; 41(4):437–441.
96. Gerding DN. Foot infections in diabetic patients: The role of anaerobes. Clin Infect Dis 1995; 20(suppl 2):S283–S288.
97. Hartemann-Heurtier A, Robert J, Jacqueminet S, et al. Diabetic foot ulcer and multidrug-resistant organisms: Risk factors and impact. Diabet Med 2004; 21(7):710–715.
98. Tentolouris N, Jude EB, Smirnof I, et al. Methicillin-resistant Staphylococcus aureus: An increasing problem in a diabetic foot clinic. Diabet Med 1999; 16(9):767–771.
99. Tentolouris N, Petrikkos G, Vallianou N, et al. Prevalence of methicillin-resistant Staphylococcus aureus in infected and uninfected diabetic foot ulcers. Clin Microbiol Infect 2006; 12(2):186–189.
100. Dang CN, Prasad YD, Boulton AJ, et al. Methicillin-resistant Staphylococcus aureus in the diabetic foot clinic: A worsening problem. Diabet Med 2003; 20(2):159–161.
101. Wagner A, Reike H, Angelkort B. Erfahrungen im Umgang mit hochresistenten Keimen bei Patienten mit diabetischem Fuβ-Syndrom unter besonderer Bercksichtigung von MRSA-Infektionen. Dtsch Med Wochenschr 2001; 126(48):1353–1356.
102. Moran GJ, Krishnadasan A, Gorwitz RJ, et al. Methicillin-resistant S. aureus infections among patients in the emergency department. N Engl J Med 2006; 355(7):666–674.
103. Kandemir O, Akbay E, Sahin E, et al. Risk factors for infection of the diabetic foot with multi-antibiotic resistant microorganisms. J Infect 2007; 54(5):439–445.
104. Hinchliffe RJ, Valk GD, Apelqvist J, et al. A systematic review of the effectiveness of interventions to enhance the healing of chronic ulcers of the foot in diabetes. Diabetes Metab Res Rev 2008; 24(suppl 1):S119–S144.
105. Apelqvist J, Ragnarson Tennvall G. Cavity foot ulcers in diabetic patients: A comparative study of cadexomer iodine ointment and standard treatment: An economic analysis alongside a clinical trial. Acta Derm Venereol 1996; 76(3):231–235.
106. Apelqvist J, Larsson J, Stenstrom A. Topical treatment of necrotic foot ulcers in diabetic patients: A comparative trial of DuoDerm and MeZinc. Br J Dermatol 1990; 123(6):787–792.
107. Bennett LL, Rosenblum RS, Perlov C, et al. An in vivo comparison of topical agents on wound repair. Plast Reconstr Surg 2001; 108(3):675–687.
108. Bergin SM, Wraight P. Silver based wound dressings and topical agents for treating diabetic foot ulcers. Cochrane Database Syst Rev 2006; (1):CD005082.
109. Gibbons GW. Lower extremity bypass in patients with diabetic foot ulcers. Surg Clin North Am 2003; 83(3):659–669.
110. Berendt AR, Peters EJ, Bakker K, et al. Diabetic foot osteomyelitis: A progress report on diagnosis and a systematic review of treatment. Diabetes Metab Res Rev 2008; 24(suppl 1):S145–S161.

111. Armstrong DG, Salas P, Short B, et al. Maggot therapy in "lower-extremity hospice" wound care: Fewer amputations and more antibiotic-free days. J Am Podiatr Med Assoc 2005; 95(3):254–257.
112. Jaklic D, Lapanje A, Zupancic K, et al. Selective antimicrobial activity of maggots against pathogenic bacteria. J Med Microbiol 2008; 57(pt 5):617–625.
113. van der Plas MJ, Jukema GN, Wai SW, et al. Maggot excretions/secretions are differentially effective against biofilms of Staphylococcus aureus and Pseudomonas aeruginosa. J Antimicrob Chemother 2008; 61(1):117–122.
114. Barnes RC. Point: Hyperbaric oxygen is beneficial for diabetic foot wounds. Clin Infect Dis 2006; 43(2):188–192.
115. Berendt AR. Counterpoint: Hyperbaric oxygen for diabetic foot wounds is not effective. Clin Infect Dis 2006; 43(2):193–198.
116. Kranke P, Bennett M, Roeckl-Wiedmann I, et al. Hyperbaric oxygen therapy for chronic wounds. Cochrane Database Syst Rev 2004; (2):CD004123.
117. Abidia A, Laden G, Kuhan G, et al. The role of hyperbaric oxygen therapy in ischaemic diabetic lower extremity ulcers: A double-blind randomised-controlled trial. Eur J Vasc Endovasc Surg 2003; 25(6):513–518.
118. Doctor N, Pandya S, Supe A. Hyperbaric oxygen therapy in diabetic foot. J Postgrad Med 1992; 38(3):112–114.
119. Faglia E, Favales F, Aldeghi A, et al. Adjunctive systemic hyperbaric oxygen therapy in treatment of severe prevalently ischemic diabetic foot ulcer: A randomized study. Diabetes Care 1996; 19(12):1338–1343.
120. Vardakas KZ, Horianopoulou M, Falagas ME. Factors associated with treatment failure in patients with diabetic foot infections: An analysis of data from randomized controlled trials. Diabetes Res Clin Pract 2008; 80(3):344–351.
121. Nelson EA, O'Meara S, Golder S, et al. Systematic review of antimicrobial treatments for diabetic foot ulcers. Diabet Med 2006; 23(4):348–359.
122. Lipsky BA. Evidence-based antibiotic therapy of diabetic foot infections. FEMS Immunol Med Microbiol 1999; 26(3–4):267–276.
123. Seabrook GR, Edmiston CE, Schmitt DD, et al. Comparison of serum and tissue antibiotic levels in diabetes-related foot infections. Surgery 1991; 110(4):671–676.
124. Raymakers JTFJ, Heyden vd JJ, Daemen MJAP, et al. Penetration of ceftazidime in ischemic tissues. In: Proceedings of the Second International Symposiumon the Diabetic Foot. Noordwijkerhout, The Netherlands, ; 1995:Abstract P-50.
125. Storm AJ, Bouter KP, Diepersloot RJ, et al. Tissue concentrations of an orally administered antibiotic in diabetic patients with foot infections. J Antimicrob Chemother 1994; 34(3):449–451.
126. Duckworth C, Fisher JF, Carter SA, et al. Tissue penetration of clindamycin in diabetic foot infections. J Antimicrob Chemother 1993; 31(4):581–584.
127. Mueller-Buehl U, Diehm C, Gutzler F, et al. Tissue concentrations of ofloxacin in necrotic foot lesions of diabetic and non-diabetic patients with peripheral arterial occlusive disease. Vasa 1991; 20(1):17–21.
128. Kuck EM, Bouter KP, Hoekstra JB, et al. Tissue concentrations after a single-dose, orally administered ofloxacin in patients with diabetic foot infections. Foot Ankle Int 1998; 19(1):38–40.
129. Marangos MN, Skoutelis AT, Nightingale CH, et al. Absorption of ciprofloxacin in patients with diabetic gastroparesis. Antimicrob Agents Chemother 1995; 39(9):2161–2163.
130. Itani KM, Weigelt J, Li JZ, et al. Linezolid reduces length of stay and duration of intravenous treatment compared with vancomycin for complicated skin and soft tissue infections due to suspected or proven methicillin-resistant Staphylococcus aureus (MRSA). Int J Antimicrob Agents 2005; 26(6):442–448.
131. Weigelt J, Itani K, Stevens D, et al. Linezolid versus vancomycin in treatment of complicated skin and soft tissue infections. Antimicrob Agents Chemother 2005; 49(6):2260–2266.

132. Stein GE, Schooley S, Peloquin CA, et al. Linezolid tissue penetration and serum activity against strains of methicillin-resistant Staphylococcus aureus with reduced vancomycin susceptibility in diabetic patients with foot infections. J Antimicrob Chemother 2007; 60(4):819–823.
133. Lipsky BA, Stoutenburgh U. Daptomycin for treating infected diabetic foot ulcers: Evidence from a randomized, controlled trial comparing daptomycin with vancomycin or semi-synthetic penicillins for complicated skin and skin-structure infections. J Antimicrob Chemother 2005; 55(2):240–245.
134. Jauregui LE, Babazadeh S, Seltzer E, et al. Randomized, double-blind comparison of once-weekly dalbavancin versus twice-daily linezolid therapy for the treatment of complicated skin and skin structure infections. Clin Infect Dis 2005; 41(10):1407–1415.
135. Seltzer E, Dorr MB, Goldstein BP, et al. Once-weekly dalbavancin versus standard-of-care antimicrobial regimens for treatment of skin and soft-tissue infections. Clin Infect Dis 2003; 37(10):1298–1303.
136. Stryjewski ME, O'Riordan WD, Lau WK, et al. Telavancin versus standard therapy for treatment of complicated skin and soft-tissue infections due to gram-positive bacteria. Clin Infect Dis 2005; 40(11):1601–1607.
137. Doan TL, Fung HB, Mehta D, et al. Tigecycline: A glycylcycline antimicrobial agent. Clin Ther 2006; 28(8):1079–1106.
138. Noel GJ, Bush K, Bagchi P, et al. A randomized, double-blind trial comparing ceftobiprole medocaril with vancomycin plus ceftazidime for the treatment of patients with complicated skin and skin-structure infections. Clin Infect Dis 2008; 46(5):647–655.
139. Noel GJ, Strauss RS, Amsler K, et al. Results of a double-blind, randomized trial of ceftobiprole treatment of complicated skin and skin structure infections caused by gram-positive bacteria. Antimicrob Agents Chemother 2008; 52(1):37–44.
140. Lipsky BA, Giordano P, Choudhri S, et al. Treating diabetic foot infections with sequential intravenous to oral moxifloxacin compared with piperacillin-tazobactam/amoxicillin-clavulanate. J Antimicrob Chemother 2007; 60(2):370–376.
141. Edmonds M, Foster A. The use of antibiotics in the diabetic foot. Am J Surg 2004; 187(5 A):25S–28S.
142. Chantelau E, Tanudjaja T, Altenhofer F, et al. Antibiotic treatment for uncomplicated neuropathic forefoot ulcers in diabetes: A controlled trial. Diabet Med 1996; 13(2):156–159.
143. Hirschl M, Hirschl AM. Bacterial flora in mal perforant and antimicrobial treatment with ceftriaxone. Chemotherapy 1992; 38(4):275–280.
144. O'Meara S, Nelson EA, Golder S, et al. Systematic review of methods to diagnose infection in foot ulcers in diabetes. Diabet Med 2006; 23(4):341–347.
145. Lipsky BA, Berendt AR, Embil J, et al. Diagnosing and treating diabetic foot infections. Diabetes Metab Res Rev 2004; 20(suppl 1):S56–S64.
146. Senneville E. Antimicrobial interventions for the management of diabetic foot infections. Expert Opin Pharmacother 2005; 6(2):263–273.
147. Armstrong DG, Liswood PJ, Todd WF. 1995 William J. Stickel Bronze Award: Prevalence of mixed infections in the diabetic pedal wound: A retrospective review of 112 infections. J Am Podiatr Med Assoc 1995; 85(10):533–537.
148. Lipsky BA, Pecoraro RE, Larson SA, et al. Outpatient management of uncomplicated lower-extremity infections in diabetic patients. Arch Intern Med 1990; 150(4):790–797.
149. Lipsky BA, Baker PD, Landon GC, et al. Antibiotic therapy for diabetic foot infections: Comparison of two parenteral-to-oral regimens. Clin Infect Dis 1997; 24(4):643–648.
150. Grayson ML, Gibbons GW, Habershaw GM, et al. Use of ampicillin/sulbactam versus imipenem/cilastatin in the treatment of limb-threatening foot infections in diabetic patients. Clin Infect Dis 1994; 18(5):683–693.
151. Mills JL, Beckett WC, Taylor SM. The diabetic foot: Consequences of delayed treatment and referral. South Med J 1991; 84(8):970–974.
152. Peterson LR, Lissack LM, Canter K, et al. Therapy of lower extremity infections with ciprofloxacin in patients with diabetes mellitus, peripheral vascular disease, or both. Am J Med 1989; 86(6 pt 2):801–808.

153. Embil JM, Rose G, Trepman E, et al. Oral antimicrobial therapy for diabetic foot osteomyelitis. Foot Ankle Int 2006; 27(10):771–779.
154. Ramsey SD, Newton K, Blough D, et al. Incidence, outcomes, and cost of foot ulcers in patients with diabetes. Diabetes Care 1999; 22(3):382–387.
155. Newman LG, Waller J, Palestro CJ, et al. Unsuspected osteomyelitis in diabetic foot ulcers: Diagnosis and monitoring by leukocyte scanning with indium in 111 oxyquinoline. JAMA 1991; 266(9):1246–1251.
156. Lipsky BA. Osteomyelitis of the foot in diabetic patients. Clin Infect Dis 1997; 25(6):1318–1326.
157. Lavery LA, Sariaya M, Ashry H, et al. Microbiology of osteomyelitis in diabetic foot infections. J Foot Ankle Surg 1995; 34(1):61–64.
158. Zimmerli W, Fluckiger U. [Classification and microbiology of osteomyelitis]. Orthopade 2004; 33(3):267–272.
159. Game F, Jeffcoate W. MRSA and osteomyelitis of the foot in diabetes. Diabet Med 2004; 21(suppl 4):16–19.
160. Gristina AG, Costerton JW. Bacterial adherence and the glycocalyx and their role in musculoskeletal infection. Orthop Clin North Am 1984; 15(3):517–535.
161. Berendt T, Byren I. Bone and joint infection. Clin Med 2004; 4(6):510–518.
162. Ciampolini J, Harding KG. Pathophysiology of chronic bacterial osteomyelitis: Why do antibiotics fail so often? Postgrad Med J 2000; 76(898):479–483.
163. Stewart PS. Mechanisms of antibiotic resistance in bacterial biofilms. Int J Med Microbiol 2002; 292(2):107–113.
164. Donlan RM, Costerton JW. Biofilms: Survival mechanisms of clinically relevant microorganisms. Clin Microbiol Rev 2002; 15(2):167–193.
165. Whitchurch CB, Tolker-Nielsen T, Ragas PC, et al. Extracellular DNA required for bacterial biofilm formation. Science 2002; 295(5559):1487.
166. Donlan RM. Role of biofilms in antimicrobial resistance. ASAIO J 2000; 46(6):S47–S52.
167. Patel R. Biofilms and antimicrobial resistance. Clin Orthop Relat Res 2005; (437):41–47.
168. Weigel LM, Donlan RM, Shin DH, et al. High-level vancomycin-resistant Staphylococcus aureus isolates associated with a polymicrobial biofilm. Antimicrob Agents Chemother 2007; 51(1):231–238.
169. Butalia S, Palda VA, Sargeant RJ, et al. Does this patient with diabetes have osteomyelitis of the lower extremity? JAMA 2008; 299(7):806–813.
170. Dinh MT, Abad CL, Safdar N. Diagnostic accuracy of the physical examination and imaging tests for osteomyelitis underlying diabetic foot ulcers: Meta-analysis. Clin Infect Dis 2008; 47(4):519–527.
171. Enderle MD, Coerper S, Schweizer HP, et al. Correlation of imaging techniques to histopathology in patients with diabetic foot syndrome and clinical suspicion of chronic osteomyelitis: The role of high-resolution ultrasound. Diabetes Care 1999; 22(2):294–299.
172. Vesco L, Boulahdour H, Hamissa S, et al. The value of combined radionuclide and magnetic resonance imaging in the diagnosis and conservative management of minimal or localized osteomyelitis of the foot in diabetic patients. Metabolism 1999; 48(7):922–927.
173. Armstrong DG, Lavery LA, Sariaya M, et al. Leukocytosis is a poor indicator of acute osteomyelitis of the foot in diabetes mellitus. J Foot Ankle Surg 1996; 35(4):280–283.
174. Grayson ML, Balaugh K, Levin E, et al. Probing to bone in infected pedal ulcers: A clinical sign of underlying osteomyelitis in diabetic patients. JAMA 1995; 273(9):721–723.
175. Shone A, Burnside J, Chipchase S, et al. Probing the validity of the probe-to-bone test in the diagnosis of osteomyelitis of the foot in diabetes. Diabetes Care 2006; 29(4):945.
176. Lavery LA, Armstrong DG, Peters EJ, et al. Probe-to-bone test for diagnosing diabetic foot osteomyelitis: Reliable or relic? Diabetes Care 2007; 30(2):270–274.
177. Kaleta JL, Fleischli JW, Reilly CH. The diagnosis of osteomyelitis in diabetes using erythrocyte sedimentation rate: A pilot study. J Am Podiatr Med Assoc 2001; 91(9):445–450.

178. Armstrong DG, Lavery LA, Sariaya M, et al. Leukocytosis is a poor indicator of acute osteomyelitis of the foot in diabetes mellitus. J Foot Ankle Surg 1996; 34(5):280–283.
179. DeStefano F, Newman J. Comparison of coronary heart disease mortality risk between black and white people with diabetes. Ethn Dis 1993; 3:145–151.
180. Weinstein D, Wang A, Chambers R, et al. Evaluation of magnetic resonance imaging in the diagnosis of osteomyelitis in diabetic foot infections. Foot Ankle 1993; 14(1):18–22.
181. Mettler MA. Essentials of Radiology. 2nd ed. Philadelphia, PA: Elsevier Saunders, 2005.
182. Yuh WT, Corson JD, Baraniewski HM, et al. Osteomyelitis of the foot in diabetic patients: Evaluation with plain film, 99mTc-MDP bone scintigraphy, and MR imaging. AJR Am J Roentgenol 1989; 152(4):795–800.
183. Wang A, Weinstein D, Greenfield L, et al. MRI and diabetic foot infections. Magn Reson Imaging 1990; 8(6):805–809.
184. Johnson JE, Kennedy EJ, Shereff MJ, et al. Prospective study of bone, indium-111-labeled white blood cell, and gallium-67 scanning for the evaluation of osteomyelitis in the diabetic foot. Foot Ankle Int 1996; 17(1):10–16.
185. Lee SM, Lee RG, Wilinsky J, et al. Magnification radiography in osteomyelitis. Skeletal Radiol 1986; 15(8):625–627.
186. Park HM, Wheat LJ, Siddiqui AR, et al. Scintigraphic evaluation of diabetic osteomyelitis: Concise communication. J Nucl Med 1982; 23(7):569–573.
187. Shults DW, Hunter GC, McIntyre KE, et al. Value of radiographs and bone scans in determining the need for therapy in diabetic patients with foot ulcers. Am J Surg 1989; 158(6):525–529.
188. Croll SD, Nicholas GG, Osborne MA, et al. Role of magnetic resonance imaging in the diagnosis of osteomyelitis in diabetic foot infections. J Vasc Surg 1996; 24(2):266–270.
189. Keenan AM, Tindel NL, Alavi A. Diagnosis of pedal osteomyelitis in diabetic patients using current scintigraphic techniques. Arch Intern Med 1989; 149(10):2262–2266.
190. Larcos G, Brown ML, Sutton RT. Diagnosis of osteomyelitis of the foot in diabetic patients: Value of 111In-leukocyte scintigraphy. AJR Am J Roentgenol 1991; 157(3):527–531.
191. Seldin DW, Heiken JP, Feldman F, et al. Effect of soft-tissue pathology on detection of pedal osteomyelitis in diabetics. J Nucl Med 1985; 26(9):988–993.
192. Levine SE, Neagle CE, Esterhai JL, et al. Magnetic resonance imaging for the diagnosis of osteomyelitis in the diabetic patient with a foot ulcer. Foot Ankle Int 1994; 15(3):51–156.
193. Oyen WJ, Netten PM, Lemmens JA, et al. Evaluation of infectious diabetic foot complications with indium-111-labeled human nonspecific immunoglobulin G. J Nucl Med 1992; 33(7):1330–1336.
194. Harwood SJ, Valdivia S, Hung GL, et al. Use of Sulesomab, a radiolabeled antibody fragment, to detect osteomyelitis in diabetic patients with foot ulcers by leukoscintigraphy. Clin Infect Dis 1999; 28(6):1200–1205.
195. Ertugrul MB, Baktiroglu S, Salman S, et al. The diagnosis of osteomyelitis of the foot in diabetes: Microbiological examination vs. magnetic resonance imaging and labelled leucocyte scanning. Diabet Med 2006; 23(6):649–653.
196. Ledermann HP, Schweitzer ME, Morrison WB. Nonenhancing tissue on MR imaging of pedal infection: Characterization of necrotic tissue and associated limitations for diagnosis of osteomyelitis and abscess. AJR Am J Roentgenol 2002; 178(1):215–222.
197. Karchevsky M, Schweitzer ME, Morrison WB, et al. MRI findings of septic arthritis and associated osteomyelitis in adults. AJR Am J Roentgenol 2004; 182(1):119–122.
198. Kapoor A, Page S, Lavalley M, et al. Magnetic resonance imaging for diagnosing foot osteomyelitis: A meta-analysis. Arch Intern Med 2007; 167(2):125–132.
199. Newman LG, Waller J, Palestro CJ, et al. Leukocyte scanning with 111In is superior to magnetic resonance imaging in diagnosis of clinically unsuspected osteomyelitis in diabetic foot ulcers. Diabetes Care 1992; 15(11):1527–1530.
200. Craig JG, Amin MB, Wu K, et al. Osteomyelitis of the diabetic foot: MR imaging-pathologic correlation. Radiology 1997; 203(3):849–855.

201. Horowitz JD, Durham JR, Nease DB, et al. Prospective evaluation of magnetic resonance imaging in the management of acute diabetic foot infections. Ann Vasc Surg 1993; 7(1):44–50.
202. Kearney T, Pointin K, Cunningham D, et al. The detection of pedal osteomyelitis in diabetic patients. Pract Diabetes Int 1999; 16:98–100.
203. Lipman BT, Collier BD, Carrera GF, et al. Detection of osteomyelitis in the neuropathic foot: Nuclear medicine, MRI and conventional radiography. Clin Nucl Med 1998; 23(2):77–82.
204. Maas M, Slim EJ, Hoeksma AF, et al. MR imaging of neuropathic feet in leprosy patients with suspected osteomyelitis. Int J Lepr Other Mycobact Dis 2002; 70(2):97–103.
205. Morrison WB, Schweitzer ME, Batte WG, et al. Osteomyelitis of the foot: Relative importance of primary and secondary MR imaging signs. Radiology 1998; 207(3):625–632.
206. Nigro ND, Bartynski WS, Grossman SJ, et al. Clinical impact of magnetic resonance imaging in foot osteomyelitis. J Am Podiatr Med Assoc 1992; 82(12):603–615.
207. Remedios D, Valabhji J, Oelbaum R, et al. 99mTc-nanocolloid scintigraphy for assessing osteomyelitis in diabetic neuropathic feet. Clin Radiol 1998; 53(2):120–125.
208. Capriotti G, Chianelli M, Signore A. Nuclear medicine imaging of diabetic foot infection: Results of meta-analysis. Nucl Med Commun 2006; 27(10):757–764.
209. Devillers A, Moisan A, Hennion F, et al. Contribution of technetium-99 m hexamethylpropylene amine oxime labelled leucocyte scintigraphy to the diagnosis of diabetic foot infection. Eur J Nucl Med 1998; 25(2):132–138.
210. Harvey J, Cohen MM. Technetium-99-labeled leukocytes in diagnosing diabetic osteomyelitis in the foot. J Foot Ankle Surg 1997; 36(3):209–214.
211. Unal SN, Birinci H, Baktiroglu S, et al. Comparison of Tc-99 m methylene diphosphonate, Tc-99 m human immune globulin, and Tc-99 m-labeled white blood cell scintigraphy in the diabetic foot. Clin Nucl Med 2001; 26(12):1016–1021.
212. Williamson BR, Teates CD, Phillips CD, et al. Computed tomography as a diagnostic aid in diabetic and other problem feet. Clin Imaging 1989; 13(2):159–163.
213. Keidar Z, Militianu D, Melamed E, et al. The diabetic foot: Initial experience with 18 F-FDG PET/CT. J Nucl Med 2005; 46(3):444–449.
214. Berendt AR, Peters EJ, Bakker K, et al. Specific guidelines for treatment of diabetic foot osteomyelitis. Diabetes Metab Res Rev 2008; 24(suppl 1):S190–S191.
215. Senneville E, Morant H, Descamps D, et al. Needle puncture and transcutaneous bone biopsy cultures are inconsistent in patients with diabetes and suspected osteomyelitis of the foot. Clin Infect Dis 2009; 48(7):888–893.
216. Slater RA, Lazarovitch T, Boldur I, et al. Swab cultures accurately identify bacterial pathogens in diabetic foot wounds not involving bone. Diabet Med 2004; 21(7):705–709.
217. Kessler L, Piemont Y, Ortega F, et al. Comparison of microbiological results of needle puncture vs. superficial swab in infected diabetic foot ulcer with osteomyelitis. Diabet Med 2006; 23(1):99–102.
218. Byren I, Peters EJ, Hoey C, et al. Pharmacotherapy of diabetic foot osteomyelitis. Expert Opin Pharmacother 2009; 10(18):3033–3047.
219. Lazzarini L, Lipsky BA, Mader JT. Antibiotic treatment of osteomyelitis: What have we learned from 30 years of clinical trials? Int J Infect Dis 2005; 9(3):127–138.
220. Stengel D, Bauwens K, Sehouli J, et al. Systematic review and meta-analysis of antibiotic therapy for bone and joint infections. Lancet Infect Dis 2001; 1(3):175–188.
221. Tan JS, Friedman NM, Hazelton-Miller C, et al. Can aggressive treatment of diabetic foot infections reduce the need for above-ankle amputation? Clin Infect Dis 1996; 23(2):286–291.
222. Ha Van G, Siney H, Danan JP, et al. Treatment of osteomyelitis in the diabetic foot: Contribution of conservative surgery. Diabetes Care 1996; 19(11):1257–1260.
223. Pittet D, Wyssa B, Herter-Clavel C, et al. Outcome of diabetic foot infections treated conservatively: A retrospective cohort study with long-term follow-up. Arch Intern Med 1999; 159(8):851–856.

224. Simpson AH, Deakin M, Latham JM. Chronic osteomyelitis: The effect of the extent of surgical resection on infection-free survival. J Bone Joint Surg Br 2001; 83(3):403–407.
225. Henke PK, Blackburn SA, Wainess RW, et al. Osteomyelitis of the foot and toe in adults is a surgical disease: Conservative management worsens lower extremity salvage. Ann Surg 2005; 241(6):885–892.
226. Venkatesan P, Lawn S, Macfarlane RM, et al. Conservative management of osteomyelitis in the feet of diabetic patients. Diabet Med 1997; 14(6):487–490.
227. Senneville E, Yazdanpanah Y, Cazaubiel M, et al. Rifampicin-ofloxacin oral regimen for the treatment of mild to moderate diabetic foot osteomyelitis. J Antimicrob Chemother 2001; 48(6):927–930.
228. Murdoch DP, Armstrong DG, Dacus JB, et al. The natural history of great toe amputations. J Foot Ankle Surg 1997; 36(3):204–208.
229. Quebedeaux TL, Lavery LA, Lavery DC. The development of foot deformity and ulcers after great toe amputation in diabetes. Diabetes Care 1996; 19(2):165–167.
230. Lavery LA, Lavery DC, Quebedeaux TL. Increased foot pressures after great toe amputation in diabetes. Diabetes Care 1995; 18(11):1460–1462.
231. Peters EJ, Lavery LA. Effectiveness of the diabetic foot risk classification system of the International Working Group on the Diabetic Foot. Diabetes Care 2001; 24(8):1442–1447.
232. Hosch J, Quiroga C, Bosma J, et al. Outcomes of transmetatarsal amputations in patients with diabetes mellitus. J Foot Ankle Surg 1997; 36(6):430–434.
233. Yamaguchi Y, Yoshida S, Sumikawa Y, et al. Rapid healing of intractable diabetic foot ulcers with exposed bones following a novel therapy of exposing bone marrow cells and then grafting epidermal sheets. Br J Dermatol 2004; 151(5):1019–1028.
234. Kumagi SG, Mahoney CR, Fitzgibbons TC, et al. Treatment of diabetic (neuropathic) foot ulcers with two-stage debridement and closure. Foot Ankle Int 1998; 19(3):160–165.
235. Kerstein MD. Osteomyelitis associated with vascular insufficiency. Curr Ther Res Clin Exp 1974; 16(4):306–310.
236. Cohen M, Roman A, Malcolm WG. Panmetatarsal head resection and transmetatarsal amputation versus solitary partial ray resection in the neuropathic foot. J Foot Surg 1991; 30(1):29–33.
237. Walenkamp GH, Kleijn LL, de LM. Osteomyelitis treated with gentamicin-PMMA beads: 100 patients followed for 1–12 years. Acta Orthop Scand 1998; 69(5):518–522.
238. Klemm K. [Gentamicin-PMMA-beads in treating bone and soft tissue infections] [author's transl]. Zentralbl Chir 1979; 104(14):934–942.
239. Blaha JD, Calhoun JH, Nelson CL, et al. Comparison of the clinical efficacy and tolerance of gentamicin PMMA beads on surgical wire versus combined and systemic therapy for osteomyelitis. Clin Orthop Relat Res 1993; (295):8–12.
240. Jerosch J, Lindner N, Fuchs S. [Results of long-term therapy of chronic, post-traumatic osteomyelitis with gentamycin PMMA chains]. Unfallchirurg 1995; 98(6):338–343.
241. Norden CW. Lessons learned from animal models of osteomyelitis. Rev Infect Dis 1988; 10(1):103–110.
242. Andros G, Armstrong DG, Attinger CE, et al. Consensus statement on negative pressure wound therapy (V.A.C. Therapy) for the management of diabetic foot wounds. Ostomy Wound Manage 2006; (suppl):1–32.

9 Offloading the diabetic foot

Sicco A. Bus

INTRODUCTION

The management of foot ulceration in patients with diabetes mellitus remains a complicated matter. This is related to the complex pathogenesis of these skin injuries (1). Neuropathic, ischemic, as well as biomechanical factors act together to cause trauma of both the plantar and dorsal foot surfaces. Most plantar foot ulcers occur in the forefoot and toe areas (2). The principle factors in the development of these plantar lesions are loss of protective sensation caused by peripheral neuropathy in combination with mechanical trauma caused by the repetitive application of increased levels of foot pressure (3,4). Accordingly, the site of a foot ulcer most often corresponds with the site of the highest measured plantar pressure (5). These elevated plantar pressures are associated with the presence of foot deformities, such as claw toes and Charcot midfoot deformity, and other structural abnormalities, such as limited joint mobility, abundant callus formation, and prominent metatarsal heads (4,6–8). Therefore, proper management of plantar diabetic foot ulcers should include interventions that accommodate these structural abnormalities and that reduce plantar pressures at the site of ulceration.

The reduction of plantar foot pressures, also known as "offloading," is considered by many as one of the most important components in the treatment of plantar foot ulcers and is probably the primary component in the healing of non-complicated neuropathic ulcers. Our early knowledge on offloading treatment of foot ulcers was based mainly on experience in the management of foot problems in Hansen's disease (leprosy). Dr. Paul Brand first introduced the concept that the repetitive application of high levels of plantar pressure was causative in the development of neuropathic foot ulceration (9), and he also popularized the total contact cast (TCC) as a custom device for foot ulcer treatment. Since the early 1980s, our knowledge of the biomechanical aspects of diabetic foot disease has further improved in terms of the role elevated plantar pressure plays in the etiology of diabetic foot ulceration as well as on the use of different modalities designed to offload diabetic foot ulcers.

Many different approaches for offloading the diabetic foot are available and used in everyday clinical practice. In this chapter, first the different mechanisms to achieve offloading will be summarized. Then, the many different modalities will be discussed regarding their efficacy to relief plantar foot pressure and to heal plantar foot ulcers in diabetic patients. Subsequently, important aspects related to offloading treatment, which require consideration in clinical practice, will be discussed. Finally, conclusions will be drawn and recommendations made as to what entails proper offloading treatment. This will be based on the currently available scientific evidence which has recently been reviewed and translated into specific guidelines on footwear and offloading by the International Working Group on the Diabetic foot (10–12).

OFFLOADING MECHANISMS

The central principle in offloading is the redistribution of pressure over a larger surface area or the transfer of pressure to regions that are less at risk for ulceration. There are several mechanisms that can be employed to achieve this goal. Some act locally, others change the gait of the patient and have effect on the whole foot. These offloading mechanisms are

- Change of gait (e.g. reduction of walking speed)
- Use of walking aids
- Cushioning of forces with different materials
- Accommodation of the sole of the foot (i.e. total contact)
- Correction of foot regions
- Limitation of joint mobility
- Redistribution of pressure to proximal regions

The Reduction of Walking Speed and Change in Gait Pattern

Plantar foot pressures have been shown to be significantly positively associated with walking speed (13). Therefore, an effective way of reducing plantar foot pressures can be the reduction of walking speed. This can be achieved voluntarily by the patient or forced by the device that the patient wears. Furthermore, plantar pressures, in particular those in the forefoot, can be significantly reduced using a different gait style, such as a shuffling gait or a "step-to" gait (14,15). Despite these positive effects of gait changes on offloading, voluntary changes in walking style are not methods commonly employed or recommended in clinical practice, likely because they require tremendous discipline from the patient and may interfere with normal functioning.

The Use of Walking Aids

With the use of a wheelchair or walking aid, much of the load that is normally applied to the foot is then carried by the buttocks or by the upper extremity. Although a significant degree of offloading or even complete offloading of the foot may be achieved with these methods, they are not very practical in their use. A foot ulcer may take weeks or months to heal and these methods require a significant amount of upper body strength. Furthermore, these methods limit the ambulatory activity of the patient over a prolonged time, which is not desirable in diabetic patients with a sedentary life style.

Cushioning of Forces with Different Materials

Forces acting between the foot and the ground or shoe can be cushioned and distributed depending on the materials used in a device. Open and closed cell rubbers and foams are examples of materials that act locally through the distribution of forces over a larger surface contact area. Despite the use of many different materials and combinations of materials in offloading practice, little is known about the in vivo pressure-relieving capabilities of these materials. Clearly, more research is needed to facilitate the choice for certain (combinations of) materials in offloading treatment.

Accommodating the Foot (Total Contact)

The human foot is a contoured structure of which many plantar regions do not make (full) contact with the floor while standing or while ambulant. Accommodation of the plantar foot surface is achieved by creating a total contact interface between the foot and the device. The goal of this approach is to increase the surface area over which the acting forces on the foot can be distributed so that locally peak pressures can be reduced. The "total contact" principle is applied in most of the custom devices discussed in this chapter. Accommodative insoles are often manufactured based on impressions of the three-dimensional foot shape using plaster cast, foam techniques or 3D foot scanning. In casting techniques, layers of fiberglass or plaster are wrapped around the foot following the foot contours and creating total contact with the plantar surface. Surprisingly, little is known about the in vivo effect of foot accommodation on pressure relief in the diabetic foot since most studies investigate the combined effect of accommodation and added corrective elements on pressure relief.

Correcting the Foot

Pressure redistribution by foot correction is a mechanism that is based on changing the mechanics of the foot by incorporating specific corrective elements in the device, insole, or shoe. This is achieved by intentionally increasing pressure at a location on the foot, which is at low risk for ulceration (most often a proximal location), thereby transferring load from the ulcer site to this secondary region providing pressure relief at the ulcer site. Metatarsal pads or bars, hallux pads, and elevated longitudinal arch supports are examples of corrective elements that can be included in an insole for this purpose. Foot correction can also be applied during cast molding where the technician manually applies pressure on the cast material proximal or lateral to the ulcer region to create what is effectively a pad or bar in order to relief pressure at the ulcer site. Another way to correct the foot is to modify the outsole of the shoe or device with which the roll-over process of the foot can be influenced. A common example is the rocker bottom shoe, which limits active dorsiflexion of the toes, thereby limiting forefoot contribution in propulsion, providing pressure relief in this area. Another example is the negative heel construction of a shoe or device, where the forefoot is elevated with respect to the heel. This moves the center of pressure proximally, which alters ankle dynamics during roll-over and limits push-off from the ground. The result is reduced forefoot pressures. Many offloading devices incorporate one or more of these corrective features, which are among the most effective pressure-relieving mechanisms for the diabetic foot (16).

Pressure Redistribution to the Lower Leg or Contralateral Foot

To offload the foot beyond the redistribution of pressure between plantar foot regions, load can be transferred to more proximal regions such as the lower leg or to the contralateral extremity. Any below-the-knee device that provides full contact with the lower leg has the ability to carry a percentage of the total load exerted on the lower extremity through the shaft of the device. This mechanism works by virtue of the inverted cone shape of the lower leg with a relatively broad upper part just below the knee and a more lean part at the ankle. Shaw et al. (16) have shown that the shaft of a TCC is capable of taking up more than 30% of the total load exerted on the lower extremity during walking, which illustrates the effect of this mechanism. Transfer of load to the contralateral extremity can be achieved by inducing asymmetry in the walking pattern, for example, by creating a leg length discrepancy often seen with the use of a TCC or offloading shoe. The effect is pressure reduction in the ipsilateral foot. One should be aware of though the potential increase in pressures in the contralateral foot and discomfort in walking using this approach, although to date such a pressure increase has not been found present with the use of a TCC (18,19).

Limitation of Joint Mobility

Limiting mobility at the joints of the foot and ankle is another mechanism for forefoot offloading. In the previous section on foot correction metatarso-phalangeal joint limitation was discussed within the context of the use of rocker bottom shoes. The same concept applies to limiting motion of the ankle by immobilizing the joint with a rigid below-the-knee device such as a TCC. This serves to limit the propulsive phase of gait and reduce push-off forces, which are normally applied through the plantar flexion movement of the ankle. As a result, forefoot plantar pressures can be significantly reduced. Despite these positive effects, one must be aware that this approach does affect patient mobility and therefore may reduce patient acceptance or cause atrophy of the calf muscles when used for prolonged periods of times.

OFFLOADING MODALITIES

In the last several decades different kinds of modalities have been introduced for offloading treatment of plantar foot ulcers in patients with diabetes. These modalities can be categorized as follows:

- Casting techniques
- Prefabricated below-the-knee devices
- Prefabricated offloading shoes
- Customized footwear
- Other offloading modalities

Casting Techniques

Casting of the foot has become a widely used and accepted treatment modality throughout the world for offloading diabetic foot ulcers. Clinical experience with the use of casting dates back to the early 1960s when foot ulcers in patients with leprosy were treated with TCCs. The first studies on the use of casting techniques for treatment of the diabetic foot emerged in the 1980s.

Total Contact Casting

Total contact casting is the most widely reported casting technique for treatment of diabetic foot ulcers. This technique involves a custom molded and minimally padded below-the-knee device made of plaster or fiberglass material (or a combination of both) that maintains contact with the entire plantar aspect of the foot and the lower leg (i.e., total contact) (Fig. 1). Traditionally, TCCs were made of plaster. Although still commonly used in clinical practice, casts made of plaster are quite bulky and heavy and they generally require the patient to remain non–weight bearing for a substantial amount of time in order for the plaster to dry and maintain its structure. Nowadays, fiberglass is used more as the base material for

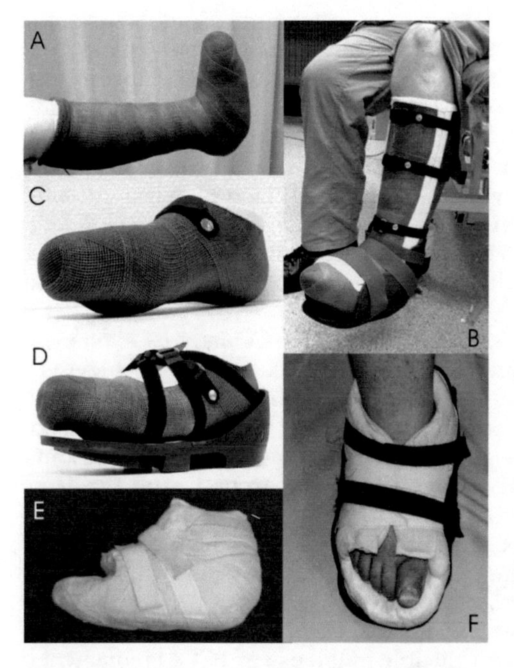

Figure 1 Several casting techniques used for offloading treatment of diabetic foot ulcers. These include the TCC made from fiberglass (**A**), the removable (bivalved) fiberglass TCC with a walking sole attached to facilitate walking (**B**), the Mabal cast shoe made from fiberglass (**C**), the Mabal cast shoe with a rubber walking sole attached (**D**), the plaster cast Scotchcast boot (**E**), and the Scotchcast boot shown with an open toe box and a walking sole attached (**F**). *Source:* Parts E and F courtesy Dr. D. G. Armstrong.

TCCs. Fiberglass is a lightweight material that sets almost immediately following its application and can be instantly molded to the foot or ankle for offloading purposes. The first reported description of the TCC for use in diabetic patients was by Coleman et al. (20) in 1984 and many still use this technique as reference although variation exists in final presentation. Several centers have the experience of making the TCC removable, mainly for wound inspection and dressing change purposes, by splitting (bivalving) the anterior and posterior parts of the cast which are then reconnected using Velcro straps (Fig. 1).

Plantar pressure relief. The TCC has been investigated for its effect on foot pressure in several cross-sectional studies in which a standard shoe was often used as control condition (level B). Fleischli et al. (21) showed reductions of 80% in forefoot peak pressure in diabetic patients walking in a plaster cast TCC when compared with a canvas control shoe. Similar degrees of offloading were found in two other studies on plaster cast TCCs in diabetic patients from the same research group (22,23). Mean peak pressures measured at the metatarsal heads and the great toe using a Novel Pedar pressure-measuring system in these studies were below 100 kPa, which is considered a very low level in comparison to the barefoot (600–1300 kPa) and in-shoe (300–600 kPa) pressures that are commonly measured in this patient group. Hartsell et al. (24) compared the pressure-relieving effect of a plaster TCC with a fiberglass TCC in healthy subjects and did not find significant differences in measured peak pressures between these two techniques.

Foot pressure studies on the removable (bivalved) TCC are infrequent. Beuker et al. (25) tested the offloading efficacy of a bivalved fiberglass TCC in a group of healthy subjects and found peak pressure reductions at the metatarsal head of 66% compared to a control shoe condition. Mean peak pressures measured in the cast were approximately 100 kPa. These pressure values are comparable to those found with the nonremovable TCC. Also in other foot regions, the pressure relieving effect of the TCC has been measured. Armstrong and Stacpoole-Shea (26) showed that peak pressures at the heel can be reduced by 33% in a TCC when compared to standard footwear. However, Shaw et al. (17) found in healthy subjects that most of the load with use of the TCC was transferred from the forefoot to the heel and they did not find lower peak pressures at the heel compared to standard footwear. Therefore, more data on the effect of the TCC in proximal foot regions is needed.

The excellent forefoot offloading capacity of the TCC may be explained by many, if not all, of the offloading mechanisms discussed in the previous subchapter. The TCC accommodates the plantar foot surface through the total contact interface. Correction to the foot may be achieved by cast molding. Load is transferred from the foot to the lower leg through the cast wall. The ankle joint is immobilized preventing an active push-off from the ground. And the TCC causes a reduction in walking speed, which also contributes to offloading (27). Nevertheless, peak pressures may be reduced even further using the TCC when the ulcer is isolated by the use of foam material between the wound and the cast (28). Metatarsal head peak pressures measured in a group of healthy subjects reduced from a mean 98 kPa to a mean 60 kPa using this approach. This led the authors to argue that the total contact principle in the use of TCCs is somewhat of a misnomer, as would isolation (i.e., loss of total contact) further improves offloading in this device.

Clinical efficacy. The efficacy of TCCs in healing plantar diabetic foot ulcers has been assessed in many studies, including several randomized controlled trials (RCTs; level A). Most of the controlled studies have compared the TCC to some other type of offloading modality or to standard treatment alone (see Appendix). In the first RCT on this topic, Mueller et al. (29) showed that the TCC heals neuropathic plantar forefoot ulcers (Wagner grade 1) more effectively and at a faster rate with fewer complications (19 of 21 ulcers healed in a mean 42 days, no infections) when compared with standard treatment consisting of dressing treatment, a healing sandal, and accommodative footwear (6/19 ulcers healed in a mean 65 days, 5 infections). Caravaggi et al. (30) compared treatment of neuropathic plantar forefoot ulcers between a windowed fiberglass TCC and therapeutic footwear and showed a significantly higher healing proportion using the TCC (13/26 versus 5/24, respectively) after only a short follow-up time of 30 days, after which the study was discontinued for ethical reasons. Comparing commonly used offloading devices for the treatment of University of Texas (UT) grade 1A neuropathic plantar forefoot ulcers, Armstrong et al. (31) showed that a fiberglass TCC was superior to a prefabricated removable walker and a half-shoe, both in terms of percentage healed ulcers within 12 weeks and in the time to healing. The proportion of healed ulcers in 12 weeks was 17/19 for the TCC, 13/20 for the removable walker, and 14/24 for the half-shoe. Mean time to healing was 34, 50, and 61 days, respectively. Daily activity level of patients was also assessed in this study using step-count monitors. Interestingly, patients wearing a TCC were considerably less active than patients wearing half-shoes (mean 600 vs. 1462 steps per day). Apparently, the TCC significantly affects the walking capacity of patients, which may have contributed to an improved ulcer healing found in this device.

Many predominantly prospective and retrospective noncontrolled studies (level C) have evaluated healing proportions and time to healing of neuropathic plantar foot ulcers in diabetic patients wearing a TCC (32–50). Generally, between 70% and 100% of ulcers healed using the TCC and mean healing times roughly ranged between 30 and 60 days. These outcomes correspond well with the findings from the controlled trials and demonstrate a consistent effect of the TCC in healing neuropathic plantar foot ulcers in diabetic patients. However, it should be kept in mind that almost all studies refer to the treatment of nonischemic and noninfected UT grade 1A or Wagner grade 1 or 2 neuropathic plantar foot ulcers. Healing percentages may be lower for ulcers of greater depth. The treatment of ischemic and infected diabetic foot ulcers using TCCs will be discussed separately in the Discussion section.

Several factors have been found to influence the success in healing of plantar foot ulcers in diabetes using TCCs. Armstrong et al. (35) showed that these factors include the duration an ulcer was present prior to treatment, baseline barefoot peak pressure level at the ulcer site, and ulcer size. Ulcers in patients with barefoot peak pressure greater than 990 kPa take longer to heal than ulcers in patients with pressures below this level, although the patients with high barefoot peak pressures were also the patients that had their ulcers for a longer period of time prior to treatment (mean 180 days vs. 50 days in patients with lower pressures). Furthermore, larger ulcers (>8 cm^2) took longer to heal than smaller ulcers (<8 cm^2): 50 versus 29 days, respectively. These influential factors should be considered when treating individual patients and when comparing the results from different studies.

In conclusion, the TCC shows to be a very effective offloading device for healing neuropathic plantar foot ulcers in the diabetic patient, which is likely a function of the excellent offloading properties of this device.

Advantages and disadvantages of the TCC. On the basis of the excellent pressure-relieving and ulcer healing capacity of the TCC, it is considered by many diabetic foot specialists as the "gold standard" offloading treatment for plantar diabetic foot ulcers. However, the use of the TCC for offloading treatment has several drawbacks. The advantages and disadvantages of the use of the TCC can be summarized as follows:

Advantages of TCC:

- Effective in offloading and healing plantar foot ulcers
- May reduce or control edema to improve microcirculation
- Protects the foot/lower leg from further external trauma and potentially protects the foot from infection or osteomyelitis
- Immobilizes the ankle, which may reduce plantar shear stress
- Provides the ability to force treatment adherence
- Allows preservation of ambulatory status and work ability when compared to complete offloading modalities such as bed rest or the use of a wheelchair or crutches

Disadvantages of TCC:

- Requires skilled and trained personnel for safe application
- Requires frequent reapplication for wound control and to maintain a total contact fit
- Prevents the ability to assess and treat the wound on a daily basis limiting the use of certain wound healing dressings
- Can cause skin abrasions or even ulcers if not applied correctly
- May give problems with activities of daily life, such as bathing, sleeping, and driving a car, which is generally not permitted
- May exacerbate postural instability
- Contraindicated for wounds with soft-tissue infections or osteomyelitis
- Costs may be high with weekly replacements
- Limits movement of the ankle joint, which significantly alters the gait of the patient
- May cause atrophy of calf muscles, joint stiffness, and bone demineralization with prolonged use
- Patient acceptance may be low, as the TCC is relatively heavy, bulky, unattractive, and not very practical in everyday use

These drawbacks may be (part of) the explanation that TCCs are not widely used in clinical practice nowadays (48,49). Some of these disadvantages are overcome by using the bivalved TCC. The bivalved TCC has been for many years the standard in TCC treatment in the diabetic foot clinic in Almelo in the Netherlands. Although good healing results seem to follow the use of this device, this does require confirmation in controlled studies. In addition, for successful healing the use of a removable TCC requires a committed patient who adheres to treatment. In many cases this cannot be guaranteed, and the nonremovable TCC should be used. The listed advantages and disadvantages should be considered for proper clincial decision making in offloading treatment for each individual patient.

Cast Shoes

Cast shoes are commonly used, at least in parts of western Europe, for treatment of plantar diabetic foot ulcers. An early description of a cast shoe was a molded double rocker plaster shoe used successfully for the treatment of a patient with a chronic neuropathic plantar ulcer (53). More recent descriptions of cast shoes include the Mabal cast shoe, the Scotchcast boot, and the Ransart boot. The Mabal cast shoe was developed in the late 1990s at the diabetic foot clinic in Almelo. It was first developed as a temporary device to overcome the period between healing of a foot ulcer in a TCC and the provision of therapeutic footwear but later as a device for the offloading treatment of plantar foot ulcers. The Mabal cast shoe is a below-the-ankle fiberglass combicast shoe that uses minimal padding. It has a rigid total contact sole and a semirigid soft cast upper (54). The shoe is used in combination with a walking sole to facilitate ambulation (Fig. 1). The shoe is easy to put on and leaves the ankle joint mobile to improve walking ability and patient acceptance. The Mabal shoe is a removable device allowing daily wound inspection and treatment without the need for weekly reapplications. The Ransart boot is quite similar to the Mabal cast shoe, although it has a window cut out in the cast over the ulcerated area (52). The Scotchcast boot is another below-the-ankle cast shoe that has been introduced in the United Kingdom for the treatment of diabetic forefoot ulcers (56,57). The Scotchcast boot is a well-padded cast cut away at the ankle making it removable for wound inspection. It is worn in combination with a sandal to improve ambulation and mobility of the patient (Fig. 1). Only few studies have been conducted on the biomechanical and clinical efficacy of these cast shoes.

Plantar pressure relief. Studies on the pressure-relieving effect of the Scotchcast boot or Ransart boot have not been found in the literature. In a study by Beuker et al. (25), the effect of the Mabal cast shoe on forefoot pressure relief was tested in a group of healthy subjects. The results showed that the Mabal cast shoe reduced peak pressures at the metatarsal heads by approximately 50% compared with a control shoe condition. This offloading effect was significantly better than with a customized insole but not as good as with a bivalved TCC or removable walker. This is likely explained by the inability of the Mabal cast shoe to transfer pressure to proximal regions (i.e., lower leg) and to limit push-off though ankle immobilization. These findings were confirmed in at risk neuropathic patients in a recent study by Bus et al. (58) who showed a 50% reduction in forefoot peak pressure using the Mabal cast shoe compared with a control shoe condition. Perceived walking comfort was assessed in this study using a visual analogue scale. Comfort was found to be significantly higher with the Mabal cast shoe than with a forefoot offloading shoe and close to the comfort perceived in a standard flexible control shoe. This may explain the good patient acceptance experienced with the use of the Mabal cast shoe.

Clinical efficacy. The clinical efficacy of cast shoes has only been evaluated in retrospective and prospective case series (level C). Hissink et al. (54) assessed the efficacy of the Mabal cast shoe to heal neuropathic plantar forefoot ulcers (UT grade 1A) and found 91% of foot ulcers to heal in a mean 34 days. These results are comparable to findings reported for the TCC. Recently, a clinical study on the Ransart boot by Dumont et al. showed that 82 of 117 diabetic plantar foot ulcers (70%) healed in a median 60 days (52). A study on the first, nonremovable, model of the Scotchcast boot by Burden et al. (56) found diabetic plantar foot ulcers to heal in a mean three months (range one to eight months) with ulcers of patients lacking pedal pulses taking the longest time to heal. In a study by Knowles et al. (57), diabetic patients with forefoot ulcers treated with a removable Scotchcast boot were found to have healed in 81% of cases. Time to healing was on average 130 days, with superficial ulcers healing quicker than deeper ulcers. Although the healing rate in this device is similar to that reported for the TCC, the average time to healing is substantially longer than with the TCC. These retrospective analyses on cast shoes have, quite surprisingly, not been followed by prospective (controlled) studies. These are needed if these devices are to become widely accepted as treatment modalities for healing plantar diabetic foot ulcers.

Prefabricated Techniques

Over the last 10 to 15 years, prefabricated off-the-shelf devices have been introduced as alternative offloading modalities for casting in the treatment of plantar foot ulcers in diabetic patients. These prefabricated devices include below-the-knee walkers and ankle-high modalities (Fig. 2). Prefabricated devices have several advantages over TCCs and cast shoes. They are relatively easy to apply,

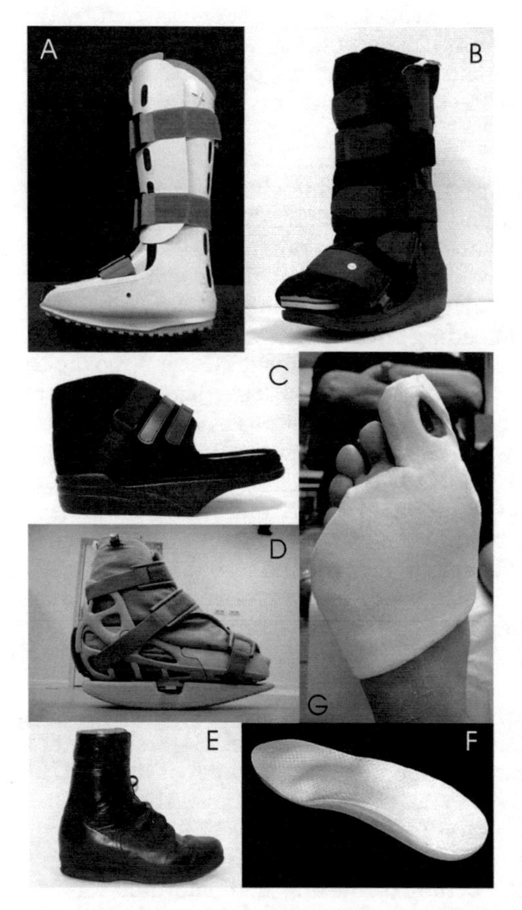

Figure 2 Prefabricated offloading modalities used for offloading diabetic foot ulcers. These devices include a pneumatic walking brace (**A**), a pressure relief walker (**B**), a forefoot offloading shoe (**C**), a low-cut vacuum cushioned system (**D**), low-cut fully customized therapeutic footwear (**E**), custom molded insoles (**F**), and felt applied to the forefoot of a patient with a hallux ulcer (**G**). *Source:* Part A courtesy Dr. R. W. van Deursen and Part B courtesy H. A. Manning.

even by the patient, they often have to be applied only once during the course of treatment, and they are removable, which makes it easier to inspect and treat the wound, and more practical in daily use. However, this advantage is at the same time also a major drawback. Since patients can remove these devices, adherence to treatment may be impaired. To overcome this drawback, recently, several solutions have aimed at making these walkers nonremovable for the patient.

Removable and Nonremovable Walkers

Removable below-the-knee walkers have originally been used for treatment of lower extremity trauma. Later, they have been modified to be used as offloading modality for diabetic foot ulcers. Different (commercial) systems are available. In the Aircast pneumatic walker (DJO, Vista, CA) an anterior and posterior shell are applied over the lower leg and foot and secured with Velcro straps. A standard insert of medium density is most often used as interface between the foot and the device. Air bladders in different parts of the device are inflated in a certain sequence to create an intermittent pneumatic compression on the skin, which provides edema control and total contact for pressure reduction. The shell incorporates a rocker bottom outsole (Fig. 2). The DH pressure relief walker

(Royce Medical, Camarillo, CA) utilizes a short leg walker in conjunction with a tri-laminated pressure relief insole. The ankle is fixated at 90 degrees by the device. The insole allows the removal of numerous independent shock-absorbing hexagons to accommodate ulcers of variable size and shape. A rocker bottom sole is attached to the device to provide additional relief of pressure (Fig. 2). More recently, a vacuum-cushioned cast replacement system (VacoDiaped) has been developed (Oped GmbH, Valley, Germany). It comprises a lightweight frame structure with a vacuum cushion (bean bag) that can be remodeled instantly to accommodate for foot deformities before the air is drawn out of the cushion to make the system rigid. The system is used together with a detachable roller outsole to facilitate walking. The first two devices have been extensively tested both for their pressure relieving and ulcer healing capacity. The vacuum-cushioned device has currently only been tested for its offloading capacity.

Plantar pressure relief. Several well-conducted cross-sectional studies have investigated the effect of removable walkers on plantar pressure relief at (previous) ulcer sites or sites at risk for ulceration. Most often, they were compared with a TCC or other offloading modalities (level B). Fleischli et al. (21) and Lavery et al. (23) showed that a removable pressure relief walker was as effective as a TCC in reducing forefoot peak pressures in patients with a current or previously healed forefoot ulcer. Peak pressure reductions compared to control between 70% and 80% were found, which was more than the level of pressure relief found in half shoes and extra-depth footwear. The offloading mechanisms that contribute to such a significant pressure relief using these devices are not exactly known. Baumhauer et al. (27) and Beuker et al. (25) confirmed these results in groups of healthy subjects tested using a pneumatic walker. These groups found reductions in forefoot peak pressure of 80% and 67%, respectively, when compared with control. For offloading other foot regions such as the heel, removable walkers were found to be less effective than the TCC but more effective than depth-inlay shoes (26). Nagel et al. (59) tested the pressure-relieving efficacy of a high-cut vacuum-cushioned system in at risk diabetic patients. They found this device to reduce peak pressures in the forefoot with 62% and in the rearfoot with 43% compared with a standard control shoe, and found this to be as effective as a forefoot offloading shoe which was included in the study.

Clinical efficacy. The efficacy of removable walkers in healing plantar diabetic foot ulcers has been compared with the efficacy of several other devices, such as the TCC and therapeutic footwear, in a number of controlled studies (Appendix). The earlier discussed RCT by Armstrong et al. (31) (level A) demonstrated that a removable walker was less effective than a TCC in healing plantar forefoot ulcers as measured by the proportion ulcers healed and time to healing. Since both devices relief pressure to a similar extent, this difference is likely related to the use of the device, which is forced with the TCC but not with the walker. This effect of adherence proves the value of continuous pressure relief during the course of treatment. However, recently a RCT from Ezio et al. (29) (level A), showed similar healing rates in neuropathic plantar foot ulcers between a removable walker boot and a TCC, which the authors ascribe to the likelihood of good adherence in their patients group. To overcome the drawback or removability of the device by the patient, Armstrong and coworkers have experimented with making the device nonremovable by wrapping coband around the shaft of the device, naming this device the "instant TCC." In two RCTs, the efficacy of the nonremovable walker in healing UT grade 1A ulcers was tested in comparison with a removable walker and a TCC (level A). Armstrong et al. (61) showed that the nonremovable walker performed significantly better than the removable walker in terms of the proportion healed ulcers in 12 weeks time (19/23 vs. 14/27) and time to healing (mean 42 vs. 58 days). Katz et al. (62) found no significant differences in the proportion healed ulcers between the nonremovable walker and the TCC: 17/21 vs. 15/20, respectively, in 12 weeks time. In a more recent RCT, Piaggesi et al. (63) confirmed these results. These authors demonstrated comparable healing rates of UT grade 1A plantar foot ulcers between a walking boot, which was made nonremovable by a simple tie rap, and a TCC: 85% and 95%, respectively. Also time to healing (mean 6.7 and 6.5 weeks, respectively) and the number of adverse events (4 and 6, respectively) were similar between the devices. Although adherence to treatment was not directly measured in these studies, the positive effects of making a walker nonremovable stresses the importance of continuous offloading for promoting wound healing in this patient group.

Offloading Shoes

Originally designed to decrease pressure under the forefoot after elective surgery, half shoes were later used as offloading treatment device for plantar foot ulcers in diabetic patients. This shoe consists of only a heel and midfoot support surface leaving the entire forefoot unsupported (64). The device is easy to use and inexpensive. However, patient acceptance may not be high due to the significant effect the shoe has on the patients' gait. Furthermore, the small support area may increase pressure in the midfoot to a level that increases risk for fracture or ulceration. Later versions of this offloading shoe had an extended support of the forefoot to facilitate walking and to overcome some of the disadvantages of the half-shoe and were named "forefoot offloading shoes" (Fig. 2). Many different models of the forefoot offloading shoe are commercially available but all have a similar design, including a rocker bottom outsole and, most often, a negative heel construction. As a particular kind of offloading shoe, the low-cut version of the vacuum-cushioned cast replacement system that was discussed in the section on walkers is also used for offloading treatment of the diabetic foot (Fig. 2).

Plantar pressure relief. Forefoot offloading shoes were found by Fleischli et al. (21) to be more effective than accommodative felt and foam dressings (worn in a postoperative shoe) or postoperative shoes alone in reducing forefoot peak pressures in diabetic patients. Reductions of 50%, 34%, and 24%, respectively, compared with a control shoe condition were found for these modalities. Bus et al. (58) tested different models of forefoot offloading shoes and compared them with a Mabal cast shoe and control shoe in a group of high-risk diabetic patients. Forefoot peak pressure reductions between 50% and 55% compared to control were found in each of the forefoot offloading shoes. The shoe was also found to be more effective in offloading the forefoot than the Mabal cast shoe. Most likely, this is achieved through the action of the negative heel and rocker bottom outsole construction, which transfers weight proximally and limits active plantar flexion of the ankle and dorsiflexion of the toes during push-off. Biomechanical analyses of walking show a significantly reduced ankle power in late stance and a significant correlation between reduced ankle power and forefoot pressure relief ($r = 0.6$) using this shoe (65). Two recent studies in high-risk diabetic patients on the efficacy of a low-cut vacuum-cushioned system showed that the offloading capacity of this system is comparable to that of a forefoot offloading shoe and Mabal cast shoe with forefoot peak pressures being reduced between 45% and 54% compared to a control shoe condition (59,66).

Clinical efficacy. Studies on the clinical efficacy of offloading shoes are scant. In the RCT from Armstrong et al. (31) (level A), discussed in previous sections, the forefoot offloading shoe (which the authors called a "half shoe") was found to be less effective in healing UT grade 1A foot ulcers than a TCC or removable walker (Appendix). In a cohort study, Ha Van et al. (67) (level A) showed that a half-shoe or heel relief shoe was less effective than a TCC in healing neuropathic plantar foot ulcers. Healing percentages were 70% and 81%, respectively, and time to healing mean 134 and 69 days, respectively in the shoe and TCC conditions (Appendix). A number of level C studies have tested the effect of offloading shoes on ulcer healing. These studies suggest that offloading shoes can be effective in treating plantar diabetic foot ulcers (37,64,68). So, although patients may benefit from the use of offloading shoes for ulcer healing, their effect is smaller than with the use of below-the-knee devices.

Footwear

Customized Footwear

The effects of footwear have not been studied extensively in the context of offloading foot ulcers in patients with diabetes. More commonly, footwear studies have focused on ulcer prevention. This is somewhat surprising since two large descriptive studies in the United States and Europe have shown that therapeutic shoes and footwear modifications are the most commonly used modality for ulcer treatment in clinical practice (51,52). Customized footwear is a generic term for interventions that range from custom inlays worn in off-the-shelf or extra-depth shoes, single or multiple footwear modifications such as the addition or adjustment of a metatarsal pad or a rocker bottom outsole configuration, to fully customized therapeutic footwear (Fig. 2).

Plantar pressure relief. The efficacy of customized footwear in reducing plantar foot pressures has been tested in one controlled study (level A). Viswanathan et al. (69) reported reductions of plantar pressures between 10% and 19% over time in patients wearing therapeutic sandals when compared with patients wearing standard footwear. However, inconsistencies in this paper shed doubt on the accuracy of these results. Most other studies are cross-sectional in design and most often include footwear with a customized insole (level B). Generally, this footwear provides significant reductions in plantar pressure between 10% and 45% when compared with standard footwear (22,23,70–76), although the pressure relief obtained is not as large as with several other offloading modalities.

Clinical efficacy. The effects of customized footwear on ulcer healing have been tested mainly in studies where this footwear was a comparisons condition to other modalities such as the TCC (Appendix). Only one recent small RCT was found in which the efficacy to heal foot ulcers was tested in custom footwear as primary intervention compared with the TCC (level A) (77). Fully customized (temporary) footwear is used frequently in the Netherlands for ulcer healing purposes. The results showed an overall low proportion healed ulcers in both treatment groups and no significant difference were found between conditions (6/21 vs. 6/22 ulcers healed). Time to healing was, however, longer in the footwear group (mean 90 days) than in the TCC group (mean 52 days). Clearly, more data from larger controlled studies are required before meaningful conclusions can be drawn. The RCT from Mueller et al. (29), discussed previously, showed that ulcer healing efficacy using a healing sandal in combination with accommodative footwear is lower than when using a TCC. These data were confirmed by Caravaggi et al. (30) who showed that a specialized cloth shoe with a rigid sole and an unloading insole was not as effective as a TCC in healing plantar diabetic foot ulcers. Evidence for the use of customized footwear in ulcer healing includes a number of level C studies. These studies suggest that molded and EVA boots can play a role in ulcer healing (78,79), and that various types of shoes and insoles can, under some circumstances, result in healing (80–83). Overall, these findings show that there is (still) insufficient evidence to support the use of this type of offloading in the treatment of diabetic plantar foot ulcers. Therefore, the frequent use of customized footwear in clinical practice stresses the need for the adoption of specific guidelines on footwear and offloading which have been developed in 2007 (14), but also a different expectation with practitioners regarding the time it should take for a diabetic foot ulcer to heal (85). Additionally, prospective controlled studies of sufficient size are needed so that sound conclusions on the use of footwear for ulcer healing purposes can be drawn.

Standard Footwear

Standard footwear includes running shoes and other prefabricated off-the-shelf shoes and insoles. Studies on the efficacy of standard footwear interventions in healing diabetic foot ulcers seem nonexistent. In terms of pressure relief, studies have been consistent in showing that standard footwear solutions provide less pressure relief than customized footwear solutions (see previous section). Only for the use of running shoes, comparable offloading percentages with custom footwear have been found: a 30% to 50% pressure reduction compared to Oxford style leather shoes (85,86). Nevertheless, standard footwear, including running shoes, is generally not considered the choice of treatment for healing diabetic foot ulcers, as many more effective modalities exist.

Other Offloading Modalities

Felted Foam

Felt or felted foam is an inexpensive and easy to use material that is widely applied in diabetic foot practice throughout the world, mostly in combination with casts, walkers, or (therapeutic) footwear (Fig. 2). Felted foam comes in different configurations ranging from pure felt sheets to combinations of felt and foam in a multilaminar fashion to provide durability. Often an aperture corresponding to the ulcer site is created to provide pressure relief for the ulcer, although edge effects with increased pressures at the wound's periphery are possible (87). Felt has the additional functionality that it absorbs wound exudate and fluid. However, felt requires frequent replacement, often several times per week, as functionality reduces in a few days. Despite the widespread use of felted foam in clinical practice, few studies of sufficient quality have dealt with its pressure relieving and ulcer healing effects.

Plantar pressure relief. In a study by Piaggesi et al. (88), double-layered polyurethane foam sheets applied at forefoot ulcer locations and tested inside the patients' own shoes showed a significant 38% reduction in peak pressure compared with wearing shoes alone. Fleischli et al. (21) showed that in diabetic patients with forefoot ulcers, a combination of $^1/_4$ inch felt and $^1/_4$ inch polyethylene foam, worn in a postoperative shoe, significantly reduced peak pressure compared to wearing postoperative shoes alone. However, neither study tested the pressure-relieving effect of these foams over the course of several days. This data is needed to establish guidelines for the frequency of replacement of this material.

Clinical efficacy. The efficacy of felted foam in treating plantar foot ulcers in diabetic patients has been tested in two similar RCTs (level A; Appendix) and in a few uncontrolled studies (level C). The two RCTs by Zimny et al. (89,90) showed that felted foam worn in a postoperative shoe led to significantly shorter healing times of plantar forefoot ulcers than the use of forefoot offloading shoes. Surprisingly, no information was provided on the proportion of ulcers healed. In addition, the type of footwear worn was different between study groups and this may have influenced the results. Furthermore, adherence to treatment was not measured. In a retrospective study by Birke and colleagues (37), the offloading method was selected based on location of ulcer, age of the patient, and duration of ulceration. Felted foam worn in a surgical shoe, healing shoe, or walking splint was shown to be as effective as a TCC, both in the proportion ulcers healed (ranging from 81% to 93%) and in the mean time to healing (ranging from 36 to 51 days). Because of the low methodological quality of both these studies, definite conclusions cannot be drawn. Therefore, high-quality controlled studies are needed, as felted foam may be a cost-effective treatment option that can be applied in many regions of the world.

Bed Rest, Crutches, and Wheelchair Use

Complete offloading of a foot ulcer can be achieved with bed rest or the use of crutches or a wheelchair. These modalities have not received much attention in the scientific literature, which is likely because none of these interventions are considered practical in the context of ulcer healing. They may be effective for offloading treatment, but at the same time they limit patient mobility and autonomy. As many ulcers take several weeks or longer to heal, such a limitation is not desirable. Crutches have the additional disadvantage that they are cumbersome to use in patients with a foot ulcer, of which many have obesity, limited cardiovascular reserves, poor upper body strength, or a combination of these complications. Wheelchairs are often impractical because of an inadequate access in the patient's home for maneuvering. Because patients do not easily see the benefit of these interventions, they have little motivation to accept the stringent discipline that they require. The goal should be to keep the patient ambulant while offloading. Previous subchapters have shown that many modalities are available with which both sufficient offloading and patient mobility can be guaranteed, and these are therefore preferred.

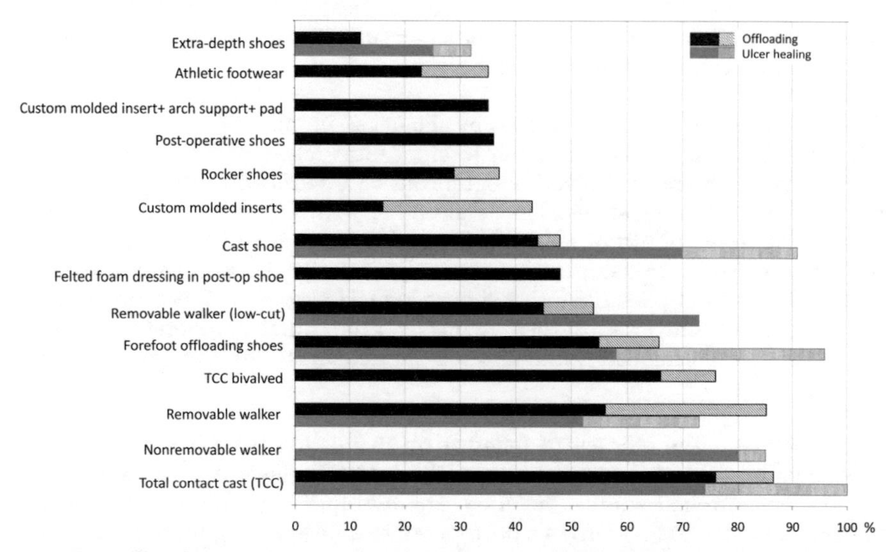

Figure 3 Offloading capacity and efficacy in ulcer healing of different modalities used in the treatment of the diabetic foot. Offloading capacity is shown in dark grey bars and expressed as percentage peak pressure reduction at the first metatarsal head region compared to a control condition. Angle striped bars show the range in percentage peak pressure reduction found in different studies. Healing efficacy for non-complicated neuropathic ulcers is shown in light grey bars and expressed as percentage of ulcers healed. Vertical striped bars show the range in percentage of healed ulcers found in different studies.

Figure 3 summarizes the pressure-relieving and ulcer healing efficacy of most discussed modalities in this chapter. The histogram shows that devices that best relieve pressure in the diabetic foot are also the devices that show best ulcer healing rates.

DISCUSSION

In the previous section different offloading modalities have been discussed regarding their capacity to relieve foot pressure and heal plantar foot ulcers in diabetic patients. Apart from the discussion of these biomechanical and clinical aspects of offloading, several important issues require consideration to fully understand the potential, application range, and limitations of using these offloading modalities in everyday clinical practice.

Pressure Relief Vs. Clinical Efficacy

Most studies on the use of offloading treatment in the diabetic foot have focused either on the pressure-relieving capacity of these interventions or on their clinical efficacy. Pressure studies can be seen as a good starting point in the evaluation of (new) offloading devices since their primary mechanism is to reduce pressure at a certain location under the foot. However, without clinical evaluation of these devices, these data do not seem very meaningful since the intended purpose is to promote healing of foot ulcers. Similarly, modalities that have been evaluated only on their clinical efficacy, lack the biomechanical framework that explains their capacity to heal foot ulcers. The degree of pressure relief with a certain modality may vary substantially across patients and therefore may affect success of healing or time to healing. Therefore, the most optimal design for intervention studies of offloading devices is a combination of foot pressure measurement and assessment of clinical efficacy in the same group of patients. Only few studies have used this study design. Armstrong et al. (35) showed that the level of measured forefoot peak pressure in diabetic patients treated with a TCC is associated with time to healing of the ulcer, higher peak pressures giving longer healing times. Similar studies are needed for other offloading modalities so that their clinical efficacy can be linked directly to their pressure relieving capacity, both on a group and individual patient level.

Pressure Threshold

Successful offloading of plantar foot ulcers implies that the pressure exerted on the ulcer is below a certain threshold required for wound closure. As the previous sections show, pressure reductions compared with control vary greatly between devices (20% to 80%). The amount of foot pressure relief needed to heal a foot ulcer is not known and, therefore, a common pressure threshold for ulcer healing has not been identified to date. This may be because most clinical efficacy studies do not incorporate the measurement of plantar pressure, required to define a threshold of pressure relief. However, even with this data available, it would still be uncertain whether a threshold for ulcer healing can be defined. As comparison, a common pressure threshold for the development of foot ulcers in at-risk diabetic feet has also never been identified, despite several attempts to do so (91). Many other factors influence the healing process of foot ulcers and likely interfere with the association between pressure level and success of healing. These factors may include, patient behavioral factors such as adherence to treatment or daily activity level shear pressure, a component that cannot be measured with the currently available equipment, the local wound environment, and presence of infection or arterial disease. As a result, the definition of a pressure relief threshold in offloading treatment for the diabetic foot remains an elusive goal so far.

Removable Vs. Nonremovable: The Issue of "Adherence"

Much debate is often heard on the issue of using removable or nonremovable devices for offloading treatment in the diabetic patient. Removable devices have several practical advantages but one major disadvantage compared to nonremovable devices, namely, the risk of nonadherence with the patient in wearing the device, posing a threat to the success of healing. Within this context, it is self-evident that even the most effective device will not be successful if it is not worn. Illustrative for this issue of nonadherence is the study by Armstrong et al. (92) who used activity monitors on the patient and the offloading device to show that patients who were prescribed a removable walker to heal their foot ulcer wore the device only 28% of the time that they were walking. In addition, Ha Van et al. (67) found adherence to treatment, assessed using questionnaires, to be much lower in patients wearing removable half shoes (10%) than in patients wearing a nonremovable cast (98%). Another self-report study on the use of prescribed footwear showed that patients wore their footwear for only 25% of the time they were walking (93). Clearly, adherence to treatment is a major problem in this patient group. Nonremovable offloading treatment can overcome this problem, although at the expense of several practical disadvantages associated with the use of nonremovable devices. Not all patients require nonremovable devices and adherence to treatment may even vary between centers or regions. Furthermore it is important to realize that the period of ulcer treatment normally represents only a small portion of the time that patients require continuous pressure relief. After healing of the ulcer, offloading the foot is just as important and for this nonremovable offloading can not be used. For which nonremovable devices are not available. Clearly, there is still much to learn regarding ways to encourage patients to adhere to offloading treatment and to persuade practitioners to prescribe nonremovable modalities when adherence is low.

Neuroischemic Wounds

The vast majority of offloading studies discussed in this chapter have focused on the treatment of noninfected, nonischemic, neuropathic plantar ulcers. These purely neuropathic foot ulcers seem to represent a continuously dropping percentage of diabetic foot ulcers seen in professional settings. A recent study on foot care in 14 specialized foot centers in Europe (Eurodiale) showed that of a total of 1232 treated foot ulcers the portion of foot ulcers that was complicated with ischemia or infection was 76%. Treatment of these ulcers is more complicated than neuropathic foot ulcers and the effects of offloading may be smaller. Sinacore et al. (42) showed only slightly longer healing times using TCC in patients with severe vascular compromise than in the total group of treated patients. However, Laing et al. (94) reported that most of their 46 patients with neuropathic ulceration treated in a TCC healed within 6 weeks, but ischemic ulcers did not heal. In a prospective analysis by Nabuurs-Franssen et al. (40), neuropathic, neuroischemic, as well as infected ulcers were treated using different casting techniques including TCCs and cast shoes. The results showed an expected 90% healing rate for the neuropathic ulcers, a 69% healing rate for the neuro-ischemic ulcers, and only a 30% healing rate for the neuro-ischemic ulcers that were infected. Clearly, ulcers complicated with infection or ischemia pose a much larger challenge to treatment than neuropathic foot ulcers and show that additional interventions to manage the infection and vascular status are required for these complicated ulcers. The limited number of offloading studies dealing with these wounds clearly indicates that more research is needed on the effects and potential pitfalls of offloading treatment in complex diabetic foot ulcers.

Do We Practice What We Preach?

One of the goals of studies on the efficacy or effectiveness of offloading interventions to heal diabetic foot ulcers is to provide evidence for the use of these interventions in clinical practice. This raises the question: does clinical practice follow the currently available evidence in offloading treatment? In a recent article on the use of pressure offloading devices with the sub-title "Do we practice what we preach?" Wu et al. (51) report on a survey they conducted in the US among 900 medical centers regarding their practice in offloading treatment of diabetic foot ulcers. The results, quite impressively, showed that footwear modifications were the most commonly applied offloading modality for treating foot ulcers. The TCC was used in only 2% of cases. Furthermore, most centers did not regard the TCC as the "gold standard" treatment option for offloading diabetic foot ulcers. In Europe, the Eurodiale study showed results in the same direction. In a subgroup of 139 patients with a plantar neuropathic forefoot or midfoot ulcer, only 18% of patients was prescribed with a TCC, with marked differences in the use of the TCC between countries, ranging from 0% to 68% (52). Also in this large descriptive study, the majority of foot ulcers were treated with footwear modalities. Apparently, there is a lack of association between the available scientific evidence on offloading treatment and the use of offloading techniques in everyday clinical practice, both in general hospitals and in specialized foot clinics. This discrepancy is likely related to personal beliefs and preferences of practitioners regarding the type of offloading used for ulcer treatment, patient acceptance of offloading treatment, available resources such as time and skilled technicians, and reimbursement issues. Clearly, the existing gap between scientific evidence and clinical practice needs to be bridged. Severel measures can be taken to achieve this goal (79). The 2007 international guidelines on footwear and offloading (10,11) are specific and evidence-based and should be adopted and implemented in clincial practice. Previous sections show that uncomplicated ulcers can heal in approximately 6–8 weeks.Therefore, expectations with practitioners regarding the time it takes for a diabetic foot ulcer to heal should change to promote quick, safe, and uncomplicated healing. Finally, prospective controlled studies should be conducted to prove the effectiveness of currently used offloading devices for which no evidence base exist.

Quality of Life and Economic Factors

Health-related quality-of-life issues and economic factors should be considered in diabetic foot ulcer treatment, as both quality of life and treatment costs may vary significantly depending on the type and duration of treatment and whether complications develop or not. Diabetic patients with a foot ulcer, especially those patients of whom the foot ulcer does not heal rapidly, experience a marked decline in their quality of life (95,96). When infection or amputation is the result of an ulcer episode, quality of life further declines. Therefore, adequate and rapid ulcer healing is important for the well being of the patient. For this reason, clinicians should be encouraged to use successful offloading approaches. The costs related to offloading treatment of foot ulcers can be substantial. Trained personnel and frequent reapplications are often needed and devices can be quite expensive in cost, in particular when they have to be paid (partly) by the patient. However, such costs have to be viewed in relation to the total cost of care for a foot ulcer and the inherent increased risk of amputation. Also, the indirect costs have to be taken into account. With more severe complications, these indirect costs increase. Since the vast majority of all lower-extremity amputations in diabetes are preceded by a foot ulcer (97), effective treatment of an ulcer can not only prevent further complications, it can also substantially reduce costs. Cost-effectiveness studies should eventually facilitate clinical decisions made for offloading treatment of foot ulcers in diabetic patients.

CONCLUSIONS AND RECOMMENDATIONS

Adequate pressure relief or offloading is an essential component in the successful treatment of plantar foot ulcers in patients with diabetes. Many different devices and mechanisms have been developed and used for this purpose and these have been discussed in this chapter. These studies should be viewed in light of their methodological limitations. There is a dominance of uncontrolled studies, the level A studies mostly involve small numbers of patients, studies generally lack the assessment of treatment adherence and activity profiles of patients, and do not combine the assessment of pressure and clinical outcomes with which mechanisms of (un)successful offloading can be determined. Nevertheless, several relevant conclusions can be drawn and recommendations for practical use can be made.

TCCs appear very effective in reducing plantar pressure at ulcer sites (level B) and they appear more effective than many types of removable modalities in healing diabetic plantar foot ulcers (level A). The use of the TCC for treating neuropathic plantar foot ulcers is recommended, although one should be aware though of the potential disadvantages of using the TCC that may limit its application in clinical practice. Cast shoes have the capacity to relieve plantar pressures to a substantial degree and these devices may heal close to the same percentage of neuropathic plantar foot ulcers at a similar rate as the TCC (level C). However, this will require confirmation in prospective controlled trials. In patients with adequate treatment adherence, cast shoes may be considered as easy to use modalities for offloading plantar diabetic foot ulcers.

Removable walkers appear to offload an area of interest under the foot to a similar degree as a TCC, but they do not seem as effective as the TCC in healing diabetic plantar foot ulcers (level A). However, when made nonremovable, the clinical efficacy of this device increases to levels comparable to the TCC (level A). This comparison clearly demonstrates the positive effect of continued pressure relief on the successful healing of forefoot ulcers in diabetes. For patients who have a low suspected treatment adherence, it is recommended to make the device nonremovable to improve healing. Offloading shoes and systems appear effective in reducing plantar pressures when compared with other ankle-high footwear modalities (level B), but they appear less effective than the TCC for healing plantar neuropathic foot ulcers (level A). In cases where TCCs or nonremovable walkers cannot be prescribed to the patient to heal an ulcer, forefoot offloading shoes are recommended. Certainly, a stronger evidence, base for these removable devices is required.

Surveys show that therapeutic footwear is often used in clinical practice for offloading treatment of diabetic plantar foot ulcers. Footwear that includes a custom molded insole or a rocker bottom outsole appears to offload the foot better than standard footwear (level B). However, the wide diversity of therapeutic footwear designs and the lack of standardization prevent clear recommendations to reduce plantar pressures. Therapeutic footwear seems less effective than other modalities for healing plantar neuropathic foot ulcers (level A). Therefore, the use of therapeutic footwear for the treatment of plantar neuropathic foot ulcers in diabetic patients should be considered only when other modalities are not available, when patient adherence can be ensured, and when patients decline treatment with other modalities.

The evidence base for the use of many other offloading modalities is small or nonexistent. Bed rest, crutches, and wheelchair use seem impractical for offloading treatment purposes and are therefore not recommended. Felted foam, when worn in shoes, appears to be effective in reducing forefoot plantar pressures when compared with wearing shoes alone (level B). The use of felted foam in offloading treatment of neuropathic plantar forefoot ulcers may be effective, although the evidence is not convincing yet (levels A and C). However, as felt is an easy to use and cheap solution, its use in combination with other offloading modalities is recommended. More studies are needed to confirm the effectiveness of felted foam as offloading modality in the treatment of neuropathic plantar foot ulcers.

Finally, the discussion of factors that determine the potential, the limitations, and the need for offloading the diabetic foot demonstrates that several issues remain to be solved. It also shows that choices made in clinical practice are still just as much a matter of experience, beliefs, patients' preferences, and available resources than the result of the application of available scientific evidence. It is hoped that the adoption and implementation of specific evidence based guidelines will bridge the large gap currently present between evidence and clinical practice. Future research will hopefully lead to the establishment of a framework within which well-informed clinical decisions can be made for the offloading treatment of foot ulcers in diabetic patients. This should rely on (a) high-quality scientific evidence, (b) knowledge on which factors determine outcome in healing, and (c) information regarding important factors which may determine the choice for a given treatment such as health-related quality of life, treatment adherence, and treatment costs.

REFERENCES

1. Boulton AJ, Kirsner RS, Vileikyte L. Clinical practice. Neuropathic diabetic foot ulcers. N Engl J Med 2004; 351(1):48–55.
2. Prompers L, Huijberts M, Apelqvist J, et al. High prevalence of ischaemia, infection and serious comorbidity in patients with diabetic foot disease in Europe. Baseline results from the Eurodiale study. Diabetologia 2007; 50(1):18–25.
3. Boyko EJ, Ahroni JH, Stensel V, et al. A prospective study of risk factors for diabetic foot ulcer. The Seattle Diabetic Foot Study. Diabetes Care 1999; 22(7):1036–1042.
4. Pham H, Armstrong DA, Harvey C, et al. Screening techniques to identify people at high risk for diabetic foot ulceration. Diabetes Care 2000; 23(5):606–611.
5. Veves A, Murray HJ, Young MJ, et al. The risk of foot ulceration in diabetic patients with high foot pressure: a prospective study. Diabetologia 1992; 35(7):660–663.
6. Ahroni JH, Boyko EJ, Forsberg RC. Clinical correlates of plantar pressure among diabetic veterans. Diabetes Care 1999; 22(6):965–972.
7. Bus SA, Maas M, de Lange A, et al. Elevated plantar pressures in neuropathic diabetic patients with claw/hammer toe deformity. J Biomech 2005; 38(9):1918–1925.
8. Armstrong DG, Lavery LA. Elevated peak plantar pressures in patients who have Charcot arthropathy. J Bone Joint Surg Am 1998; 80(3):365–369.
9. Bauman JH, Girling JP, Brand PW. Plantar pressures and trophic ulceration: an evaluation of footwear. J Bone Joint Surg Br 1963; 45:652–673.
10. Bus SA, Valk GD, van Deursen RW, et al. The effectiveness of footwear and offloading interventions to prevent and heal foot ulcers and reduce plantar pressure in diabetes: a systematic review. Diabetes Metab Res Rev 2008; 24 (Suppl 1):S162–S180.
11. International Working Group on the Diabetic Foot. International Consensus on the Diabetic Foot. Specific Guidelines on Footwear and Offloading 2007. Amsterdam, the Netherlands, on DVD (www.idf.org/bookshop).
12. Bus SA, Valk GD, van Deursen RW, et al. Specific guidelines of footwear and offloading. Diabetes Metab Res Rev 2008; 24 (Suppl 1):S192–S193.
13. Rosenbaum D, Hautmann S, Gold M, et al. Effects of walking speed on plantar pressure patterns and hindfoot angular motion. Gait Posture 1994; 2:191–197.
14. Brown HE, Mueller MJ. A "step-to" gait decreases pressures on the forefoot. J Orthop Sports Phys Ther 1998; 28(3):139–145.
15. Zhu HS, Wertsch JJ, Harris GF, et al. Foot pressure distribution during walking and shuffling. Arch Phys Med Rehabil 1991; 72(6):390–397.

16. Bus SA. Foot structure and footwear prescription in diabetes mellitus. Diabetes Metab Res Rev 2008; 24 (Suppl 1):S90–S95.
17. Shaw JE, Hsi WL, Ulbrecht JS, et al. The mechanism of plantar unloading in total contact casts: implications for design and clinical use. Foot Ankle Int 1997; 18(12):809–817.
18. Lavery LA, Vela SA, Lavery DC, et al. Total contact casts: pressure reduction at ulcer sites and the effect on the contralateral foot. Arch Phys Med Rehabil 1997; 78:1268–1271.
19. Hartsell HD, Brand RA, Saltzman CL. Total contact casting: its effect on contralateral plantar foot pressure. Foot Ankle Int 2002; 23(4):330–334.
20. Coleman WC, Brand PW, Birke JA. The total contact cast. A therapy for plantar ulceration on insensitive feet. J Am Podiatry Assoc 1984; 74(11):548–552.
21. Fleischli JG, Lavery LA, Vela SA, et al. Comparison of strategies for reducing pressure at the site of neuropathic ulcers. J Am Podiatr Med Assoc 1997; 87(10):466–472.
22. Lavery LA, Vela SA, Lavery DC, et al. Reducing dynamic foot pressures in high-risk diabetic subjects with foot ulcerations. A comparison of treatments. Diabetes Care 1996; 19(8):818–821.
23. Lavery LA, Vela SA, Fleischli JG, et al. Reducing plantar pressure in the neuropathic foot. A comparison of footwear. Diabetes Care 1997; 20(11):1706–1710.
24. Hartsell HD, Brand RA, Frantz RA, et al. The effects of total contact casting materials on plantar pressures. Foot Ankle Int 2004; 25(2):73–78.
25. Beuker BJ, van Deursen RW, Price P, et al. Plantar pressure in off-loading devices used in diabetic ulcer treatment. Wound Repair Regen 2005; 13(6):537–542.
26. Armstrong DG, Stacpoole-Shea S. Total contact casts and removable cast walkers. Mitigation of plantar heel pressure. J Am Podiatr Med Assoc 1999; 89(1):50–53.
27. Baumhauer JF, Wervey R, McWilliams J, et al. A comparison study of plantar foot pressure in a standardized shoe, total contact cast, and prefabricated pneumatic walking brace. Foot Ankle Int 1997; 18(1):26–33.
28. Petre M, Tokar P, Kostar D, et al. Revisiting the total contact cast: maximizing off-loading by wound isolation. Diabetes Care 2005; 28(4):929–930.
29. Mueller MJ, Diamond JE, Sinacore DR, et al. Total contact casting in treatment of diabetic plantar ulcers. Controlled clinical trial. Diabetes Care 1989; 12(6):384–388.
30. Caravaggi C, Faglia E, De GR, et al. Effectiveness and safety of a nonremovable fiberglass off-bearing cast versus a therapeutic shoe in the treatment of neuropathic foot ulcers: a randomized study. Diabetes Care 2000; 23(12):1746–1751.
31. Armstrong DG, Nguyen HC, Lavery LA, et al. Off-loading the diabetic foot wound: a randomized clinical trial. Diabetes Care 2001; 24(6):1019–1022.
32. Wukich DK, Motko J. Safety of total contact casting in high-risk patients with neuropathic foot ulcers. Foot Ankle Int 2004; 25(8):556–560.
33. Borssen B, Lithner F. Plaster casts in the management of advanced ischaemic and neuropathic diabetic foot lesions. Diabet Med 1989; 6(8):720–723.
34. Birke JA, Novick A, Patout CA, et al. Healing rates of plantar ulcers in leprosy and diabetes. Lepr Rev 1992; 63(4):365–374.
35. Armstrong DG, Lavery LA, Bushman TR. Peak foot pressures influence the healing time of diabetic foot ulcers treated with total contact casts. J Rehabil Res Dev 1998; 35(1):1–5.
36. Birke JA, Novick A, Graham SL, et al. Methods of treating plantar ulcers. Phys Ther 1991; 71(2):116–122.
37. Birke JA, Pavich MA, Patout CA Jr, et al. Comparison of forefoot ulcer healing using alternative off-loading methods in patients with diabetes mellitus. Adv Skin Wound Care 2002; 15(5):210–215.
38. Boulton AJ, Bowker JH, Gadia M, et al. Use of plaster casts in the management of diabetic neuropathic foot ulcers. Diabetes Care 1986; 9(2):149–152.
39. Nabuurs-Franssen MH, Huijberts MS, Sleegers R, et al. Casting of recurrent diabetic foot ulcers: effective and safe? Diabetes Care 2005; 28(6):1493–1494.

40. Nabuurs-Franssen MH, Sleegers R, Huijberts MS, et al. Total contact casting of the diabetic foot in daily practice: a prospective follow-up study. Diabetes Care 2005; 28(2):243–247.
41. Saltzman CL, Zimmerman MB, Holdsworth RL, et al. Effect of initial weight-bearing in a total contact cast on healing of diabetic foot ulcers. J Bone Joint Surg Am 2004; 86-A(12):2714–2719.
42. Sinacore DR, Mueller MJ, Diamond JE, et al. Diabetic plantar ulcers treated by total contact casting. A clinical report. Phys Ther 1987; 67(10):1543–1549.
43. Lin SS, Bono CM, Lee TH. Total contact casting and Keller arthoplasty for diabetic great toe ulceration under the interphalangeal joint. Foot Ankle Int 2000; 21(7):588–593.
44. Matricali GA, Deroo K, Dereymaeker G. Outcome and recurrence rate of diabetic foot ulcers treated by a total contact cast: short-term follow-up. Foot Ankle Int 2003; 24(9):680–684.
45. Lin SS, Lee TH, Wapner KL. Plantar forefoot ulceration with equinus deformity of the ankle in diabetic patients: the effect of tendo-Achilles lengthening and total contact casting. Orthopedics 1996; 19(5):465–475.
46. Walker SC, Helm PA, Pullium G. Total contact casting and chronic diabetic neuropathic foot ulcerations: healing rates by wound location. Arch Phys Med Rehabil 1987; 68(4):217–221.
47. Helm PA, Walker SC, Pullium G. Total contact casting in diabetic patients with neuropathic foot ulcerations. Arch Phys Med Rehabil 1984; 65(11):691–693.
48. Lavery LA, Armstrong DG, Walker SC. Healing rates of diabetic foot ulcers associated with midfoot fracture due to Charcot's arthropathy. Diabet Med 1997; 14(1):46–49.
49. Myerson M, Papa J, Eaton K, et al. The total-contact cast for management of neuropathic plantar ulceration of the foot. J Bone Joint Surg Am 1992; 74(2):261–269.
50. Sinacore DR. Healing times of diabetic ulcers in the presence of fixed deformities of the foot using total contact casting. Foot Ankle Int 1998; 19(9):613–618.
51. Wu SC, Jensen JL, Weber AK, et al. Use of pressure offloading devices in diabetic foot ulcers: do we practice what we preach? Diabetes Care 2008; 31(11):2118–2119.
52. Prompers L, Huijberts M, Apelqvist J, et al. Delivery of care to diabetic patients with foot ulcers in daily practice: results of the Eurodiale study, a prospective cohort study. Diabet Med 2008; 25(6):700–707.
53. Diamond JE, Sinacore DR, Mueller MJ. Molded double-rocker plaster shoe for healing a diabetic plantar ulcer. A case report. Phys Ther 1987; 67(10):1550–1552.
54. Hissink RJ, Manning HA, van Baal JG. The MABAL shoe, an alternative method in contact casting for the treatment of neuropathic diabetic foot ulcers. Foot Ankle Int 2000; 21(4):320–323.
55. Dumont IJ, Lepeut MS, Tsirtsikolou DM, et al. A proof-of-concept study of the effectiveness of a removable device for offloading in patients with neuropathic ulceration of the foot: the Ransart boot. Diabetic Med 2009; 26:778–782.
56. Burden AC, Jones GR, Jones R, et al. Use of the "Scotchcast boot" in treating diabetic foot ulcers. Br Med J (Clin Res Ed) 1983; 286(6377):1555–1557.
57. Knowles EA, Armstrong DG, Hayat SA, et al. Offloading diabetic foot wounds using the scotchcast boot: a retrospective study. Ostomy Wound Manage 2002; 48(9):50–53.
58. Bus SA, van Deursen RW, Kanade RV, et al. Plantar pressure relief in the diabetic foot using forefoot offloading shoes. Gait Posture 2009; 29(4):618–622.
59. Nagel A, Rosenbaum D. Vacuum cushioned removable cast walkers reduce foot loading in patients with diabetes mellitus. Gait Posture 2009; 30(1):11–15.
60. Ezio F, Caravaggi C, Giacomo, et al. Effectiveness of removable walker cast versus non-removable fiberglass off-bearing cast in the healing of diabetic plantar foot ulcera randomized controlled trial. Diabetes Care 2010; DOI 10.2337/dc09-1708.
61. Armstrong DG, Lavery LA, Wu S, et al. Evaluation of removable and irremovable cast walkers in the healing of diabetic foot wounds: a randomized controlled trial. Diabetes Care 2005; 28(3):551–554.
62. Katz IA, Harlan A, Miranda-Palma B, et al. A randomized trial of two irremovable off-loading devices in the management of plantar neuropathic diabetic foot ulcers. Diabetes Care 2005; 28(3):555–559.

63. Piaggesi A, Macchiarini S, Rizzo L, et al. An off-the-shelf instant contact casting device for the management of diabetic foot ulcers: a randomized prospective trial versus traditional fiberglass cast. Diabetes Care 2007; 30(3):586–590.
64. Chantelau E, Breuer U, Leisch AC, et al. Outpatient treatment of unilateral diabetic foot ulcers with 'half shoes'. Diabet Med 1993; 10(3):267–270.
65. Bus SA, Maas J, Otterman NM. Lower extremity dynamics of walking neuropathic diabetic patients wearing a forefoot offloading shoe (Abstract). In: Book of Abstracts of the 21st Congress of the International Society of Biomechanics, July 1–5, 2007, Taipei, Taiwan.
66. Bus SA, Waaijman R, Arts M, et al. The efficacy of a removable vacuum-cushioned cast replacement system in reducing plantar forefoot pressures in diabetic patients. Clin Biomech (Bristol, Avon) 2009; 24(5):459–464.
67. Ha Van G, Siney H, Hartmann-Heurtier A, et al. Nonremovable, windowed, fiberglass cast boot in the treatment of diabetic plantar ulcers: efficacy, safety, and compliance. Diabetes Care 2003; 26(10):2848–2852.
68. Chantelau E, Haage P. An audit of cushioned diabetic footwear: relation to patient compliance. Diabet Med 1994; 11(1):114–116.
69. Viswanathan V, Madhavan S, Gnanasundaram S, et al. Effectiveness of different types of footwear insoles for the diabetic neuropathic foot: a follow-up study. Diabetes Care 2004; 27(2):474–477.
70. Albert S, Rinoie C. Effect of custom orthotics on plantar pressure distribution in the pronated diabetic foot. J Foot Ankle Surg 1994; 33(6):598–604.
71. Ashry HR, Lavery LA, Murdoch DP, et al. Effectiveness of diabetic insoles to reduce foot pressures. J Foot Ankle Surg 1997; 36(4):268–271.
72. Bus SA, Ulbrecht JS, Cavanagh PR. Pressure relief and load redistribution by custom-made insoles in diabetic patients with neuropathy and foot deformity. Clin Biomech 2004; 19(6):629–638.
73. Kato H, Takada T, Kawamura T, et al. The reduction and redistribution of plantar pressures using foot orthoses in diabetic patients. Diabetes Res Clin Pract 1996; 31(1–3):115–118.
74. Lord M, Hosein R. Pressure redistribution by molded inserts in diabetic footwear: a pilot study. J Rehabil Res Dev 1994; 31(3):214–221.
75. Raspovic A, Newcombe L, Lloyd J, et al. Effect of customized insoles on vertical plantar pressures in sites of previous neuropathic ulceration in the diabetic foot. FOOT 2000; 10(3):133–138.
76. Tsung BYS, Zhang M, Mak AFT, et al. Effectiveness of insoles on plantar pressure redistribution. J Rehabil Res Dev 2004; 41(6A):767–774.
77. Van De Weg FB, Van Der Windt DA, Vahl AC. Wound healing: total contact cast vs. custom-made temporary footwear for patients with diabetic foot ulceration. Prosthet Orthot Int 2008; 32(1):3–11.
78. Maland E, Walker C, Dalton J. Use of an EVA boot in a patient with a foot ulcer. J Wound Care 1997; 6(7):319–320.
79. Singleton EE, Cotton RS, Shelman HS. Another approach to the long-term management of the diabetic neurotrophic foot ulcer. J Am Podiatry Assoc 1978; 68(4):242–244.
80. Downs DM, Jacobs RL. Treatment of resistant ulcers on the plantar surface of the great toe in diabetics. J Bone Joint Surg Am 1982; 64(6):930–933.
81. Davies S, Gibby O, Phillips C, et al. The health status of diabetic patients receiving orthotic therapy. Qual Life Res 2000; 9(2):233–240.
82. Holstein P, Larsen K, Sager P. Decompression with the aid of insoles in the treatment of diabetic neuropathic ulcers. Acta Orthop Scand 1976; 47(4):463–468.
83. Larsen K, Fabrin J, Holstein PE. Incidence and management of ulcers in diabetic Charcot feet. J Wound Care 2001; 10(8):323–328.
84. Cavanagh PR, Bus SA. Off-loading the diabetic foot for ulcer prevention and healing. JA Am Podiatric Med Assoc 2010; In press.
85. Kastenbauer T, Sokol G, Auinger M, et al. Running shoes for relief of plantar pressure in diabetic patients. Diabet Med 1998; 15(6):518–522.

86. Perry JE, Ulbrecht JS, Derr JA, et al. The use of running shoes to reduce plantar pressures in patients who have diabetes. J Bone Joint Surg Am 1995; 77(12):1819–1828.
87. Armstrong DG, Liswood PJ, Todd WF. Potential risks of accommodative padding in the treatment of neuropathic ulcerations. Ostomy Wound Manage 1995; 41(7):44–49.
88. Piaggesi A, Romanelli M, Fallani E, et al. Polyurethane foam sheets for relieving pressure from diabetic neuropathic plantar ulcers: a pilot study. J Dermatolog Treat 2000; 11(1):39–42.
89. Zimny S, Meyer MF, Schatz H, et al. Applied felted foam for plantar pressure relief is an efficient therapy in neuropathic diabetic foot ulcers. Exp Clin Endocrinol Diabetes 2002; 110(7):325–328.
90. Zimny S, Schatz H, Pfohl U. The effects of applied felted foam on wound healing and healing times in the therapy of neuropathic diabetic foot ulcers. Diabet Med 2003; 20(8):622–625.
91. Armstrong DG, Peters EJ, Athanasiou KA, et al. Is there a critical level of plantar foot pressure to identify patients at risk for neuropathic foot ulceration? J Foot Ankle Surg 1998; 37(4):303–307.
92. Armstrong DG, Lavery LA, Kimbriel HR, et al. Activity patterns of patients with diabetic foot ulceration: patients with active ulceration may not adhere to a standard pressure off-loading regimen. Diabetes Care 2003; 26(9):2595–2597.
93. Knowles EA, Boulton AJ. Do people with diabetes wear their prescribed footwear? Diabet Med 1996; 13(12):1064–1068.
94. Laing PW, Cogley DI, Klenerman L. Neuropathic foot ulceration treated by total contact casts. J Bone Joint Surg Br 1992; 74(1):133–136.
95. Goodridge D, Trepman E, Sloan J, et al. Quality of life of adults with unhealed and healed diabetic foot ulcers. Foot Ankle Int 2006; 27(4):274–280.
96. Ribu L, Hanestad BR, Moum T, et al. A comparison of the health-related quality of life in patients with diabetic foot ulcers, with a diabetes group and a nondiabetes group from the general population. Qual Life Res 2007; 16(2):179–189.
97. Pecoraro RE, Reiber GE, Burgess EM. Pathways to diabetic limb amputation. Basis for prevention. Diabetes Care 1990; 13(5):513–521.

Appendix: Evidence Tables for Controlled Studies on Offloading Treatment of Foot Ulcers and Plantar Pressure Relief in Diabetic Patients

Reference	Study Design + level of evidence#	Study population and characteristics	Intervention (I) and control (C) conditions	Results on primary/secondary outcomes + statistic
Armstrong et al., 2001 (31)	RCT A	Patients: I: 25, C1: 25, C2: 25 Superficial neuropathic plantar foot ulcers (UT grade 1 A) Study duration: 12 weeks or healing Lost to study: 12 (I:6, C1:5, C2:1)	I: TCC C1: Removable walker C2: Half shoe	Healing proportions: I :17/19; C1 :13/20; C2 :14/24 Statistic: I vs. C1 + C2: $P = 0.026$, OR = 5.4 (95% CI = 1.1–26.1) Average time to healing (days): I: 33.5, C1: 50.4, C2: 61.0 Statistic: I vs. C1: $P = 0.07$; I vs. C2: $P = 0.005$ Average number of daily steps: I: 600, C1: 768, C2: 1462 Statistic: I vs. C2: $P = 0.04$
Armstrong et al., 2005 (61)	RCT A	Patients: I: 23, C: 27 Superficial neuropathic plantar foot ulcers (UT grade 1 A) Study duration: 12 weeks or healing Lost to study: 4	I: Non-removable walker C: Removable walker	Healing proportions: I: 19/23, C: 14/27 Statistic: $P = 0.02$, OR = 1.8 (95% CI = 1.1–2.9)
Caravaggi et al., 2000 (30)	RCT A	Patients: I: 26, C: 24 neuropathic plantar foot ulcers Study duration: 30 days Lost to study: not reported	I : TCC C: Therapeutic shoe (rocker bottom, extradepth + 8 mm plastazote insoles)	Healing proportions: I: 13/26, C: 5/24 Statistic: $P = 0.03$
Ezio et al., 2010 (60)	RCT A	Patients: I: 25, C: 23 Neuropathic plantar foot ulcers (UT grade 1A) Study duration: 90 days Lost to study: 3 (I: 1, C:2)	I: Removable walking boot C: TCC	Healing proportions: I: 16/22, C: 17/23 Statistic: P = 0.794 Average time to healing (days): I:39.7, C:35.3 Statistic: P = 0.708 Ulcer surface reduction (cm^2): I: 2.18 to 0.45, C: 1.41 to 0.21 Statistic: P = 0.722

Ha Van et al., 2003 (67)	CBA B	Patients: I: 42, C: 51 Neuropathic plantar foot ulcers (UT grade 1A) Study duration: until healing/complications Lost to study: not reported	I: TCC C: Half shoe or heel-relief shoe	Healing percentages: I: 81%, C: 70% Statistic: $P = 0.017$, Hazard ratio: 1.68 (95% CI: 1.04–2.70) Average time to healing (days): I: 69, C: 134 No statistics Adherence: I: 98%, C: 10% Statistic: $P = 0.001$
Katz et al., 2005 (62)	RCT A	Patients: I: 21, C: 20 Neuropathic plantar foot ulcers (UT grade 1A or 2A) Study duration: 12 weeks or healing Lost to study: 7 (I: 4, C: 3)	I: Nonremovable walker C: TCC	Healing proportions: I: 17/21 (80%), C: 15/20 (74%) Statistic: $P = 0.65$
Mueller et al., 1989 (29)	RCT A	Patients: I: 21, C: 19 Noninfected neuropathic plantar foot ulcers (Wagner 1 and 2) Study duration: not reported Lost to study: not reported	I: TCC C: Accommodative footwear (i.e. healing sandal + extra depth shoe with a plastazote insole)	Healing proportions: I: 19/21, C: 6/19 Statistic: $P < 0.05$ Mean time to healing (days): I: 42, C: 65 Statistic: $P < 0.05$
Piaggesi et al., 2007 (63)	RCT A	Patients: I: 20, C: 20 Noninfected, nonischemic neuropathic plantar foot ulcers (UT grade 1A or 2A) Study duration: 12 weeks Lost to study: 0	I: Nonremovable medium high walker C: TCC	Healing percentages: I: 85%, C: 95% Statistic: not significant Mean time to healing (weeks): I: 6.7, C: 6.5 Statistic: not significant Number of adverse events: I: 4, C: 6 Statistic: not significant

(*Continued*)

Appendix: Evidence Tables for Controlled Studies on Offloading Treatment of Foot Ulcers and Plantar Pressure Relief in Diabetic Patients (*Continued*)

Reference	Study Design + level of evidence#	Study population and characteristics	Intervention (I) and control (C) conditions	Results on primary/secondary outcomes + statistic
Viswanathan et al., 2004 (69)	Cohort B	Patients: I1: 100; I2: 59; I3: 32; C: 50 Study duration: 9 months Lost to study: not reported All patients had a history of ulceration Group I3 had foot deformities (not defined)	I1: MCR insoles in customized sandals I2: Polyurethane insoles in customized sandals I3: Molded insoles in customized sandals C: Usual sandals with hard leather board insole	Change in plantar pressure (9 months vs. baseline): I1: −57.4%, I2: −62.0%, I3: −58.0%, C: +39.4% Statistic: $P < 0.01$
Van de Weg et al., 2008 (77)	RCT A	Patients: I: 20; C: 20 Noninfected neuropathic plantar foot ulcers (Wagner 1 or 2) Study duration: 16 weeks Lost to study: 2 (I: 0, C: 2)	I: Fully customized temporary orthopaedic footwear C: TCC	Healing proportion: I: 6/20, C: 6/20 Statistic: not significant Mean time to healing (days): I: 90, C: 59 Statistic: not significant Wound surface area reduction in 16 weeks: I: from 1.9 to 0.4 cm^2, C: from 3.6 to 0.4 cm^2 Statistic: not significant
Zimny et al., 2003 (90)	RCT A	Patients: I: 24, C: 30 Noninfected, nonischemic neuropathic plantar forefoot ulcers (Wagner 1 or 2) Study duration: 10 weeks Lost to study: not reported	I: Felted foam in post-operative shoe C: Pressure relief half shoe	Mean time to healing (days): I: 75, C: 85 Statistic: $P = 0.03$ Ulcer radius reduction per week (mm): I: 0.48, C: 0.39 Statistic: $P = 0.005$ Survival analysis: $P = 0.06$ between groups

#Based on system of the Oxford Center for Evidence Based Medicine.

10 Surgical approach to the diabetic foot ulcer

Nathan A. Hunt* and Douglas P. Murdoch

SURGICAL APPROACH TO THE DIABETIC FOOT ULCER

The discovery of and ability to manufacture insulin in 1922 drastically changed the prognosis of patients diagnosed with diabetes (1). This discovery turned a fatal, untreatable disease into a chronic, treatable disease, which has presented new and equally challenging health concerns in this unique patient population that include retinopathy, nephropathy, peripheral vascular disease, and peripheral neuropathy (2). Not only do these comorbidities pose significant challenges to the surgeon but also are becoming more and more prevalent as people live longer with the disease. The Centers for Disease Control and Prevention (CDC) estimates that 7.8% of the U.S. population, or 23.6 million people, have diabetes, and it estimates that another 57 million people in the United States have impaired fasting glucose level and are at significant risk of developing diabetes (3). This trend means there will be a greater percentage of the general population living with this disease with more foot wounds, infections, and amputations.

The prognosis for diabetic foot ulcers (DFUs) is often poor (4). Surgically correcting structural deformity or improving the range of motion is controversial in this high-risk patient population. The objective of this chapter is to discuss the rationale and evidence for elective surgery to treat DFUs and prevent recurrence. Before considering any surgical procedure the patient's vascular status and comorbidities (hypertension, cardiovascular, and renal disease) must be assessed and optimized. Once this has been done, surgical treatment of DFUs should be considered for patients who have failed proper off-loading and wound care, or who have recurrent ulcers with appropriate preventative care.

Diverting the Causal Pathway

The etiology of neuropathic foot ulcers involves limited joint mobility and deformity in the setting of sensory neuropathy, which leads to abnormal pressure and shear forces. This commonly exceeds the soft tissue's ability to absorb and dissipate the repetitive forces of ambulation resulting in full-thickness ulceration. These superficial wounds are significant medical risks because an ulcer precedes 84% of all atraumatic amputations (5). Reiber et al. reported that minor trauma, neuropathy, and deformity were the most common causes of foot ulceration (6). Likewise, Armstrong and Lavery reported an association between the presence and the number of foot deformities and elevated foot pressures in patients with diabetes (7).

The rationale for surgical intervention is to correct the structural deformity and/or increase motion and interrupt the causal pathway to foot ulceration.

**Current affiliation*: Orthopaedic Center of the Rockies, Fort Collins, Colorado, U.S.A.

Table 1 Risk-based Classification for Diabetic Foot Surgery

Class		Example
Class 1 ELECTIVE	Relief of PAINFUL deformity—intact neurovascular system	Bunion, hammertoe
Class 2 PROPHYLACTIC	Treat RISK FACTORS for ulcers—peripheral sensory neuropathy and deformity	No active ulcer (or has healed ulcer) but has potential to occur/reoccur
Class 3 CURATIVE	Addresses an ACTIVE pathology (ulcer) that failed conservative care	Flexor tenotomy, arthroplasty, metatarsal head resection etc.
Class 4 EMERGENT	ACUTE limb/foot salvage	Abscess, osteotomy, necrosis/gangrene

Armstrong et al. Diabet Med 2003; 20:329–331.

Surgical treatment of the diabetic foot can be classified in one of four groups: elective, prophylactic, curative, and emergent (see Table 1). This supports the premise that there may be opportunities to intervene in the pathway to deformity, ulceration, and infection before amputation becomes the only surgical option.

Risk Versus Benefit

Knowing the probability of obtaining and maintaining a healed, functional foot after surgical intervention is difficult to determine for patients with diabetes because they have greater complication rates than age-matched, nondiabetic patients. However, a patient recently diagnosed with diabetes or who has controlled the disease since diagnosis may have normal or near-normal healing parameters. On the other hand, patients with chronically elevated blood glucose level, peripheral neuropathy, peripheral vascular disease, pedal deformities, or end-stage renal disease; or, those whose duration of diabetes has been more than 10 years, which correlates with high prevalence of said comorbidities, have greater risk for complications (8).

The surgeon must consider and discuss the risks and benefits of treatment with the patient. First, the risk of a chronic open wound must be discussed. The patient should understand the incidence of soft tissue and bone infection, and foot or leg amputation is high. More than 50% of foot ulcers are treated for infection and 20% develop osteomyelitis (9–11). In cohort studies of patients with foot wounds, 56% of patients develop infections and 6% to 15% of foot ulcers end in amputation (12,13). Adequate assessment of patients' neurovascular status and medical condition will give the surgeon an opportunity to discuss the patients' individual risk of surgically treating their condition.

Ulcer Risk Assessment

Ulcer recurrence is common after DFUs heal. With every recurrent wound, the risk of infection and amputation looms. Even with standard preventative care such as therapeutic shoes and insoles, education, and regular foot care, 25% to 33% of patients will develop another foot ulcer within the next year (14–17). Without standard preventative care, 58% to 83% of patients with a healed foot ulcer develop another wound (14–16). When an ulcer has healed with proper treatment and later recurs, surgical care must be considered if the etiology relates to a deformity that causes repetitive stresses on the tissues. There are elements that affect wound healing that can fluctuate (bacterial load, blood glucose levels, and nutritional status), whereas others can remain static but unrecognized or underappreciated (deformity, limited joint mobility, anemia, peripheral vascular disease, etc.). All factors must be evaluated and addressed to heal the ulcer and prevent recurrence.

When a patient with diabetes presents with a foot wound, the patient should be evaluated thoroughly to accurately understand the risk of surgical and nonsurgical treatment. The patient's cardiovascular, neurologic, and renal status should be assessed on initial presentation. Some of these assessments may be done with a thorough chart review; however, if the patient has not seen an internist or endocrinologist recently, then appropriate laboratory tests along with a detailed physical examination should be performed. We will briefly discuss cardiovascular, neurologic, and renal evaluation as it pertains to patients with diabetes and increased risk of wound healing complications. Then, we will discuss specific pedal problems common to this patient population.

Cardiovascular Risk Assessment

The Trans-Atlantic Inter-Society Consensus (TASC II) on management of peripheral arterial disease (PAD) estimates that 15% to 20% of patients aged 70 years or older have PAD (18). A European study showed that one in four patients with diabetes and no known vascular disease had subclinical PAD (2), and TASC II states that for every symptomatic patient, there are three or four asymptomatic patients with PAD (18,19). With an aging population and an increasing prevalence of diabetes mellitus, PAD will become increasingly more common; therefore, surgeons should have a high index of suspicion when evaluating a patient with diabetes.

Other known risk factors for PAD include male sex, smoking, increasing age, non-Hispanic blacks, hypertension, hyperglycemia, dyslipidemia, elevated C-reactive protein level, hypercoagulable state, hyperhomocysteinemia, and chronic renal insufficiency (18,20–25). Therefore, standard blood chemistry, complete blood cell count, prothrombin time, partial thromboplastin time, creatinine phosphokinase level, hemoglobin A1c level, erythrocyte sedimentation rate, and lipid profile are useful laboratory tests to consider when assessing healing potential and cardiovascular risk preoperatively (18,26). These risk factors also emphasize the importance of routinely obtaining blood pressure when evaluating a patient with diabetes.

Assessing perfusion is a primary concern for a surgeon contemplating treatment for a patient with diabetes. A recent history of healing is probably the best indicator of healing potential. A patient who has already proven that he can heal a foot ulcer with wound care and off-loading has a good prognosis for healing a surgical procedure that reduces the deforming force responsible for the ulcer recurring.

PAD is a clinical diagnosis that can usually be assessed with noninvasive inexpensive methods. First, all peripheral pulses of the lower extremity should be manually palpated: femoral, popliteal, dorsalis pedis, and posterior tibial arteries. When any of these are difficult to palpate, a ratio between the systolic pressure in the ankle divided by the systolic pressure of the brachial artery should be obtained (ankle brachial index, ABI). The systolic pressure of the dorsalis pedis and the posterior tibial artery of each leg, as well as the systolic pressure of brachial artery in each arm, should be obtained, and the higher pressure in the leg should be divided by the higher of the two brachial pressures. An ABI less than 0.9 is an independent risk factor for cardiovascular events, including death (27). A decreased ABI also increases the patient's risk for complications in wound healing; however, several authors have reported successful wound healing rates approaching 90% if the ABI is greater than 0.45 (28,29). These results were more recently reproduced with an ABI equal to or greater than 0.5 in patients with diabetes (30).

Patients with diabetes can have a unique pattern of atherosclerosis that causes vascular calcifications that limit the effectiveness of the ABI. An ABI greater than 1.4 is suspect of this condition, and these patients may be at greater risk for cardiovascular events (27). In this instance, pulse volume recordings, skin perfusion pressure, and transcutaneous oxygen tensions are valuable noninvasive examinations (14,31,53). If peripheral vascular disease is detected, a vascular surgeon should be consulted for more thorough cardiovascular workup and treatment. A noninvasive vascular examination can often result in normal large vessel perfusion and significant microvascular disease. These patients are at a greater risk for a complicated healing course and should be advised of this increased risk and referred to vascular surgery.

Neurologic Risk Assessment

Peripheral neuropathy is also a clinical diagnosis that can be made with a focused physical examination. Many detailed clinical examinations have been proposed to detect diabetic peripheral neuropathy (32–34). These have not been used widely in clinical practice because they are time consuming and use expensive equipment. Inability to feel a Semmes-Weinstein 5.07, 10 g monofilament at 4 of the following 10 sites: plantar first, third, and fifth toes and metatarsal heads; medial and lateral plantar midfoot, plantar heel and dorsum of the foot; and inability to feel the vibration at the pulp of the great toe with a biothesiometer vibrating at 100 Hz and 25 V, have been shown to effectively diagnose peripheral neuropathy sufficient for pedal ulcerations to develop (35).

Once the examination is complete, it is important to assist patients in receiving the appropriate care by referring them to the primary care physician, endocrinologist, or vascular surgeon as necessary.

Benefits of Surgery

Several authors have reported the results of planned surgical procedures to heal foot ulcers. These studies suggest a relatively low infection rate (4.4%–40%); although 40% is quite high, it did not differ from the nonoperative group, which had a 38% infection rate. Even with a relatively high infection rate, 91% to 96% of the wounds went on to heal and only 2.4% to 6.6% of those surgically treated had recurrence of the ulcer (36–38).

Armstrong et al. (38) retrospectively examined 31 diabetic and 33 nondiabetic patients who underwent a single lesser-digit arthroplasty for hammertoe deformity. This would be considered "prophylactic" surgery (see Table 1) (39). They further divided the diabetic group into risk group 2 (peripheral neuropathy and deformity) and risk group 3 (peripheral neuropathy, deformity, and history of ulcer) (38,40). They examined postoperative infection rates and dehiscence rates with an average follow-up of 3 years. Their results showed that there was no significant difference in overall complications between diabetic and nondiabetic patients with this procedure, but there was a significantly higher risk of postoperative infection in patients who had a history of neuropathic ulcers. The long-term outcome of this "prophylactic" surgery in high-risk diabetic patients (risk group 3) was uniformly good, with approximately 96% remaining ulcer-free at a mean of 3 years follow-up (38).

The overall goal of surgical care is to reduce the long-term risk for ulceration by preserving motion and reducing abnormal pressure and shear forces. Understanding pathologic structural and biomechanical abnormalities is essential to plan appropriate surgical procedures. Both static and dynamic components of the deformities must be evaluated. We will now discuss clinical evaluation of specific pathologic deformities by anatomic location and the evidence-based procedures currently used to correct these deformities.

HALLUX AND FIRST METATARSOPHALANGEAL JOINT ULCERS

More than 50% of plantar foot ulcers occur on either the hallux or the first metatarsal head (41,42). Therefore, ulcers at these locations have been the topic of much discussion, and surgical correction has been controversial (36,38,43,44). We will address this pathology separate from lesser toe and metatarsal deformities.

Distal Hallux Ulcer

An ulcer at this location usually occurs because of a flexion deformity at the interphalangeal joint causing excessive stress to the distal aspect of the hallux (45). This deformity should be evaluated and classified as either rigid (unable to manually reduce the deformity) or flexible (manually reducible). A flexible deformity can be treated with a flexor tenotomy (46). Rigid deformities can be addressed with an interphalangeal joint arthroplasty (36) (level B).

Plantar Hallux Interphalangeal Joint Accessory Bone

Interphalangeal joint sesamoid: An ulcer that occurs at the plantar aspect of the hallux interphalangeal joint with adequate first metatarsophalangeal joint range of motion should alert the clinician to the possibility of an accessory sesamoid. This is done by close inspection of the appropriate radiographs. Surgical removal of the sesamoid could effectively decrease the pressure, which leads to wound healing. There are no published data on the long-term outcomes of this isolated procedure in patients with diabetes (level D). However, there are data to support ulcerations of the plantar aspect of the interphalangeal joint of the hallux healing with an arthroplasty of the metatarsophalangeal or interphalangeal joint (36,37,47,48) (level B).

Hallux Rigidus and Hallux Valgus

Structural deformity and limited joint mobility of the first metatarsophalangeal joint is often associated with ulcers under the metatarsal head and interphalangeal joint of the great toe. Hallux rigidus and hallux valgus can present individually or combined. Both compromise first metatarsophalangeal joint function.

Arthroplasty of the base of the proximal phalanx of the great toe (Keller arthroplasty) is the most common procedure described (Fig. 1). The surgical options to heal and prevent recurrence include arthroplasty of the interphalangeal joint of the great toe, metatarsophalangeal joint arthroplasty, or metatarsophalangeal joint arthroplasty with implant (total or hemi-implant). Total and

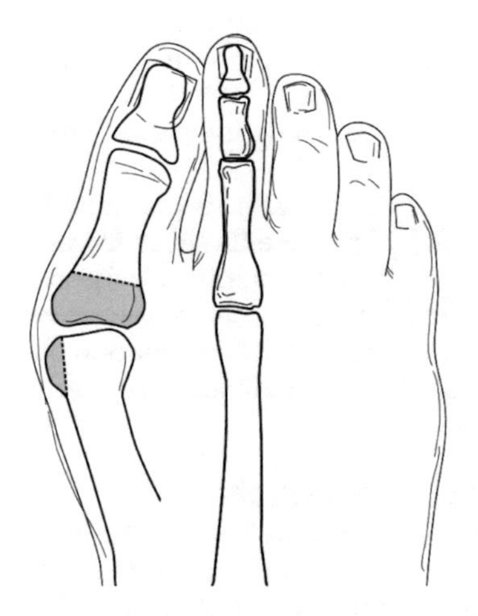

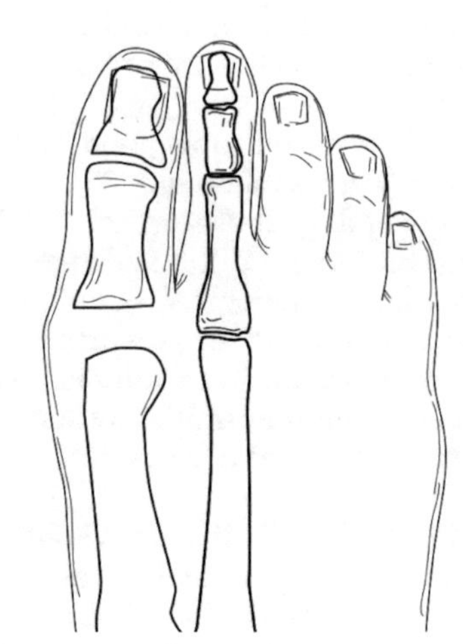

Figure 1 Keller arthroplasty.

hemi-implants are avoided in this patient population because the ulceration causes increased risk of infection with retained implants.

Keller arthroplasty is a procedure that improves the motion and alignment of the first metatarsophalangeal joint by removing the proximal aspect of the proximal phalanx of the hallux (Fig. 1). One of the most important technical aspects of the procedure is to maintain the insertion of the flexor hallucis brevis tendon, which can be accomplished with a limited resection of the base of the proximal phalanx (49). If the tendon insertion is damaged, suturing the tendon into the residual phalangeal base will help maintain the integrity of the flexor hallucis brevis tendon and the stability of the great toe. If the brevis tendon is damaged, a dynamic imbalance is induced about the first metatarsophalangeal joint involving the flexor hallucis longus tendon and the extensor tendons that may cause a hammertoe deformity to develop.

Stewart and Reed (50) reported that patients with diabetes were four times more likely to have the base of the proximal phalanx of the hallux resected than a metatarsophalangeal joint arthrodesis or implant arthroplasty. He used the 1996-through-2000 national Hospital Discharge Survey to identify 14,043 patients who had the base of the proximal phalanx of the hallux resected and 12,010 patients who had either a first metatarsophalangeal joint arthrodesis or an implant arthroplasty (50). This study design prohibits analysis of efficacy of the procedures or complications. They concluded that resection of the base of the proximal phalanx of the hallux is being done more frequently in patients with diabetes than those without diabetes who are admitted to the hospital. This number is likely overrepresented because all three of these procedures are often performed on an outpatient basis in healthy individuals. Inpatient cases would be more likely to have an infection, peripheral vascular disease, or uncontrolled chronic diseases, which are more prevalent in patients with diabetes than in their age-matched cohort.

Armstrong et al. (37) found that performing an arthroplasty of the first metatarsophalangeal joint resulted in a faster healing time, fewer recurrent ulcers, and no increase in infection rate for patients with plantar interphalangeal joint ulcers of the hallux.

Lin et al. (47) reported that 14 of 14 recalcitrant plantar hallux wounds healed in 23 days or less after resecting the base of the proximal phalanx of the hallux and off-loading in a total contact cast (TTC) group compared with 15 randomly selected controls. All of the controls healed in an average of 47 days with TCC immobilization. All of the surgical candidates had toe brachial indices of at least 0.65 and initially failed 40 days of TCC therapy before surgery. There were no recurrences or other complications 26 weeks after surgery (47).

Downs and Jacobs reported six cases of recalcitrant plantar hallux wounds healing with resection of the base of the proximal phalanx. These wounds initially failed nonoperative treatment. This case series had a 100% healing rate after vascular status was improved/declared adequate for healing per a vascular surgeon. One of the six had delayed surgical wound healing that went on to complete healing with local wound care. One patient had a second lesion at the distal aspect of the second toe of the ipsilateral foot that required a partial amputation of this toe that healed uneventfully. There were no other complications documented with at least 2 years of follow-up (48) (level B).

TOE ULCERS

Toe deformities are common in people who have had diabetes for more than 10 years (51–55). They are thought to develop in some cases because of motor neuropathy that first affects the intrinsic muscles in the foot. One of the functions of the intrinsic muscles is to stabilize the toes against the metatarsals. Thus, weak intrinsic muscles allow the long flexors and extensors to become imbalanced, causing toe contractures. This type of deformity may cause pathologic pressure on the distal aspect of the toe when weight-bearing, dorsal aspect of the head of the proximal phalanx from rubbing the toe box in shoe gear, and plantar aspect of the corresponding metatarsal head from ground force when weight-bearing.

Ulcers of the toes are usually associated with structural deformity (56). In many cases, toe ulcers are associated with a high rate of recurrence (14,37). The definitions of toe deformities should facilitate discussion of the level and the severity of pathology; however, considerable ambiguity exists in the literature regarding the exact definitions (57–59). In this chapter, we will define a hammertoe deformity as a dorsal contracture (extension) of the proximal phalanx at the metatarsophalangeal joint and plantar contracture (flexion) of the middle phalanx at the proximal interphalangeal joint. A claw toe deformity is a dorsal contracture (extension) of the proximal phalanx at the metatarsophalangeal joint and plantar contractures (flexion) at both the proximal and distal interphalangeal joints. A mallet toe deformity is a plantar contracture at the distal interphalangeal joint and does not involve the other joints of the toe (57).

It is crucial to perform a thorough clinical examination of the involved digit(s) to plan the appropriate surgical procedure(s). This involves a close correlation of what is seen when the patient is sitting compared with when standing and walking. There may appear to be soft tissue contractures at the metatarsophalangeal joint at rest, but when the patient stands, this joint may align normally. Similarly, when gait is observed, deformities at each level may be present that do not occur in stance or sitting. The clinical examination and weight-bearing pedal radiographs are necessary to develop an effective surgical plan.

Ulcers on the Tip of the Toe

If the long flexor tendon becomes overpowering, flexion deformity at the distal interphalangeal joint level can occur, placing the normally distal-facing end of the toe plantarward, bearing weight when standing and walking. The distal tip of the toe has very little fat pad to absorb the shock and shear of standing, walking, and running. The increased pressure to this skin results in excessive hyperkeratotic buildup, which exacerbates the pathologic pressure on the distal toe. If left unchecked, this repetitive cycle can lead to hemorrhagic callosities, skin breakdown, and a full-thickness ulcer. This commonly results in soft tissue infection and osteomyelitis of the distal phalanx through direct extension.

If regular debridement and off-loading (toe crest pads, shock-attenuating insole materials, casting, etc.) do not resolve the ulcer or the ulcer recurs and the deformity is reducible, then surgical release of the long flexor should be considered (Fig. 2) (46,55).

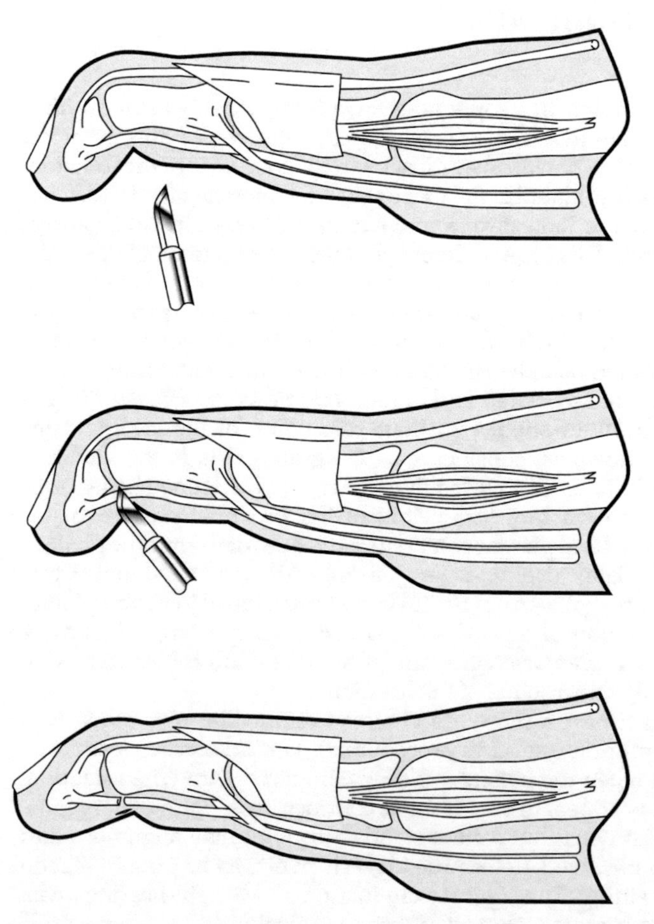

Figure 2 Long flexor tenotomy.

Laborde (46) retrospectively evaluated 28 toe ulcers that were treated with a percutaneous flexor tenotomy with at least 20 months of follow-up. Seventeen (61%) of the toes with ulceration were the great toe. All of the deformities were flexible (manually reducible), and all 28 ulcers healed in 2 months or less (46).

Tamir et al. (55) retrospectively assessed the results of flexor tenotomy and hyperextension of rigid joint (osteoclasis) in 34 toes (14 patients with diabetes). Twenty-four (71%) digits had a concomitant ulceration at the time of tenotomy. The other digits had a claw toe deformity and had the tenotomy performed prophylactically. Three of the ulcerations had osteomyelitic changes of the tuft of the distal phalanx on radiographs. These ulcerations healed in 8 weeks; all of the other ulcers healed in 3 weeks. They concluded that this procedure is effective for healing wounds penetrating to bone with osteomyelitis (with appropriate antibiotic therapy) but the wound healing will be prolonged (55) (level B).

Dorsal Ulcers of the Proximal or Distal Interphalangeal Joint

When there is a rigid deformity that cannot be manually reduced, resecting the head of the phalanx is usually necessary. The procedure can be performed at the proximal or distal interphalangeal joint, depending on where the deformity lies. If there are accompanying soft tissue contractures at the metatarsophalangeal joint, additional procedures may be required to reduce these deformities (Fig. 3).

We were able to identify only two retrospective studies that report outcomes and complications of arthroplasties in persons with diabetes. Armstrong et al. evaluated a cohort of patients with arthroplasty of the proximal interphalangeal joint for hammertoe deformity and stratified them by the presence of diabetes (31 with diabetes and 33 without diabetes). He found that 14.3% of patients who

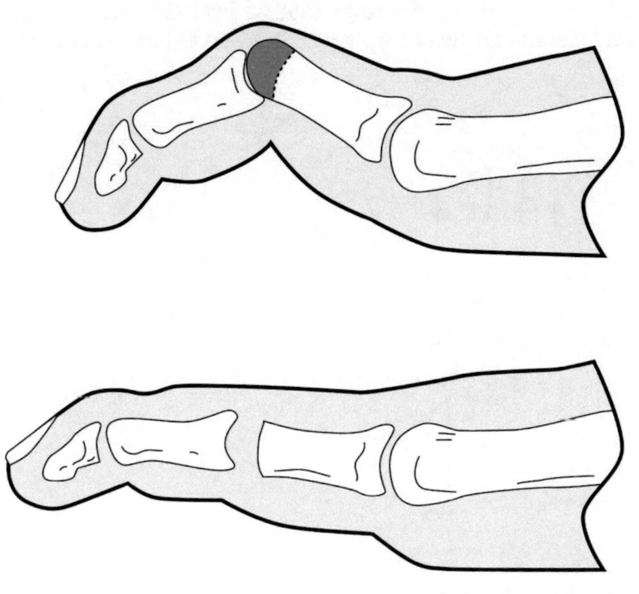

Figure 3 Proximal interphalangeal joint resection arthroplasty.

had diabetes and a history of ulceration had a postoperative infection. Ultimately 96.3% of these patients went on to heal the ulcer and remained ulcer-free for at least 12 months (38).

Kim et al. (60) reported results of a cohort of patients with diabetes with ulcers and osteomyelitis. They reviewed 72 lesser toe arthroplasties performed because of ulceration and underlying osteomyelitis. They removed devitalized tissue and infected bone, and 79% of the toes went on to complete healing in 32 days (60).

These studies show that an arthroplasty at the site of the deformity is effective at reducing the deformity with favorable healing rates (96% for wounds without osteomyelitis and 79% for wounds with osteomyelitis) (38,60) (level B).

Metatarsal Head Ulcers

Some ulcers persist or recur plantar to a metatarsal head despite addressing the digital deformities mentioned earlier. This is likely due to focal plantar pressure from a prominent/deformed metatarsal. Concomitantly, ankle joint equinus could be contributing to these local deformities in the forefoot (see "Ankle Joint Equinus"). This must be thoroughly evaluated clinically and radiographically to determine the etiology and effective surgical intervention. The causes of such ulcers are often due to the following deformities: hammertoe, hallux valgus, forefoot arthropathy, soft tissue atrophy, and compensated or uncompensated forefoot varus or valgus (61,62).

When custom orthoses with accommodations for the aforementioned deformities fail to heal the ulcer and maintain intact skin, then surgical correction should be considered. Surgeons have performed isolated metatarsal surgery at the apex of the deformity (63); however, some have advocated for removal of all metatarsal heads because of a relatively high rate of peak pressure being transferred to an adjacent metatarsal head and causing a secondary ulceration (Fig. 4) (18).

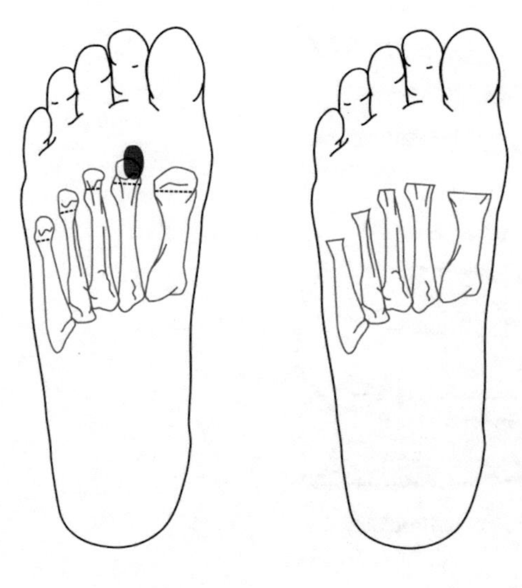

Figure 4 Pan-metatarsal head resection.

Metatarsal Surgery

This can be divided into two classes of surgery: isolated metatarsal surgery and panmetatarsal head resection.

Blume et al. conducted at retrospective study of 67 diabetic patients who had peripheral neuropathy and ulcer without osteomyelitis. All patients underwent a single-stage osseous procedure (arthroplasty, exostectomy, phalangectomy, planing, etc.) of the forefoot, midfoot, or rearfoot, with primary closure with local flaps. Ultimately, 97% of the ulcers healed after surgery, and 96% were healed 20 weeks after surgery. The most common complications were wound dehiscence (18%), infection (12%), skin slough (9%), and fracture/Charcot collapse (6%). They report a low rate of transfer or recurrence 11.9% (8/67) after at least 22 months of follow-up (64).

Rosenblum et al. excised 22 metatarsal heads and performed 15 metatarsal osteotomies and 5 panmetatarsal head resections in 42 feet that had recently undergone lower extremity revascularization procedures [aortobifemoral bypass (1), bypass to the popliteal (8), tibial/peroneal (20), dorsalis pedis/plantar artery (13)]. Eighty-three percent (35/42) healed primarily and maintained an ulcer-free foot and patent bypass grafts during the 21-month follow-up period. Two patients (5%) required a revision of the original foot surgery to heal, and three patients (7%) experienced transfer lesions and had a secondary procedure to obtain an ulcer-free foot. One patient required a below-knee amputation secondary to a thrombosed graft and ischemia, and one patient died 6 months after foot surgery and before his ulcer had healed. Ultimately, 40 (95%) went on to heal with no recurrence in the follow-up period (65).

Giurini et al. retrospectively analyzed 34 panmetatarsal head resections in patients with diabetes and a forefoot ulcer (66). Thirty-two feet healed primarily, 1 healed slowly with secondary intention, and 1 had a recurrent ulcer. Ultimately, 97% of the ulcers healed and remained ulcer-free for an average of 20.9 months.

Patients with neuropathic diabetic ulcers and peripheral vascular disease can successfully undergo therapeutic surgical procedures to heal foot ulcers if they undergo distal bypass grafts to improve pedal perfusion (level B).

ANKLE JOINT EQUINUS

Equinus deformity (reduced dorsiflexion) at the ankle joint has been associated with high pressures on the plantar aspect of the foot and increased risk of foot ulceration in persons with diabetes (67). For instance, diabetic patients with equinus were three times more likely to have elevated foot pressures compared with diabetic patients without equinus (67,68).

Grant et al. (69) noted a disorganized structure of the Achilles tendon in patients with diabetes compared with persons without diabetes, by using electron microscopy. He identified increased packing density of collagen fibrils, decreases in fibrillar diameter, and abnormal fibril morphology (69). A recent study confirmed Achilles tendinopathy in 89% of patients with diabetes mellitus, via ultrasound evaluation (70). Advanced glycation end products have been suggested to alter the biomechanical properties of soft tissues, resulting in stiffness and reduced flexibility (71). Reddy demonstrated that glycation of the tendon contributes to abnormal biomechanical properties by increasing tensile strength, Young's modulus of elasticity, energy absorption, and toughness in an in vitro study with New Zealand white rabbit Achilles tendons (72). If this same

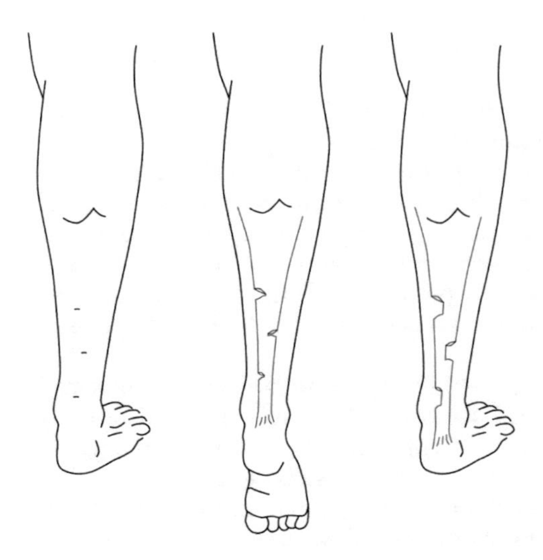

Figure 5 Percutaneous Achilles tendon lengthening.

process occurs in humans with diabetes, advanced glycation end products could shorten and stiffen the Achilles tendon. In gait, this would reduce the time of heel contact and subsequently increase the duration of peak forefoot pressure.

Achilles Tendon Lengthening

To address this deformity in patients with recalcitrant forefoot ulcers, several authors have surgically lengthened the Achilles tendon. Several approaches can be used to lengthen the Achilles tendon: endoscopic or open gastrocnemius recession, Z-lengthening of the Achilles tendon, and percutaneous Achilles tendon lengthening (ATL).

The most common procedure described in the medical literature in patients with diabetes is the percutaneous ATL. Percutaneous ATL is simple to perform and can be done with local anesthesia (Fig. 5). Many patients who would be considered for the procedure have severe neuropathy, and regional pain during the procedure is obscured by neuropathy. The incisions are small and performed on the posterior aspect of the leg, so difficulty healing the surgical incisions because of poor perfusion is uncommon.

Lengthening the Achilles tendon is indicated when reduced ankle joint dorsiflexion is limited by a short Achilles tendon. Ankle joint motion is measured with the long axis of the goniometer along the fibula and the fifth metatarsal bone. The patient should be supine with the knee extended. The subtalar joint should be in neutral position, and the foot should be dorsiflexed on the lower leg (Figure 6). Ankle joint equinus deformity has been defined in different ways from, "a plantarflexed sagittal plane attitude of foot to leg with maximum ankle joint dorsiflexion" to, less than 15° of "normal" dorsiflexion (73–75). While few people would argue an inability to bring the foot out of a plantarflexed position is normal function of the ankle joint, there is no evidence that suggests how much ankle dorsiflexion is necessary to avoid a pathologic condition. In our practice, we usually consider patients with less than 5° of dorsiflexion as candidates for Achilles tendon lengthening procedures (level D).

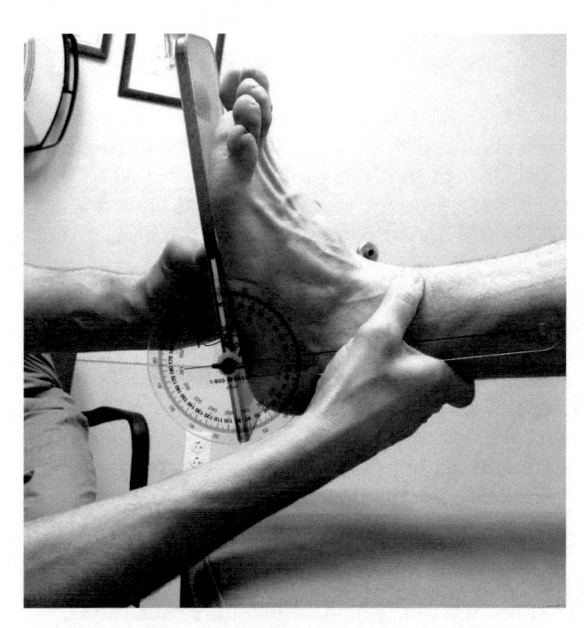

Figure 6 Ankle joint dorsiflexion measurement.

It is crucial to determine the etiology of the ankle joint equinus deformity, because it may be due to osteoarthritis. In this situation, the osseous structures of the ankle limit its motion. Clearly, an ATL will not improve ankle joint dorsiflexion for these patients.

Holstein et al. stressed the importance of evaluating the severity of sensory neuropathy particularly of the heel pad before proceeding with an ATL. They defined complete anesthesia of the heel as the inability to feel the 10 g monofilament or a sharp or dull instrument firmly applied to the heel and suggested that an ATL is contraindicated in such patients. They came to this conclusion because 47% of their patients who met the criteria of complete anesthesia developed heel ulcers postoperatively (76).

The ATL procedure has a growing body of evidence that supports its clinical effectiveness and documents potential complications. The surgical approach has been shown to have low morbidity in selected patients, to be an effective procedure to heal recalcitrant forefoot ulcers, and to reduce the high rate of reulceration observed in persons with diabetes. The procedure is especially valuable in patients who have failed conservative therapy or have recurrent ulcers with contracture of the Achilles.

Mueller and colleagues performed the only randomized clinical trial assessing the effectiveness of ATL versus a TCC control in healing DFUs (68). The criterion for the surgery was ankle dorsiflexion less than 5°, recurrent or nonhealing Wagner grade II ulceration, palpable ankle pulse, and neuropathy. All of the ATL patients healed in an average of 58 ± 47 days and 88% healed in a mean time of 41 ± 28 days in the TCC group. Average ankle joint dorsiflexion increased 15.2°, with the knee extended in the ATL group, and patients maintained this motion at their 7-month follow-up visit. There was no change in range of motion of ankle in subjects treated with casting.

Patients with an ATL have fewer recurrent foot ulcers than do controls. For instance, Mueller's randomized clinical trial showed the ulcer recurrence rate after 7 and 24 months was 15% and 38% in the ATL group and 59% and 83% in the TCC group. In addition, the average time for reulceration was significantly longer in patients who had an ATL (431 days) compared with the TCC group (131 days) (68) (level A).

Armstrong et al. reported a 27% reduction in forefoot pressures in 10 patients with diabetes and a healed foot ulcer after ATL (77). The average increase in ankle dorsiflexion was 9°. This reduced forefoot pressure helps explain the higher rates of DFU healing and lower rates of reulceration after an ATL compared with off-loading with TCCs and accommodative shoe gear.

However, an ATL is not without its complications. In addition to the completely neuropathic patients mentioned earlier, Holstein et al. reported that 18% of patients with more than 10° of ankle dorsiflexion after surgery developed a heel ulcer (76). Barry and Mueller report heel ulcers in 16% and 13% of patients after undergoing an Achilles tendon lengthening procedure (68,78). Decreasing the strength of the ankle joint plantarflexors effectively reduces the pressure on the forefoot and redistributes the pressure to the heel, which may cause an ulcer on the heel. This has been attributed to overlengthening the Achilles tendon; however, in Mueller's study, none of the patients who sustained a heel ulcer had excessive motion (9°–12° of dorsiflexion) (68).

Other potential risks associated with lengthening the Achilles tendon include infection, rupture of the tendon, and Charcot neuroarthropathy.

Postoperative care is critical to minimize these complications. If neuropathic patients are not compliant with non–weight-bearing or protected weight-bearing, they can tear or rupture the Achilles and over-lengthen the tendon. Immobilization in a TCC after Achilles tendon lengthening accomplishes several important goals. It reduces patients' activity, and it forces them to be compliant with off-loading. Armstrong et al. used activity monitors in patients treated with casts, removable cast walkers, and healing sandals to demonstrate a significant reduction in the number of steps taken in the TCC group compared with the healing sandal group. In addition, patients in the removable cast walker group removed their off-loading device, so the majority of their activities were full–weight-bearing on the ulcerated extremity (79). Crutches, walkers, and wheelchairs should be encouraged after surgery to assist appropriate healing of the Achilles tendon and the ulcer (level B).

SUMMARY

Successfully treating patients with diabetes and foot ulcers will become more important as the incidence of young people diagnosed with type 2 diabetes increases. This trend will prolong the duration in which patients will live with the long-term effects of the disease (80). The deformed insensate foot with recalcitrant or recurrent ulcers deserves consideration and evaluation for surgical care after ensuring that the medical condition is optimized. Understanding which clinical factors put this patient population at risk for complications is central to developing effective treatment and referral protocols that will keep this patient population active and productive.

REFERENCES

1. Banting FG, Best CH. The internal secretion of the pancreas. J Lab Clin Med 1922; 7:251–266.
2. Mostaza JM, Suarez C, Manzano L, et al. Sub-clinical vascular disease in type 2 diabetic subjects: Relationship with chronic complications of diabetes and the presence of cardiovascular disease risk factors. Eur J Intern Med 2008; 19:255–260.
3. Centers for Disease Control and Prevention. National Diabetes Fact Sheet, 2007. Atlanta, Georgia: Department of Health and Human Services, 2007.
4. Margolis DJ, Kantor J, Berlin JA. Healing of diabetic neuropathic foot ulcers receiving standard treatment: A meta-analysis. Diabetes Care 1999; 22:692–695.
5. Pecoraro RE, Reiber GE, Burgess EM. Pathways to diabetic limb amputation: Basis for prevention. Diabetes Care 1990; 13:513–521.
6. Reiber GE, Vileikyte L, Boyko EJ, et al. Causal pathways for incident lower-extremity ulcers in patients with diabetes from two settings. Diabetes Care 1999; 22:157–162.
7. Armstrong DG, Lavery LA. Elevated peak plantar pressures in patients who have Charcot arthropathy. J Bone Joint Surg Am 1998; 80:365–369.
8. The effect of intensive treatment of diabetes on the development and progression of long-term complications in insulin-dependent diabetes mellitus: The Diabetes Control and Complications Trial Research Group. N Engl J Med 1993; 329:977–986.
9. Lavery LA, Harkless LB, Ashry HR, et al. Infected puncture wounds in adults with diabetes: Risk factors for osteomyelitis. J Foot Ankle Surg 1994; 33:561–566.
10. Lavery LA, Armstrong DG, Wunderlich RP, et al. Risk factors for foot infections in individuals with diabetes. Diabetes Care 2006; 29:1288–1293.
11. Lavery LA, Armstrong DG, Wunderlich RP, et al. Diabetic foot syndrome: Evaluating the prevalence and incidence of foot pathology in Mexican Americans and non-Hispanic whites from a diabetes disease management cohort. Diabetes Care 2003; 26:1435–1438.
12. Winkley K, Stahl D, Chalder T, et al. Risk factors associated with adverse outcomes in a population-based prospective cohort study of people with their first diabetic foot ulcer. J Diabetes Complications 2007; 21:341–349.
13. Jeffcoate WJ, Chipchase SY, Ince P, et al. Assessing the outcome of the management of diabetic foot ulcers using ulcer-related and person-related measures. Diabetes Care 2006; 29:1784–1787.
14. Dargis V, Pantelejeva O, Jonushaite A, et al. Benefits of a multidisciplinary approach in the management of recurrent diabetic foot ulceration in Lithuania: A prospective study. Diabetes Care 1999; 22:1428–1431.
15. Edmonds ME, Blundell MP, Morris ME, et al. Improved survival of the diabetic foot: The role of a specialized foot clinic. Q J Med 1986; 60:763–771.
16. Uccioli L, Faglia E, Monticone G, et al. Manufactured shoes in the prevention of diabetic foot ulcers. Diabetes Care 1995; 18:1376–1378.
17. Lavery LA, Peters EJ, Williams JR, et al. Reevaluating the way we classify the diabetic foot: Restructuring the diabetic foot risk classification system of the International Working Group on the Diabetic Foot. Diabetes Care 2008; 31:154–156.
18. Norgren L, Hiatt WR, Dormandy JA, et al. Inter-Society Consensus for the Management of Peripheral Arterial Disease (TASC II). J Vasc Surg 2007; 45(suppl S): S5–S67.
19. Fowkes FG, Housley E, Cawood EH, et al. Edinburgh Artery Study: Prevalence of asymptomatic and symptomatic peripheral arterial disease in the general population. Int J Epidemiol 1991; 20:384–392.
20. O'Hare AM, Vittinghoff E, Hsia J, et al. Renal insufficiency and the risk of lower extremity peripheral arterial disease: Results from the Heart and Estrogen/Progestin Replacement Study (HERS). J Am Soc Nephrol 2004; 15:1046–1051.
21. Ridker PM, Stampfer MJ, Rifai N. Novel risk factors for systemic atherosclerosis: A comparison of C-reactive protein, fibrinogen, homocysteine, lipoprotein(a), and standard cholesterol screening as predictors of peripheral arterial disease. JAMA 2001; 285:2481–2485.

22. Senti M, Nogues X, Pedro-Botet J, et al. Lipoprotein profile in men with peripheral vascular disease: Role of intermediate density lipoproteins and apoprotein E phenotypes. Circulation 1992; 85:30–36.
23. Criqui MH, Vargas V, Denenberg JO, et al. Ethnicity and peripheral arterial disease: The San Diego Population Study. Circulation 2005; 112:2703–2707.
24. Muntner P, Wildman RP, Reynolds K, et al. Relationship between HbA1c level and peripheral arterial disease. Diabetes Care 2005; 28:1981–1987.
25. Selvin E, Marinopoulos S, Berkenblit G, et al. Meta-analysis: Glycosylated hemoglobin and cardiovascular disease in diabetes mellitus. Ann Intern Med 2004; 141: 421–431.
26. Brem H, Sheehan P, Rosenberg HJ, et al. Evidence-based protocol for diabetic foot ulcers. Plast Reconstr Surg 2006; 117:193S–209S, discussion 1910S–1911S.
27. Fowkes FG, Murray GD, Butcher I, et al. Ankle brachial index combined with Framingham Risk Score to predict cardiovascular events and mortality: A meta-analysis. JAMA 2008; 300:197–208.
28. Dickhaut SC, DeLee JC, Page CP. Nutritional status: Importance in predicting wound-healing after amputation. J Bone Joint Surg Am 1984; 66:71–75.
29. Wagner FW Jr. Amputations of the foot and ankle: Current status. Clin Orthop Relat Res 1977; (122):62–69.
30. Pinzur MS, Stuck RM, Sage R, et al. Syme ankle disarticulation in patients with diabetes. J Bone Joint Surg Am 2003; 85-A:1667–1672.
31. Hirsch AT, Haskal ZJ, Hertzer NR, et al. ACC/AHA 2005 guidelines for the management of patients with peripheral arterial disease (lower extremity, renal, mesenteric, and abdominal aortic): Executive summary a collaborative report from the American Association for Vascular Surgery/Society for Vascular Surgery, Society for Cardiovascular Angiography and Interventions, Society for Vascular Medicine and Biology, Society of Interventional Radiology, and the ACC/AHA Task Force on Practice Guidelines (Writing Committee to Develop Guidelines for the Management of Patients With Peripheral Arterial Disease) endorsed by the American Association of Cardiovascular and Pulmonary Rehabilitation; National Heart, Lung, and Blood Institute; Society for Vascular Nursing; TransAtlantic Inter-Society Consensus; and Vascular Disease Foundation. J Am Coll Cardiol 2006; 47:1239–1312.
32. Bril V. NIS-LL: The primary measurement scale for clinical trial endpoints in diabetic peripheral neuropathy. Eur Neurol 1999; 41(suppl 1):8–13.
33. Dyck PJ, Melton LJ III, O'Brien PC, et al. Approaches to improve epidemiological studies of diabetic neuropathy: Insights from the Rochester Diabetic Neuropathy Study. Diabetes 1997; 46(suppl 2):S5–S8.
34. Olaleye D, Perkins BA, Bril V. Evaluation of three screening tests and a risk assessment model for diagnosing peripheral neuropathy in the diabetes clinic. Diabetes Res Clin Pract 2001; 54:115–128.
35. Armstrong DG, Lavery LA, Vela SA, et al. Choosing a practical screening instrument to identify patients at risk for diabetic foot ulceration. Arch Intern Med 1998; 158: 289–292.
36. Rosenblum BI, Giurini JM, Chrzan JS, et al. Preventing loss of the great toe with the hallux interphalangeal joint arthroplasty. J Foot Ankle Surg 1994; 33:557–560.
37. Armstrong DG, Lavery LA, Vazquez JR, et al. Clinical efficacy of the first metatarsophalangeal joint arthroplasty as a curative procedure for hallux interphalangeal joint wounds in patients with diabetes. Diabetes Care 2003; 26:3284–3287.
38. Armstrong DG, Lavery LA, Stern S, et al. Is prophylactic diabetic foot surgery dangerous? J Foot Ankle Surg 1996; 35:585–589.
39. Armstrong DG, Frykberg RG. Classifying diabetic foot surgery: Toward a rational definition. Diabet Med 2003; 20:329–331.
40. Armstrong DG, Lavery LA, Harkless LB. Treatment-based classification system for assessment and care of diabetic feet. J Am Podiatr Med Assoc 1996; 86:311–316.
41. Birke JA, Sims DS. Plantar sensory threshold in the ulcerative foot. Lepr Rev 1986; 57:261–267.

42. Armstrong DG, Lavery LA, Harkless LB. Validation of a diabetic wound classification system: The contribution of depth, infection, and ischemia to risk of amputation. Diabetes Care 1998; 21:855–859.
43. Gudas CJ. Prophylactic surgery in the diabetic foot. Clin Podiatr Med Surg 1987; 4:445–458.
44. Armstrong DG, Lavery LA, Frykberg RG, et al. Validation of a diabetic foot surgery classification. Int Wound J 2006; 3:240–246.
45. Boffeli TJ, Bean JK, Natwick JR. Biomechanical abnormalities and ulcers of the great toe in patients with diabetes. J Foot Ankle Surg 2002; 41:359–364.
46. Laborde JM. Neuropathic toe ulcers treated with toe flexor tenotomies. Foot Ankle Int 2007; 28:1160–1164.
47. Lin SS, Bono CM, Lee TH. Total contact casting and Keller arthoplasty for diabetic great toe ulceration under the interphalangeal joint. Foot Ankle Int 2000; 21:588–593.
48. Downs DM, Jacobs RL. Treatment of resistant ulcers on the plantar surface of the great toe in diabetics. J Bone Joint Surg Am 1982; 64:930–933.
49. Vallier GT, Petersen SA, LaGrone MO. The Keller resection arthroplasty: A 13-year experience. Foot Ankle 1991; 11:187–194.
50. Stewart J, Reed JF III. An audit of Keller arthroplasty and metatarsophalangeal joint arthrodesis from national data. Int J Low Extrem Wounds 2003; 2:69–73.
51. Reiber GE, Boyko EJ, Smith DG. Lower extremity foot ulcers and amputations in diabetes. In: Harris M, ed. Diabetes in America. 2nd ed. Bethesda, MD: National Institutes of Health, 1995:409–428.
52. Singh N, Armstrong DG, Lipsky BA. Preventing foot ulcers in patients with diabetes. JAMA 2005; 293:217–228.
53. Young MJ, Breddy JL, Veves A, et al. The prediction of diabetic neuropathic foot ulceration using vibration perception thresholds: A prospective study. Diabetes Care 1994; 17:557–560.
54. Boyko EJ, Ahroni JH, Stensel V, et al. A prospective study of risk factors for diabetic foot ulcer: The Seattle Diabetic Foot Study. Diabetes Care 1999; 22:1036–1042.
55. Tamir E, McLaren AM, Gadgil A, et al. Outpatient percutaneous flexor tenotomies for management of diabetic claw toe deformities with ulcers: A preliminary report. Can J Surg 2008; 51:41–44.
56. Leung PC. Diabetic foot ulcers—A comprehensive review. Surgeon 2007; 5:219–231.
57. McGlamry ED, Jimenez AL, Green DR. Lesser ray deformities. In: Banks AS, Downey MS, Martin DE, et al., eds. McGlamry's Comprehesive Textbook of Foot and Ankle Surgery. 3rd ed. Philadelphia, PA: Lippincott Williams & Wilkins, 2001:268–269.
58. Padanilam TG. The flexible hammer toe flexor-to-extensor transfer. Foot Ankle Clin 1998; 3:259–267.
59. Schrier JC, Verheyen CC, Louwerens JW. Definitions of hammer toe and claw toe: An evaluation of the literature. J Am Podiatr Med Assoc 2009; 99:194–197.
60. Kim JY, Kim TW, Park YE, et al. Modified resection arthroplasty for infected non-healing ulcers with toe deformity in diabetic patients. Foot Ankle Int 2008; 29:493–497.
61. Mueller MJ, Minor SD, Diamond JE, et al. Relationship of foot deformity to ulcer location in patients with diabetes mellitus. Phys Ther 1990; 70:356–362.
62. Mueller MJ, Hastings M, Commean PK, et al. Forefoot structural predictors of plantar pressures during walking in people with diabetes and peripheral neuropathy. J Biomech 2003; 36:1009–1017.
63. Griffiths GD, Wieman TJ. Metatarsal head resection for diabetic foot ulcers. Arch Surg 1990; 125:832–835.
64. Blume PA, Paragas LK, Sumpio BE, et al. Single-stage surgical treatment of noninfected diabetic foot ulcers. Plast Reconstr Surg 2002; 109:601–609.
65. Rosenblum BI, Pomposelli FB Jr, Giurini JM, et al. Maximizing foot salvage by a combined approach to foot ischemia and neuropathic ulceration in patients with diabetes: A 5-year experience. Diabetes Care 1994; 17:983–987.
66. Giurini JM, Basile P, Chrzan JS, et al. Panmetatarsal head resection: A viable alternative to the transmetatarsal amputation. J Am Podiatr Med Assoc 1993; 83:101–107.

67. Lavery LA, Armstrong DG, Boulton AJ. Ankle equinus deformity and its relationship to high plantar pressure in a large population with diabetes mellitus. J Am Podiatr Med Assoc 2002; 92:479–482.
68. Mueller MJ, Sinacore DR, Hastings MK, et al. Effect of Achilles tendon lengthening on neuropathic plantar ulcers: A randomized clinical trial. J Bone Joint Surg Am 2003; 85-A:1436–1445.
69. Grant WP, Sullivan R, Sonenshine DE, et al. Electron microscopic investigation of the effects of diabetes mellitus on the Achilles tendon. J Foot Ankle Surg 1997; 36:272–278, discussion 330.
70. Batista F, Nery C, Pinzur M, et al. Achilles tendinopathy in diabetes mellitus. Foot Ankle Int 2008; 29:498–501.
71. Rosenthal AK, Gohr CM, Mitton E, et al. Advanced glycation end products increase transglutaminase activity in primary porcine tenocytes. J Investig Med 2009; 57: 460–466.
72. Reddy GK. Glucose-mediated in vitro glycation modulates biomechanical integrity of the soft tissues but not hard tissues. J Orthop Res 2003; 21:738–743.
73. DiGiovanni CW, Kuo R, Tejwani N, et al. Isolated gastrocnemius tightness. J Bone Joint Surg Am 2002; 84-A:962–970.
74. Morton DJ. The Human Foot. New York, NY: Columbia University Press, 1935.
75. Michael SD. Ankle equinus. In: Banks AS, Downey MS, Martin DE, et al., eds. McGlamry's Comprehensive Textbook of Foot and Ankle Surgery. 3rd ed. Philadelphia, PA: Lippincott Williams & Wilkins, 2001:715–760.
76. Holstein P, Lohmann M, Bitsch M, et al. Achilles tendon lengthening, the panacea for plantar forefoot ulceration? Diabetes Metab Res Rev 2004; 20(suppl 1):S37–S40.
77. Armstrong DG, Stacpoole-Shea S, Nguyen H, et al. Lengthening of the Achilles tendon in diabetic patients who are at high risk for ulceration of the foot. J Bone Joint Surg Am 1999; 81:535–538.
78. Barry DC, Sabacinski KA, Habershaw GM, et al. Tendo Achillis procedures for chronic ulcerations in diabetic patients with transmetatarsal amputations. J Am Podiatr Med Assoc 1993; 83:96–100.
79. Armstrong DG, Lavery LA, Kimbriel HR, et al. Activity patterns of patients with diabetic foot ulceration: patients with active ulceration may not adhere to a standard pressure off-loading regimen. Diabetes Care 2003; 26:2595–2597.
80. Greene S. Diabetes in the young: What are their long term health prospects? Arch Dis Child 2009; 94:251–253.

11 Charcot arthropathy

Javier La Fontaine

EPIDEMIOLOGY

In 1968, Jean-Martin Charcot described neuroarthropathy in the foot in relation to tabes dorsalis (1). He proposed the first theory in how this process may occur. In 1936, Jordan was the first to described Charcot in diabetes (2). Charcot neuroarthropathy is a disabling and devastating condition. Although the cause of this potentially debilitating condition is not known, it is generally accepted that the components of diabetic neuropathy that lead to foot complications must exist. Untreated Charcot arthropathy may lead to a rocker bottom foot, which will lead to increased plantar pressure in the neuropathic foot. This cascade will lead to an ulceration and possible amputation. A recent study shows, however, that Charcot arthropathy alone may not pose a risk for amputation, but Charcot arthropathy along with an ulceration has 12 times increased risk of having an amputation (3).

The incidence of Charcot neuroarthropathy is about 0.1 to 5% in diabetic neuropathy (4) (level B). Fabrin et al. found an incidence of 0.3% in diabetic population (5) (level B). It seems to be a relationship in the duration of diabetes and the incidence of Charcot neuroarthropathy. Eighty percent of the cases occur in patients with diabetes for more than 15 years and 60% of the cases in patients with diabetes for more than 10 years. The prevalence of Charcot arthropathy ranges from 0.08% to 8.5%. Frequently, this pathology occurs between fifth and sixth decade, with a mean age of 50.3 years (6) (level A) and no difference between genders. Although it is more common unilaterally, it can involve both extremities in up to 39% of the cases. The incidence of ulceration was 17% per year (7). Mortality in this population is comparable with the population with uncomplicated neuropathic ulcer, and it is considered high, which ranges from 42% to 63% (8).

CLASSIFICATION AND STAGING

There are different types of classifications to describe Charcot arthropathy. Most classifications are inconsistent, since they have a wide spectrum of descriptions that use radiographical changes, clinical locations, and/or patterns of destruction. None of the classifications suggests a possible treatments or prognostic factors. The first classification was described by Eichenholtz in 1966 (9). This classification uses three clinical and radiological stages of progression: the stage of development, the stage of coalescence, and the stage of reconstruction. The stage of development or stage 1 is defined by periarticular debris formation and fragmentation of subchondral bone and by joint subluxation and dislocation. Clinically, the foot is warm, erythematous, edematous, painful, and with bounding pulses. In most occasions, the affected limb needs to be compared with the contralateral limb to appreciate the erythematous changes.

During the coalescent stage, or stage 2, the large bone fragments become fused and united with bone adjacent bones. Absorption of small debris is noticeable as well. Eichenholtz suggested that the sclerotic changes at the end of bones are produced by lack of vascularity. Clinically, a stage 2 foot will present with decreased warmth and swelling, but instability of the joints may continue. Finally, the stage of reconstruction, or stage 3, is characterized by bone consolidation and rounding of bone fragments. As revascularization occurs, there is a decrease in sclerosis. Clinically, the foot will have no warmth or erythema but will continue to be swollen as the patient recovers.

In 1990, Shibata proposed a stage 0 or pre-Charcot stage (10). The authors described a sudden onset, warmth, and erythema in the neuropathic patient with diabetes. Normal anatomy or joint distention may be observed radiologically. In 1999, Sella and Barette revisited Eichenholtz classification and elaborated the classification by describing in detail the deformities through progression rather than destructive radiologic findings (11). Forty patients with 51 neuropathic feet were evaluated. They were able to identify five stages of Charcot deformities. Stage 0 is a clinical stage in which the patient presents with a locally swollen, warm, and often painful foot. Radiographs are negative (Fig. 1) and technetium-99 bone scan is markedly positive. Indium and gallium scans are normal. Stage 1, in addition to the clinical findings, demonstrates periarticular cysts, erosions, localized osteopenia, and sometimes diastases (Fig. 2). Stage 2 is marked by joint subluxations, usually starting between the second cuneiform and the base of the second metatarsal and spreading laterally (Fig. 3). Stage 3 is identified by stable joint dislocation and arch collapse and, therefore, a stable end result of the process. Clinically, there is no temperature gradient between the two feet. Radiographically, there is bony trabeculation across joint spaces indicative of mature fusion (Fig. 4).

According to Sanders and Frykberg, reporting their findings in 1991, the most common location involved in the foot are tarsometatarsal joint (30%), metatarsophalangeal joint (30%), followed by the tarsal joints (24%), ankle joint

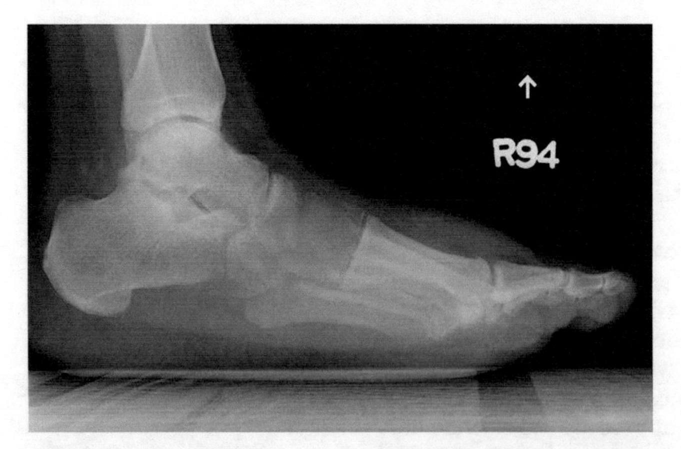

Figure 1 Stage 0 Charcot foot; note decrease osseous density in the medial cuneiform and distal aspect of navicular.

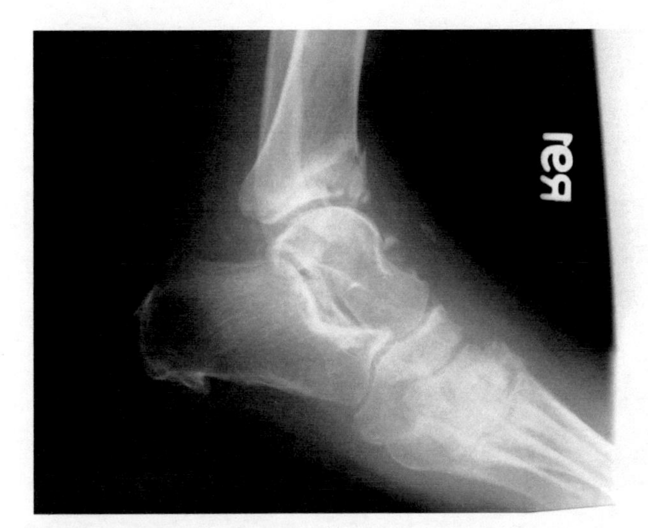

Figure 2 Stage 1 Charcot foot; fragmentation and erosive changes at the ankle joint are key findings in this stage.

(11%), and interphalangeal joint (4%) (12). In 1997, Armstrong et al. found that 48% of Charcot events were located at the Lisfranc joint, followed by 34% in the Chopart joint, 13% in the ankle joint, 3% in forefoot joints, and 2% in posterior calcaneus. This retrospective study used two treatment-oriented phases based on radiographic, dermal thermometry, and clinical signs. Another classification by location was described by Brodsky and Rouse in 1993 (13). The classification detailed four types of involvement where joint destruction may occur: the

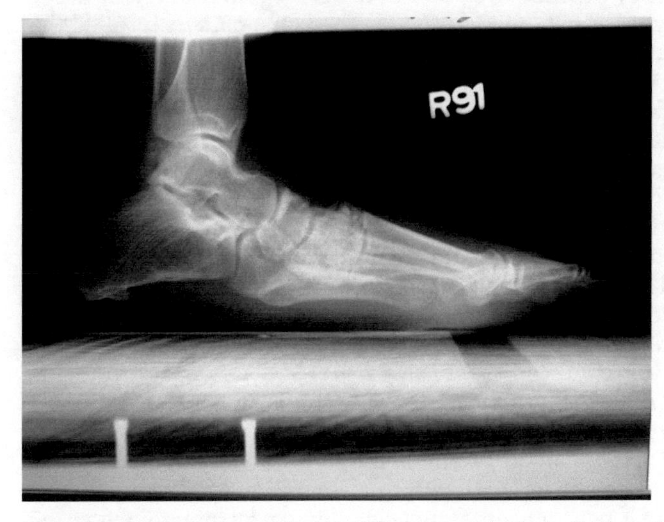

Figure 3 Stage 2 Charcot foot; bossing and periarticular fusion of osseous fragments is a clinical sign of coalescence.

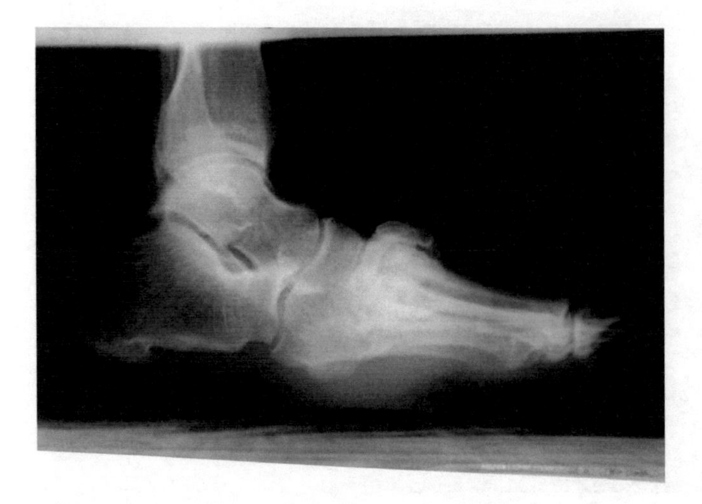

Figure 4 Stage 3 Charcot foot; note osseous bridging across the tarsometatarsal joint indicating a stable deformity.

midfoot, hindfoot, ankle, and posterior calcaneus. However, this classification resembles previous ones, and it was described in 12 subjects.

There are three classifications that describe patterns of destruction in Charcot arthropathy. The first classification was described by Harris and Brand in 1966 (14). They describe the stress distribution from the extremity leads to disintegration of different joints in the foot. The authors made the association that the insensate foot that goes under the process of "disintegration" is often warmer than the normal foot. They describe five patterns of disintegration that may occur to the insensate foot when is exposed to trauma. These are: pattern 1, called the posterior pillar with calcaneus collapse; pattern 2, central (body of talus) with collapse of the talus due to the incongruity of the subtalar joint; pattern 3, anterior pillar (medial arch), which involves medial arch collapse or forefoot collapse; pattern 4, anterior pillar (lateral arch), which authors relate that may be involved with sepsis and the most dangerous deformity; and pattern 5, cuneiforms-metatarsal base, which, in their observation, was uncommon and easily treated with immobilization. Subsequently, Schon, in 1998, describes in a complex classification the pattern of destruction of Charcot arthropathy in which detailed multiple locations and patterns involved Lisfrancs pattern, naviculocuneiform pattern, perinavicular pattern, and transverse tarsal pattern (15). This complex description resembles closely what the clinician encounter when treating this pathology. The best study describing pattern of destruction and proposing risk factors for poor outcomes is the prospective study done by Serbst et al. in 2004 (16) (level A). They followed 55 patients prospectively and classified patients by injury (fracture, dislocation, or combination) and by location (ankle, hindfoot, midfoot, and forefoot). They also measured bone mineral density (BMD) with dual-energy x-ray absorptiometry (DEXA). They found that poor outcomes associated with fracture involving the ankle and forefoot. They noticed that this pattern was associated with osteopenia as well.

CLINICAL ASSESSMENT AND IMAGING

The general consensus is that in order to develop Charcot arthropathy, the patient has to be neuropathic. Currently, diabetes is the main cause for neuropathy in the lower extremity. Factors such as osteopenia, equinus, peripheral vascular disease, and nephropathy have also been described as risk factors for Charcot arthropathy.

Although the cause of this potentially debilitating condition is not known, a number of theories have been proposed:

- Following the development of autonomic neuropathy, there is an increased blood flow to the extremity, resulting in increased bone reabsorption and osteopenia.
- Following sensor-motor neuropathy, the resulting sensory loss and muscle imbalance induces abnormal stress in the bones and joints of the affected limb, leading to bone destruction (17).
- Stretching of the ligaments due to joint effusion may lead to joint subluxation (18).

PATHOGENESIS

The pathogenesis of Charcot neuroarthropathy is not clear. There are two etiological theories to the development of Charcot arthropathy: the neurovascular theory or French theory and the neurotraumatic theory or German theory. The neurovascular theory was developed by Charcot in 1868 (1). After studying more than 5000 chronically ill patients, Charcot concluded the profound joint destruction and deformities were secondary to changes in the trophic centers of the spinal cord, specifically the diseased anterior horn cells, which resulted in neurogenic and circulatory disruption. Therefore, an autonomic nervous system dysfunction causes a hyperemic demineralization leading to osteopenia. Edelman et al. observed three cases where neuropathic osteoarthropathy developed 2 to 5 years after lower limb revascularization (19). However, Shapiro et al. conducted a study where blood flow was measured with Doppler with local skin warming in patients with Charcot arthropathy and neuropathy and in healthy patients (20). Increasing local skin temperature increased skin blood flow and vasomotion in healthy and patients with Charcot arthropathy but not in patients with diabetes and neuropathy. They concluded that blood flow in the controls and patients with Charcot arthropathy, despite the extent of neuropathy, was intact. The loss of peripheral blood flow and vasomotion in patients with diabetes and neuropathy could be protective against Charcot arthropathy.

The neurotraumatic theory or the German theory was described in 1870 by Volkman (21). The theory is based on the rationale that unperceived trauma or injuries to an insensate joint will lead to stress fractures. This results in progressive and permanent damage to the bone and joints in the foot, forming a problematic biomechanical foot.

Charcot feet develop an increase in vertical pressures and shear stress. The amount of soft tissue insult depends on the level of neuropathy, the amount of stress, and the activity level of the patient. Equinus deformity has also been noted to cause the triceps surae to plantarflex the foot and increase the pressure over the metatarsophalangeal joint and increase stress at the tarsometatarsal and midtarsal joints. In 1998, Armstrong and Lavery reviewed 21 diabetic patients who had acute Charcot arthropathy and others with neuropathic ulcers; the peak plantar pressure was noted at the level of the metatarsal heads or distally (22). Peak plantar pressures were higher in acute those with Charcot arthropathy than in those with neuropathic ulcer. The site of maximum involvement in those with Charcot arthropathy was the midfoot, but the peak plantar pressure was on the forefoot, suggesting that the forefoot may function as a lever, causing midfoot collapse.

To understand the pathogenesis of Charcot arthropathy, we need to understand that this pathology may present as acute or chronic. Most commonly, an acute presentation of the patient presents with erythematous, warm, edematous foot. The most common complaint is pain (23). Usually, patients will not recall an injury. For example, a sudden increase in activity may illicit an inflammatory response, which if not treated, will lead to Charcot arthropathy. Clinically, patients demonstrate significant neuropathy with bounding pulses. If patients do not seek treatment immediately, the foot will collapse, giving the appearance of a "rocker bottom". When presentation is chronic, a midfoot ulcer may become evident. Although the classic description of a Charcot foot is a rocker bottom foot, other deformities such as ankle dislocation, abduction of the forefoot, and dislocated metatarsophalangeal joints can be evident. Also, the chronic Charcot may present with pain as neuropathic patient often become hyperesthetic or the joint destruction may involve proximal joints, where the sensory fibers are not damaged.

DIAGNOSTIC MODALITIES

There are few diagnostic modalities that can be used to diagnose this entity. Often, Charcot arthropathy is a clinical diagnosis supported by testing to rule out other disease processes such as bone infection and deep venous thrombosis. The clinical presentation usually involves unilateral swelling of the foot, ankle, and leg with no known trauma in patients with sensory neuropathy. In many cases, ultrasound is initially performed in the emergency department to rule out a deep venous thrombosis.

Skin temperature changes are the most accurate tool to diagnosis and monitor the progression of Charcot neuropathy. Patients with acute Charcot experienced increased temperature of the affected foot compared with the contralateral foot. Skin temperature of approximately 4°F should be carefully assessed and off-loaded until normalization of temperatures (23).

Laboratory studies can be helpful when the diagnosis of Charcot arthropathy is not clear. White blood cell (WBC) count with differential count and erythrocyte sedimentation rate (ESR) can help distinguish between acute Charcot arthropathy and an acute soft tissue or bone infection, but these are nonspecific markers for inflammation (24). Kaleta et al. showed the ESR is highly predictive of osteomyelitis (25). A retrospective review of 29 diabetic patients with diagnosis of osteomyelitis or cellulitis of the foot was followed for 1 year. The ESR was the only measure that significantly differed between the groups. An optimal cut off value of 70 mm/h was a level above which osteomyelitis was present with the highest sensitivity (89.5%) and specificity (100%), along with a positive predictive value of 100% and negative predictive value of 83%. A comprehensive metabolic profile may be useful to assess the general health status of the patient. For instance, serum creatinine level will provide a reference for renal function, and increase in serum glucose level will raise concern about diabetes control. Serum levels of alkaline phophatase, calcium, phosphorous, parathyroid hormone, pyridinoline, and deoxypyridinoline can identify bone diseases. Pyridinoline and, specifically, deoxypyridinoline are the most useful markers available today in measuring bone resorption.

PATHOPHYSIOLOGY

By convention, most textbooks suggest that Charcot primarily occurs in patients with adequate blood flow to the foot. Other studies suggest that there is usually adequate large vessel perfusion to the foot with arterial venous shunting associated with autonomic neuropathy that alters the microcirculation. In addition, metabolic and vascular insulin resistance in Charcot patients is thought to lead to early changes in endothelial function. A dysfunctional endothelium compromises the regulation of blood flow and pressure, facilitates cell migration, and proliferation, and an inflammatory response ensues. Lipid deposition and formation of reactive oxygen species contribute to enhance this process and structural changes progress to plaque formation. Vascular wall atheromas may rupture, and intraluminal clotting with platelet adhesion leads to occlusion and distal ischemia.

Several authors have suggested that an exaggerated inflammatory response in diabetes may be associated with Charcot arthropathy. It has been recognized for a hundred years that sympathetic denervation is associated with distal hyperemia (inflammation) and impaired vasoconstriction in patients with Charcot neuroarthropathy. Young went a step further and suggested an association of small fiber neuropathy with increased osteoclast activity, resulting in a reduced BMD and increased Charcot fracture risk (26). Sinacore suggested that the prolonged inflammatory response observed in Charcot neuroarthropathy contributes to osteolysis and loss of BMD in the calcaneus (27). He compared 22 patients with diabetes, neuropathy, and midfoot deformities with 29 healthy controls. The control group's BMD was 13% higher than that of those with diabetes and neuropathy. Among those with diabetes, BMD was 16% lower in the involved foot compared with the uninvolved foot without deformity.

For a Charcot arthropathy to develop, significant sensory loss must exist. It has been speculated that loss of vascular tone may lead to decrease bone mineralization.

The extent to which abnormal vasodilatation and inappropriate microvascular tone control contribute to the development of the Charcot arthropathy has not yet been defined. The loss of BMD as a result of increased bone turnover, similar to that of osteoporosis, has been demonstrated in diabetic patients (26) (level B). These investigators found that there was a significant reduction in the BMD of the lower limbs with Charcot arthropathy and that this was greater in the affected limb. Also, it has been reported that patients with type 1 and type 2 diabetes have decreased BMD when compared with age- and sex-matched control subjects and that this might predispose to increased fracture risk (28) (level B). Therefore, a decrease in vascular tone and decrease in BMD may predispose neuropathic patients to develop Charcot arthropathy.

Petrova suggested that osteopenia may be found at presentation in the contralateral, unaffected foot in those with type 1, but not type 2 diabetes (29). Baumhauer and colleagues studied bone specimens from subjects with known CN for cytokine mediators interleukin 1, tumor necrosis factor (TNF)-α, and interleukin 6 (30). They observed a moderate pattern of staining for TNF-α and interleukin 1 in osteoclasts and a diffuse pattern for interleukin 6. They hypothesized that these molecules may have a regulatory effect on osteoclasts during the remodeling phase of Charcot neuroarthropathy. Mabilleau and colleagues demonstrated increase in osteoclast formation in peripheral blood monocytes from nine patients with Charcot neuroarthropathy (31). They were compared with eight diabetic controls and eight healthy controls. The addition of receptor activator of nuclear factor κ-B ligand (RANKL) to the cultures led to marked increase in osteoclastic resorption in Charcot group. However, the addition of osteoprotegerin (OPG) and RANKL in these cultures led to an incomplete suppression of osteoclastic resorption. This suggests that there is a RANKL-independent pathway. Therefore, further research is necessary to assess the role of OPG/RANKL pathway and other pathways involved in the development of Charcot neuroarthropathy.

Jeffcoate and Mabilleau have advocated using the RANKL/OPG pathway to identify and evaluate therapies for fracture complications and Charcot neuroarthropathy (31,32). Most of the work that evaluate RANKL and OPG expression in diabetic bone has been done in streptozotocin-induced type I animal models. Animal studies show increased levels of RANKL in diabetes induced animals with tibia and femur fractures compared with controls.

RANKL and its decoy receptor, OPG, were identified. The system is a key mediator of bone metabolism, and it has been used to evaluate osteoclastogenesis and osteolytic processes in a number of disease states such as rheumatoid arthritis, osteoarthritis, bone tumors, prosthetic failure, and periodontal disease. RANKL is part of the TNF-α superfamily. Proinflammatory cytokines (TNFs and interleukins) and calciotropic hormones [parathyroid hormones, calcitonin, calcitonin gene-related peptide (CGRP)] mediate RANKL and the acute inflammatory responses following fracture. The process of bone resorption and formation is controlled by the levels of RANKL and OPG. When RANKL expression is higher in relation to that of OPG, it increases osteoclastogenesis. On the other hand, if OPG concentrations are high in relation to RANKL concentration, OPG prevents binding with RANKL receptors. Thus bone resorption will not increase. In diabetes, Charcot arthropathy is exemplified by prolonged inflammation and osteolysis that may be similar to the osteolysis observed in rheumatoid arthritis, periodontal disease, and hip implant failure.

There is emerging evidence that the nervous system and neuropeptides effect bone metabolism. One such neuropeptide is CGRP. In the peripheral nervous system, CGRP can be demonstrated in motor, sensory, and autonomic nerve fibers, particularly unmyelinated C-type and small myelinated A-δ fibers. Sensory fibers contribute to the maintenance of trabecular bone integrity through mechanisms mediated by CGRP and/or substance P, another neuropeptide product of sensory nerve fibers. In addition, ablation of CGRP results in osteopenia due to reduced osteoblastic bone formation. To investigate this possibility, La Fontaine and colleagues studied bone samples from normal subjects, subjects with diabetic neuropathy, and subjects with diabetes and CN (33). He investigated the differences of cellular components (osteoblasts and osteoclasts) in hematoxylin-eosin stains and used immunohistochemical techniques to immunolocalize CGRP and endothelial nitric oxide synthase (eNOS) in bone samples. Hematoxylin-eosin stains demonstrated increased numbers of osteoblasts and osteoclasts in bone samples from subjects with Charcot and diabetic neuropathy compared with those from normal subjects. In Charcot specimens, immunolocalization of CGRP and eNOS intensifies at the margin of trabecular bone, osteocytes, and osteoclasts cytoplasm compared with normal bone. No difference of CGRP and eNOS immunolocalization was noticeable between Charcot neuroarthropathy (CN) and Diabetic neuropathy (DN) specimens.

The authors concluded that CGRP and eNOS may regulate osteoblastic and osteoclastic activity in neuropathy.

IMAGING

Advances in radiology has provided the clinician additional tools to make the correct diagnosis. Radiographs are the most useful in diagnosing the pathology, locate the area of involvement, evaluate quality of bone, and identify whether the process is acute or chronic. If an infection is suspected, foreign bodies and soft tissue emphysema can be identified. Also, radiographs are helpful in correlating the ulcer location and the area of osteomyelitis. Charcot arthropathy is commonly mistaken for osteomyelitis even when the location of the ulcer is not near a site of the bone destruction. Bone scans are a modality that can be used to assist in diagnosis. They are more sensitive and can confirm pathology earlier, but they are not required on every patient. Triphasic technetium-99 bone scan detects bone activity early in the process. It is not very helpful in differentiating between acute Charcot arthropathy and osteomyelitis, because the specificity is very low (34). Indium-111 WBC count is more specific for infection than technetium-99 scan since WBCs accumulate in the area where the infective process is present. When an infectious process is suspected in the area of chronic Charcot arthropathy, this imaging technique may be helpful. However, in the presence of acute Charcot arthropathy, the significant inflammatory response around the soft tissue will make diagnosis difficult. In addition, leukocyte imaging included long preparation time, low count rates can result in poor spatial resolution, and the absence of bone landmarks can make it difficult to differentiate soft tissue from bone infection (35). Tc-99 HMPAO (Tc-hexamethylpropyleneamine oxime, aka *Ceretech*)–labeled leukocyte scan is a noninvasive means of determining osteomyelitis. Label patient's WBCs with hexamethylpropyleneamine from venous blood and reinject it back into patient. Images are then viewed on a gamma camera. The test is positive when focal uptake is greater in bone than soft tissue when osteomyelitis is present. Blume et al. (36) found Tc-99 HMPAO WBC sensitive for osteomyelitis at 90%, with specificity at 86%. Boc et al. (37) found that false positives do occur using the Tc-99 HMPAO test.

Sulfur colloid scanning is an innovative and useful modality for the differentiation between osteomyelitis and acute Charcot arthropathy. Leukocytes scintigraphy and bone marrow scanning have been shown to be useful in cases of osteomyelitis and underlying neuroarthropathy. Labeled leukocytes will not accumulate in regions where bone infection is present as infection infarcts bone marrow elements. On the other hand, during the process of bone resorption and bone formation in acute Charcot arthropathy, labeled leukocytes will accumulate, and the diagnosis of Charcot arthropathy can be made. Palestro and colleagues evaluated the role of combined leukocyte/marrow scintigraphy in the assessment of the neuropathic or Charcot joints (38). Seventeen patients with 20 radiographically confirmed Charcot joints underwent 99mTc-sulfur colloid marrow scintigraphy. Leukocyte/marrow studies were positive for osteomyelitis in 4 of the 20 neuropathic joints. None of the 16 neuropathic joints with negative leukocyte/marrow scans were infected. The authors concluded that labeled leukocyte accumulation in the uninfected Charcot joint did occur and was related to hematopoietically active marrow. Leukocyte/marrow scintigraphy is a reliable way to differentiate between marrow and infection as the cause of labeled leukocyte accumulation in the neuropathic joint and was superior to both three-phase bone scintigraphy and combined leukocyte/bone scintigraphy.

Magnetic resonance imaging (MRI) is a modality commonly used for the diagnosis of Charcot arthropathy. The ability of this technique to detail different types of soft tissue structures, bone marrow, and articular cartilage makes it easier to use. For instance, if a patient presents with an acute Charcot arthropathy and neuropathic ulcer that probes to bone, an MRI will be helpful because the ulcer can be identified, cortical disruption will be seen in the osseous structure below the ulcer, and an abscess may be identified as well. One of the key findings to identify bone involvement in MRI is the presence of bone edema. Studies have shown that an MRI may be very specific for Charcot arthropathy as well as for osteomyelitis. Marcus et al. (39) described key radiological signs in acute and chronic Charcot arthropathy. In acute Charcot arthropathy, decreased signal is observed in T1 and in T2. In chronic Charcot arthropathy, all images will show decreased signal. Well-differentiated cystic lesions are seen as foci of decreased signal in T1 and increased signal in T2. A comparison with indium, technetium bone scans has been done in the past. Fourteen patients (16 sites) with clinical and/or radiographic evidence of neuropathic osteoarthropathy (Charcot joints) were evaluated with combined indium-111-leukocyte (111In-WBC) and technetium-99 m-methylene diphosphonate (99mTc-MDP) bone imaging for suspected osteomyelitis. MRI scans were obtained in seven patients. Using a positive bone culture as the criterion for the presence of osteomyelitis, there were four true-positive studies, six true-negative sites, and one false-negative 111In-WBC study. Five of 16 sites (31%) had false-positive 111In-WBC uptake at noninfected sites. There were four true-positive and three false-positive MRI studies. All false-positive tests showed at least moderately abnormal findings by both techniques at sites of rapidly progressing osteoarthropathy of recent onset. In this preliminary study, both techniques appear to be sensitive for detection of osteomyelitis, and a negative study makes osteomyelitis unlikely. However, the findings of 111In-WBC/99mTc-MDP and MRI scans at sites of rapidly progressing, noninfected neuropathic osteoarthropathy may be indistinguishable from those of osteomyelitis (40).

Bone biopsy with bone culture is the most definitive diagnostic procedure. By harvesting the bone in question, sampling for culture and biopsy can be performed. The area of biopsy should be obtained away from any chronic wound. Polymorphonuclear (PMN) cells are found in patients with Charcot arthropathy, and the presence of bacteria and leukocytes are found in patient with bone infection. It is not uncommon for the bone culture and bone biopsy to give different results. The clinician will have to make a diagnosis based on history and physical examination.

OFF-LOADING

On the basis of our current knowledge of the pathologic process, the goal of the treatment is to maintain a plantigrade foot, with minimal deformity and hence no areas of increased pressure. The gold standard treatment for Charcot has been immobilization (41) (level C). The total contact cast (TCC) is often advocated as the ideal gold standard to off-load and immobilize the Charcot foot. However, treatment with the TCC is lengthy and often leads to contralateral Charcot development (23,41) (level C). Despite adequate immobilization, severe and unstable deformities develop in most patients. Therefore, to improve the clinical outcome of patients with diabetes and Charcot foot, it is necessary to better understand the pathogenesis of Charcot arthropathy.

A variety of different types of treatment have been studied for this entity. As mentioned earlier, the gold standard for the treatment of acute Charcot arthropathy is immobilization with TCC. Most of the medical evidence supporting TCC for CN is retrospective and lacks significant detailed results. Armstrong treated 55 subjects for a maximum period of 92 weeks with TCCs, removable cast boots, and finally with custom shoes. The average time for TCC treatment was 18.5 weeks. Subjects returned to wearing shoes in average of 28.3 weeks (42) (level B). This is the first study to suggest a timeline of how long the clinician should immobilize patients with CN.

Recently, a prospective study by Pinzur and colleagues showed that a weight-bearing TCC is an effective method of treatment for the stage 1 acute Charcot arthropathy. Ten subjects with stage 1 Charcot arthropathy were treated as such. The weight ranges of subjects were between 160 and 275 pounds. Subjects returned to depth inlay shoes in an average of 9.2 weeks (43) (level C). A larger cohort study was studied prospectively with weight-bearing TCCs by de Souza (44). Twenty-seven patients with stage 1 or early stage 2 Charcot arthropathy of the foot and ankle were followed for 18 years, with an average follow-up of 5.5 years. Complications regarding ulcerations or progression of deformity were not observed.

Another modality used to immobilize and off-load the Charcot foot is the Charcot Restraint Orthotic Walker (CROW). The CROW is advocated mostly as a transition device from cast immobilization, and it is very effective in controlling lower extremity edema. Although it is commonly used, the evidence is minimal to support its effectiveness. A retrospective review was done on 18 patients in whom 10 patients had surgery for Charcot arthropathy and 8 patients were managed without surgery (45) (level D). All patients were immobilized with a CROW. Patients reported improvement in quality of life and felt that the CROW did not limit their activity level. However, minor adjustments, replacements, or changes in devices were done in some of the patients. Also, almost half of the population had a delayed diagnosis of 11 weeks prior to treatment, which could have contributed to the repeat surgeries.

The patellar tendon-bearing brace has been used for the management of Charcot arthropathy, mostly when the rearfoot or the ankle is involved. The evidence is limited. One study by Saltzman involved six subjects with midfoot collapse. He measured a decrease of 15% mean force to the entire foot and a 32% reduction with additional padding. The reduction of forces occurred only at the rearfoot. Thus, the author recommended that the patellar-tendon brace may be use for midfoot pathology (46) (level D).

MEDICAL MANAGEMENT

The medical management of Charcot arthropathy has been evolving in the past few years with emphasis on drugs that regulate osteoclastic activity. Historical, descriptive data demonstrated osseous changes in radiographs (47–49) (level D). These changes include vascular calcifications, fragmentations, dislocations, periarticular lytic lesions, and sclerosis. Also, osteopenia has been shown to be more prevalent in patients with diabetic neuropathy and Charcot arthropathy (26,50,51) (level B). Subsequently, Gough and colleagues demonstrated measurements of serum markers that suggested that osteoclastic activity, not osteoblastic activity, is increased in patients with acute Charcot arthropathy. Markers of osteoclast and osteoblast activity were measured in four groups of patients: 16 with an acute Charcot foot, 16 with a chronic Charcot foot, 10 diabetic controls, and 10 nondiabetic controls. Serum carboxyterminal telopeptide of type 1 collagen (ICTP) level, a marker of osteoclastic bone resorption, was significantly raised in the acute Charcot foot compared with the chronic Charcot foot, diabetic controls, and nondiabetic controls. Serum procollagen carboxyterminal propeptide (P1CP) level, an indicator of osteoblastic bone formation, was not significantly different between the feet of patients with acute Charcot neuroarthropathy and the other three groups. The authors suggested that the acute Charcot foot demonstrates excess osteoclastic activity without increase in osteoblastic function (26) (level B). Bisphosphonates are a promising treatment for this entity. Selby and colleagues demonstrated an increase in bone-specific alkaline phosphatase and dehydroxypridinoline in patients with acute Charcot arthropathy. The authors studied the action of pamidronate, in six diabetic patients with active Charcot neuroarthropathy. The treatment was associated with improvement in patients' symptoms and a reduction in Charcot activity, as measured by temperature of the affected foot, which fell from 3.4°C $\pm$ 0.7°C to 1.0°C $\pm$ 0.5°C above the intact foot (28) (level C). There was a significant reduction in bone turnover as measured by alkaline phosphatase activity. These preliminary data suggest that bisphosphonates may be indicated in the management of active Charcot neuroarthropathy and suggested controlled trials should be conducted.

Subsequently, Jude and colleagues randomized 39 patients with active Charcot arthropathy for 1year to a double-blind, controlled investigation. A single 90-mg pamidronate infusion showed decreased bone turnover and decreased alkaline phosphatase level after 8 weeks compared with that in 18.6 weeks in the control group. Also, a decrease skin temperature was accomplished after 4 weeks. It was statistically significant when compared with the baseline, but there was no difference between groups (8) (level A). In 2005, 20 patients with active Charcot arthropathy were randomized to a controlled trial and received a 70-mg dose of alendronate orally once a week for 6 months. A decrease in bone turnover and ICTP after 6 months was observed. Similar to the previous study, a decrease in skin temperature was observed in both groups. Moreover, the DEXA scan demonstrated increase bone mineralization in the foot (52) (level A).

Intranasal calcitonin has also been studied. Calcitonin may be superior to bisphosphonates in that calcitonin cause cessation of osteoclastic activity, and it does not have an effect on osteoblastic activity, which differs from bisphosphonates. Bem and colleagues studied 32 patients with active Charcot arthropathy in a randomized controlled trial. Salmon calcitonin nasal spray 200 IU and calcium supplements were given to the treatment group, and only calcium supplements were given to the control group. A decrease in 1CTP occurred during the first 3 months when compared with the control group. Similarly to the other two studies, a decrease in skin temperature was found in both groups, and DEXA scans showed an increase in bone mineralization in the foot (53) (level A).

Bone stimulation has also been studied for the treatment of acute Charcot arthropathy. A meta-analysis on 11 articles concluded that electromagnetic bone stimulation has not demonstrated significant impact on delayed unions (54) (level A). However, an in vitro study demonstrated that pulse electromagnetic fields stimulate insulin-like growth factor II, which in turn increases the rate of bone cell proliferation. They noticed an increases flux of calcium in bone cell cultures (55) (level D). Hockenberry reviewed the results of arthrodesis for Charcot ankle and hindfoot joints with an internal bone stimulator in 11 complex cases (56) (level D). Nine patients were healed at 3.7 months after surgery, and one patient developed a stable pseudarthrosis. In addition, Hanft and colleague applied combined magnetic field every day for 30 minutes in 31 patients with acute (stage 1) Charcot arthropathy. Ten subjects were randomly assigned to the control group and 21 subjects were assigned to the treatment group. They found that the treatment group ambulated sooner, and earlier consolidation was accomplished (11 weeks vs. 23.8 weeks) (57) (level B). In 2000, Grady et al. used electrostimulation in 11 patients for a period of 18 months. They showed consolidation between 2 and 5 months in patient with stage 1 and 2 Charcot arthropathy (58) (level D). In both studies, however, healing was dependent of one investigator's opinion. Therefore, randomized controlled trials need to be conducted.

SURGICAL MANAGEMENT

The surgical treatment of Charcot arthropathy has become popularized in the recent years, although it was advocated in the early 90s. Eichenholtz proposed five factors to take into consideration when operating on the Charcot foot.

- Unknown role of neuropathy in bone healing
- Compression is not indicated
- Similar Charcot processes have been observed after a fracture of a long bone
- Prolonged non–weight-bearing is required
- Bone grafting is indicated

Most published reports have been small, retrospective, descriptive studies. Often, subjects included in the studies had different stages of Charcot arthropathy that involved different locations, a variety of fixation methods were used, and patients with and without ulcerations were included. Also, the definition of success varied among studies. Some investigators defined radiographic healing as a successful outcome; others described return to ambulation as a successful outcome. Recently, the principal controversy is the use of internal fixation or external fixation.

Tendo-Achilles lengthening (TAL) is a common adjunctive procedure for the surgical management of Charcot arthropathy. In a retrospective study, Armstrong demonstrated a high peak pressures in the forefoot, even though the Charcot patient had collapsed midfoot (22). The authors suggested that the forefoot may serve as lever, forcing the collapse of the midfoot. Exostectomy or planning is commonly used by surgeons to relieve pressure in areas at risk for ulcerations especially in patients with long-standing, rigid rocker bottom deformities.

Exostectomy was first described in four cases by Leventen, in 1986 (59) (level D). In a descriptive study, Brodsky and Rouse reviewed 12 patients who underwent a total of eight medial exostectomies, and four lateral exostectomies for midfoot ulcerations with a follow up of 25 months. Eleven of 12 patients healed uneventfully, and 1 ulcer recurred and required a Symes amputation (13) (level D). A retrospective review of 27 procedures in 20 patients was performed and included a follow-up of 21.6 months. Exostectomies for 18 medial ulcers and 9 lateral ulcers were performed. Results showed healing rate for medial ulcers was 92% and that for lateral ulcers was 37.5%. Revisional surgery was required in five out of nine lateral wounds. Complications and outcomes were more unpredictable for lateral column ulcers (60) (level C).

Many surgeons have suggested internal fixation as a technique to prevent or correct severe deformities in the late stages of Charcot arthropathy (61–65) (level C). The first to describe internal fixation for Charcot arthropathy correction were Papa and colleagues. Patients included unstable or fixed deformities. He used internal fixation in 25 patients and external fixation in the other 4 patients. Even though there were 9 stable pseudarthrosis, limb salvage was accomplished in 27 patients at an average of 42-month follow-up (61) (level C). Early and Hansen reviewed 18 patients (21 feet) who underwent surgical reconstruction with 28-month follow-up. Ten of the 21 feet had ulcers. Eighteen of the 21 feet (86%) healed successfully with radiographic union by 5 months. Two patients required below-the-knee amputation secondary to osteomyelitis, and 2 patients developed new ulcers (65) (level C).

In the most recent study by Simon, 14 patients with stage 1 Charcot arthropathy underwent tarsometatarsal arthrodesis and were followed for 41 months. All arthrodesis procedures were successful. Unassisted weight-bearing was achieved in an average of 15 ± 8.8 weeks. The mean return to regular shoes was 27 ± 14.4 weeks. All patients regained the level of walking ability, and all procedures were deemed to be successful by the authors (66) (level C). However, the definition of stage 1 Charcot arthropathy was not defined clearly in the study.

Recently, external fixation has become popular and advocated as a treatment option for Charcot arthropathy in the earlier stages and/or in cases complicated with open wounds or infection. However, the medical literature is composed mostly of review articles, expert opinions, and retrospective cohort studies. The advantages of external fixation include biomechanical stability, access to soft tissue, early ability to bear weight, and the ability to make adjustments postoperatively. Early et al. in 1998 described successful use of external fixation in a young woman with bilateral Charcot arthropathy of the ankle (67) (level D). Fabrin et al. reviewed 12 feet with severe Charcot arthropathy of the ankle with a median follow-up of 48 months. Nine limbs had ankle wounds. Seven ankle arthrodesis and five tibiocalcaneal arthrodesis were performed. Results included one transtibial amputation and six asymptomatic nonunions (68) (level D).

Farber and colleagues performed a single-stage correction with external fixation in the ulcerated Charcot foot as an alternative of amputation. Eleven patients were reviewed with an average of 24-month follow-up. Patients returned to depth-inlay shoes and bracing after external fixation of 8 weeks and TCC immobilization of approximately 19 weeks (69) (level C).

The only prospective study done for surgical management was by Pinzur in 2007. His prospective study included 26 adults with midfoot, stage 2 or 3 Charcot arthropathy. Fourteen of 26 patients had osteomyelitis and wounds larger than 2 cm. Patients were followed for a minimum of 1 year. One transtibial amputation due to infection and four recurrent ulcers resulted. Patients with recurrent ulcers underwent exostectomy and healed uneventfully. Two wound complications and two tibial stress fractures were identified (70) (level B). Pinzur concluded that in patients at high risk for amputation, external fixation is an alternative for amputation.

It is important to mention that studies involving surgical correction of Charcot arthropathy often conclude that outcomes were successful, although many patients had complications such as repeat surgeries, recurrent ulcers, and nonunions. Therefore, revisiting the literature may be necessary to determine the best surgical treatment of choice.

There is only one study that compares surgical and nonsurgical treatment for CN. A total of 198 patients (201 feet) with Charcot arthropathy were followed for 6 years. Out of them, 147 feet had midfoot collapse. The endpoint for this study was time to return to extra-depth shoe with custom inlays. After a 1-year follow-up, 59.2% of patients had a plantigrade foot without surgery. Forty-two of 147 feet with midfoot involvement required corrective surgery (40.8%) (71) (level B). Therefore, more than half of the limbs were managed successfully with accommodative measures.

Combination of therapy to ease the foot into weight-bearing is a must for the successful treatment of Charcot arthropathy. In a retrospective study, Fabrin and colleagues followed 115 subjects (140 limbs) for a median of 48 months. All subjects were diabetic patients and maintained in non–weight-bearing status with protective shoes or crutches until temperature were normal. One hundred thirty-two out of the 140 feet healed. However, late complications were observed. Forty-seven percent of the subjects developed new onset of Charcot or neuropathic ulcer (72) (level B). Almost half of the population developed late complications. It is possible that the method of treatment utilized may not prevent the development of deformity and may not provide stability to the foot and ankle.

A single treatment protocol has been shown to be an effective treatment for Charcot arthropathy. In a retrospective study of 115 subjects (127 limbs), patients were treated surgically or conservatively for Charcot arthropathy to evaluate an intensive, nonoperative program for Charcot arthropathy management. The program included immediate immobilization with casting, transfer to a CROW, and then transfer to custom full-contact inserts. All types of Charcot foot deformities were included. At a median 3.8 years, the limb survivorship was 90%. Thirty-six limbs (31%) that presented initially with ulceration went into some type of amputation, compared with 6% of those without chronic ulceration. Eleven percent (15 limbs) required a below-the-knee amputation. Sixty-two limbs (49%) had ulcer recurrence. The authors suggest that improved care for patients with Charcot arthropathy is necessary (73) (level B).

REFERENCES

1. Charcot JM. Sur quelques arthropathies qui paraissent dépendre d'une lésion du cerveau ou de la moëlle épinière. Archives de physiologie normale et pathologique. Paris. 1868; 1:161–178, 379–400.

2. Jordan W. Neuritic manifestations in diabetes mellitus. Arch Intern Med 1936; 57: 307–358.
3. Sohn MW, Stuck RM, Pinzur M, et al. Lower-extremity amputation risk after Charcot arthropathy and diabetic foot ulcer [published online ahead of print October 13, 2009]. Diabetes Care 2010; 33(1):98–100.
4. Sinha S, Munichoodappa CS, Kozak GP. Neuro-arthropathy (Charcot joints) in diabetes mellitus (clinical study of 101 cases). Medicine (Baltimore) 1972; 51(3):191–210.
5. Fabrin J, Larsen K, Holstein PE. Long term follow-up in diabetic Charcot feet with spontaneous onset. Diabetes Care 2000; 23(6):796–800.
6. Lavery L, Armstrong DA, Wunderlich R, et al. Diabetic foot syndrome: Evaluating the prevalence and incidence of foot pathology in Mexican-Americans and non-Hispanic whites from a diabetes disease management cohort. Diabetes Care 2003; 26(5): 1435–1438.
7. Larsen K, Fabrin J, Holstein PE. Incidence and management of ulcers in diabetic Charcot feet. J Wound Care 2001; 10(8):323–328.
8. Jude EB, Selby PL, Burgess J, et al. Bisphosphonates in the treatment of Charcot neuroarthropathy: A double-blind randomised controlled trial. Diabetologia 2001; 44(11):2032–2037.
9. Eichenholtz SN. Charcot Joints. Springfield, IL: Charles Thomas Co., 1966.
10. Shibata K, Tada K, Hashizume C. The results of arthrodesis of the ankle for leprotic neuroarthropathy. J Bone Joint Surg Am 1990; 72-A:749–756.
11. Sella EJ, Barrette C. Staging of Charcot neuroarthropathy along the medial column of the foot in the diabetic patient. J Foot Ankle Surg 1999; 38(1):34–40.
12. Sanders LE, Frykberg RG. Diabetic neuropathic osteoarthropathy: The Charcot foot. In: Frykberg RG, ed. The High Risk Foot in Diabetes Mellitus. New York, NY: Churchill Livingstone, 1991:297–338.
13. Brodsky JW, Rouse AM. Exostectomy for symptomatic bony prominences in diabetic Charcot feet. Clin Orthop Relat Res 1993; (296):21–26.
14. Harris JR, Brand PW. Pattern of disintegration of the tarsus in the anaesthetic foot. J Bone Joint Surg 1966; 48B(1):4–16.
15. Schon LC, Easley ME, Weinfield SB. Charcot neuroarthropathy of the foot and ankle. Clin Orthop 1998; 349:116–131.
16. Serbst SA, Jones KB, Saltzman CL. Pattern of diabetic neuropathic arthropathy associated with the peripheral bone mineral density. J Bone Joint Surg Br 2004; 86(B):378–383.
17. Edmonds M, Clarke MB, Newton S, et al. Increased uptake of bone radiopharmaceutical in diabetic neuropathy. Q J Med 1985; 57(224):843–855.
18. Katz I, Rabinowitz JG, Dziadiw R. Early changes in Charcot's joints. Am J Roentgenol Radium Ther Nucl Med 1961; 86:965–974.
19. Edelman SV, Kosofsky EM, Paul RA, et al. Neuroarthropathy (Charcot's joint) in diabetes mellitus following revascularization surgery: Three case reports and a review of the literature. Arch Inter Med 1987; 147:1504–1508.
20. Shapiro SA, Stansbery KB, Hill MA, et al. Normal blood flow response and vasomotion in the diabetic Charcot foot. J Diabetes Complications 1998; 12:147–153.
21. Delano PJ. The pathogenesis of Charcot's joint. Am J Roentgenol 1946; 56:189–200.
22. Armstrong DG, Lavery LA. Elevated peak plantar pressures in patients who have Charcot arthropathy. J Bone Joint Surg 1998; 80-A(3):365–369.
23. Armstrong DG, Lavery LA. Monitoring healing of acute Charcot's arthropathy with infrared dermal thermometry. J Rehabil Res Dev 1997; 34(3):317–321.
24. Rabjohn L, Roberts K, Troiano M, et al. Diagnostic and prognostic value of erythrocyte sedimentation rate in contiguous osteomyelitis of the foot and ankle. J Foot Ankle Surg 2007; 46(4):230–237.
25. Kaleta JL, Fleischli JW, Reilly CH. The diagnosis of osteomyelitis in diabetes using erythrocyte sedimentation rate: A pilot study. J Am Podiatr Med Assoc 2001; 91(9):445–450.
26. Young MJ, Marshall A, Adams JE, et al. Osteopenia, neurological dysfunction, and the development of Charcot neuroarthropathy. Diabetes Care 1995; 18(1):34–38.

27. Sinacore DR, Fielder FA, Johnson JE. Bone mineral density during total contact cast immobilization for a patient with neuropathic (Charcot) arthropathy. Phys Ther 2005; 85(3):249–256.
28. Selby PL, Young MJ, Boulton AJ. Bisphosphonates: A new treatment for diabetic Charcot neuroarthropathy? Diabet Med 1994;11(1):28–31.
29. Petrova NL, Foster AV, Edmonds ME. Calcaneal bone mineral density in patients with Charcot neuropathic neuroarthropathy: Differences between type 1 and type 2 diabetes. Diabet Med 2005: 22(6):756–761.
30. Baumhauer JF, O'Keefe RJ, Schon LC, et al. Cytokine-induced osteoclastic bone resorption in Charcot arthropathy: An immunohistochemical study. Foot Ankle Int 2006; 27(10):797–800.
31. Mabilleau G, Petrova NL, Edmonds ME, et al. Increased osteoclastic activity in acute Charcot's osteoarthropathy: The role of receptor activator of nuclear factor-kappaB ligand. Diabetologia 2008; 51:1035–1040.
32. Jeffcoate WJ, Game F, Cavanagh P. The role of pro-inflammatory cytokines in the cause of neuropathic osteoarthropathy (acute Charcot foot) in diabetes. Lancet 2005; 366:2058–2061.
33. La Fontaine J, Harkless LB, Sylvia VL, et al. Levels of endothelial nitric oxide synthase and calcitonin gene-related peptide in the charcot foot: A pilot study [published online ahead of print July 14, 2008]. J Foot Ankle Surg 2008; 47(5):424–429
34. Jay PR, Michelson JD, Mizel MS, et al. Efficacy of three-phase bone scans in evaluating diabetic foot ulcers. Foot Ankle Int 1999; 20(6):347–355.
35. Maurer AH, Millmond SH, Knight LC, et al. Infection in diabetic osteoarthropathy: Use of indium-labeled leukocytes for diagnosis. Radiology 1986;161(1):221–225.
36. Blume PA, Dey HM, Daley LJ, et al. Diagnosis of pedal osteomyelitis with Tc-99m HMPAO labeled leukocytes. J Foot Ankle Surg 1997; 36(2):120–126, discussion 160.
37. Boc SF, Brazzo K, Lavian D, et al. Acute Charcot foot changes versus osteomyelitis: Does Tc-99m HMPAO labeled leukocytes scan differentiate? J Am Podiatr Med Assoc. 2001; 91(7):365–368.
38. Palestro CJ, Mehta HH, Patel M, et al. Marrow versus infection in the Charcot joint: Indium-111 leukocyte and technetium-99m sulfur colloid scintigraphy. J Nucl Med 1998; 39(2):346–350.
39. Marcus CD, Ladam-Marcus VJ, Leone J, et al. MR imaging of osteomyelitis and neuropathic osteoarthropathy in the feet of diabetics. Radiographics 1996;16(6):1337–1348.
40. Seabold JE, Flickinger FW, Kao SCS, et al. Indium- 111 leukocyte/technetium-99m-MDPBone and magnetic resonance imaging: Difficulty of diagnosing osteomyelitis in patients with neuropathic osteoarthropathy. J Nucl Med 1990; 31:549–556.
41. Clohisy DR, Thompson RC Jr. Fractures associated with neuropathic arthropathy in adults who have juvenile-onset diabetes. J Bone Joint Surg Am 1988; 70(8):1192–1200.
42. Armstrong DG, Todd WF, Lavery LA, et al. The natural history of acute Charcot's arthropathy in a diabetic foot specialty clinic. Diabet Med 1997; 87(6):357–363.
43. Pinzur MS, Lio T, Posner M. Treatment of Eichenholtz Stage I Charcot foot arthropathy with a weight-bearing total contact cast. Foot Ankle Int 2006; 27(5):324–329.
44. de Souza LJ. Charcot arthropathy and immobilization in a weight-bearing total contact cast. J Bone Joint Surg Am 2008; 90(4):754–759.
45. Morgan JM, Biehl WC III, Wagner FW Jr. Management of neuropathic arthropathy with the charcot restraint orthotic walker. Clin Orthop Relat Res 1993; 296:58–63.
46. Saltzman CL, Johnson KA, Goldstein RH, et al. The patellar tendon-bearing brace as treatment for neurotrophic arthropathy: A dynamic force monitoring study. Foot Ankle 1992; 13(1):14–21.
47. Geoffroy J, Hoeffel JC, Pointel JP, et al. The feet in diabetes: Roentgenologic observation in 1501 cases. Diagn Imaging 1979; 48(5):286–293.
48. Clouse ME, Gramm HF, Legg M, et al. Diabetic osteoarthropathy: Clinical and roentgenographic observations in 90 cases. Am J Roentgenol Radium Ther Nucl Med 1974; 121(1):22–34.

49. Buchman NH. Bone and joint changes in the diabetic foot. J Am Podiatry Assoc 1976; 66(4):211–226.
50. Cundy TF, Edmonds ME, Watkins PJ. Osteopenia and metatarsal fractures in diabetic neuropathy. Diabet Med 1985; 2(6):461–464.
51. Jirkovská A, Kasalick P, Boucek P, et al. Calcaneal ultrasonometry in patients with Charcot osteoarthropathy and its relationship with densitometry in the lumbar spine and femoral neck and with markers of bone turnover. Diabet Med 2001; 18(6): 495–500.
52. Pitocco D, Ruotolo V, Caputo S, et al. Six-month treatment with alendronate in acute charcot neuroarthropathy: A randomized controlled trial. Diabetes Care 2005; 28(5):1214–1215.
53. Bem R, Jirkovská A, Fejfarová V, et al. Intranasal calcitonin in the treatment of acute Charcot neuroosteoarthropathy: A randomized controlled trial. Diabetes Care 2006; 29(6):1392–1394.
54. Mollon B, da Silva V, Busse JW, et al. Electrical stimulation for long-bone fracture-healing: A meta-analysis of randomized controlled trials. J Bone Joint Surg Am 2008; 90(11):2322–2330.
55. Fitzsimmons RJ, Ryaby JT, Mohan S, et al. Combined magnetic fields increase insulin-like growth factor-II in TE-85 human osteosarcoma bone cell cultures. Endocrinology 1995; 136(7):3100–3106.
56. Hockenbury RT, Gruttadauria M, McKinney I. Use of implantable bone growth stimulation in Charcot ankle arthrodesis. Foot Ankle Int 2007; 28(9):971–976.
57. Hanft JR, Goggin JP, Landsman A, et al. The role of combined magnetic field bone growth stimulation as an adjunct in the treatment of neuroarthropathy/Charcot joint: An expanded pilot study. J Foot Ankle Surg 1998; 37(6):510–515.
58. Grady JF, O'Connor KJ, Axe TM, et al. Use of electrostimulation in the treatment of diabetic neuroarthropathy. J Am Podiatr Med Assoc 2000; 90(6):287–294.
59. Leventen EO. Charcot foot—A technique for treatment of chronic plantar ulcer by saucerization and primary closure. Foot Ankle 1986; 6(6):295–299.
60. Catanzariti AR, Mendicino R, Haverstock B. Ostectomy for diabetic neuroarthropathy involving the midfoot. J Foot Ankle Surg 2000; 39(5):291–300.
61. Papa J, Myerson M, Girard P. Salvage, with arthrodesis, in intractable diabetic neuropathic arthropathy of the foot and ankle. J Bone Joint Surg Am 1993; 75(7): 1056–1066.
62. Bono JV, Roger DJ, Jacobs RL. Surgical arthrodesis of the neuropathic foot: A salvage procedure. Clin Orthop Relat Res 1993; (296):14–20.
63. Holmes GB Jr, Hill N. Fractures and dislocations of the foot and ankle in diabetics associated with Charcot joint changes. Foot Ankle Int 1994; 15(4):182–185.
64. Sammarco GJ, Conti SF. Surgical treatment of neuroarthropathic foot deformity. Foot Ankle Int 1998; 19(2):102–109.
65. Early JS, Hansen ST. Surgical reconstruction of the diabetic foot: A salvage approach for midfoot collapse. Foot Ankle Int 1996;17(6):325–330.
66. Simon SR, Tejwani SG, Wilson DL, et al. Arthrodesis as an early alternative to nonoperative management of Charcot arthropathy of the diabetic foot. J Bone Joint Surg Am 2000; 82-A(7):939–950.
67. Prokuski LJ, Saltzman CL. External fixation for the treatment of Charcot arthropathy of the ankle: A case report. Foot Ankle Int 1998; 19(5):336–341.
68. Fabrin J, Larsen K, Holstein PE. Arthrodesis with external fixation in the unstable or misaligned Charcot ankle in patients with diabetes mellitus. Int J Low Extrem Wounds 2007; 6(2):102–107.
69. Farber DC, Juliano PJ, Cavanagh PR, et al. Single stage correction with external fixation of the ulcerated foot in individuals with Charcot neuroarthropathy. Foot Ankle Int 2002; 23(2):130–134.
70. Pinzur MS. Neutral ring fixation for high-risk nonplantigrade Charcot midfoot deformity. Foot Ankle Int 2007; 28(9):961–966.

71. Pinzur M. Surgical versus accommodative treatment for Charcot arthropathy of the midfoot. Foot Ankle Int 2004; 25(8):545–549.
72. Fabrin J, Larsen K, Holstein PE. Long-term follow-up in diabetic Charcot feet with spontaneous onset. Diabetes Care 2000; 23(6):796–800.
73. Saltzman CL, Hagy ML, Zimmerman B, et al. How effective is intensive nonoperative initial treatment of patients with diabetes and Charcot arthropathy of the feet? Clin Orthop Relat Res 2005; (435):185–190.

12 Amputation

I. M. Nordon, R. J. Hinchliffe, and K. G. Jones

INTRODUCTION

The end stage of the diabetic foot syndrome is the requirement for amputation. In the United Kingdom, 80% of all amputations carried out are due to vascular disease, of which 20% to 30% are due to diabetes (1). Patients with diabetes have a 15 times increased risk of amputation relative to the normal population (2). Sadly amputation is often seen as a failure of care in patients with diabetes; however, for some patients, it should be perceived as a positive procedure as it allows the patient to move forward in their care. Often, patients will have been suffering with chronic sepsis, ischemic pain, or open necrotic wounds which have been dominating their lives. Formal amputation will allow them to move on to a new chapter in their lives free from infection and pain (3).

The St Vincent Declaration, in 1989, highlighted the challenges facing the growing number of patients with diabetes mellitus. It identified that countries should deploy resources for the prevention, identification, and treatment of the complications for diabetes. Local, national, and European plans and investment were put in place to limit the complications including blindness, renal failure, gangrene, and amputation (4). The Istanbul commitment reiterated these plans. Empowerment and education of patients and medical personnel in combination with advances in technology are all tools of this initiative to prevent progression of disease and tissue loss.

The risk factors leading to eventual tissue loss are categorized in Table 1. The recent report of the Eurodiale registry, a prospective multicentre cohort study of more than 1200 patients, examined risk factors leading to amputation. Statistically significant predictors of amputation were ischemic rest pain [odds ratio (OR) 5.9, $p < 0.001$] and infection (OR 2.3, $p = 0.003$) (5) (level B). The startling finding of that study was that current multidisciplinary guidelines are still not being followed in a large number of patients, thus providing sub-optimal care. Optimum care of a diabetic patient facing tissue loss is the most conservative effective debridement possible. The best outcome is one of the most favorable functions.

Techniques of tissue preservation and revascularization have already been discussed. It is important to reinforce the value of preserving as much healthy native tissue as possible. This will allow the amputation level to be more distal and ensure adequate healing of the amputation wound. It is important that the new amputation wound heals to enable prompt rehabilitation. Return to function, both physical and psychological, and expedient discharge from hospital are priorities.

Despite advances in medical care, mortality from amputation in this group remain high, between 10% and 20% (6). Major amputation is high-risk surgery and

Table 1 Risk Factors for Amputation (7)

Risk factors
Neuropathy (loss of protective sensation)
Peripheral vascular disease (PVD)
Infection
Prior ulceration/amputation
Structural foot abnormality
Trauma
Charcot foot
Visual impairment
Poor glycemic control
Age
Male sex
Ethnicity (increased in black/Hispanic groups)

therefore optimization of comorbid disease is crucial to limit perioperative complications. Cardiopulmonary, diabetic, and renal disease should be optimized; sepsis should be controlled; and the patient should be psychologically ready for surgery and rehabilitation.

Once a patient has had an amputation at the level of the foot, they become 36 times more likely to develop an ulcer on that foot than an individual who did not have an amputation (8). This emphasizes the continuing risk of this patient group; ideal initial surgery should be followed by intensive care of skin, wounds, and pressure areas. Simple measures including chiropody and footwear should be used to off-load the sites of maximal pressure to encourage healing.

Plantar ulcers common in diabetic patients result from a combination of neuropathy, high plantar pressures, and foot deformity. Limited dorsiflexion of the foot on the leg is thought to be a key contributory factor in ulcer causation (9). Conservative management with immobilization in a total in contact cast has proven efficacy in primary healing of these ulcers but has a recurrence rate of 20% to 70% (10). One measure that is additive to casting is Achilles tendon lengthening. In an randomised controlled trial (RCT) published in 2003, Achilles tendon lengthening in combination with total in-contact casting was proven to be beneficial over casting alone for reduction in recurrent neuropathic ulceration (11) (level A).

DECISION MAKING

Treating patients with diabetic foot complications requires a multidisciplinary approach. It may appear that the decision to amputate would be straightforward, certainly in the place of non-reconstructible vascular insufficiency and ischemic necrosis. The efforts to preserve the limb are dependent on patient factors, including comorbidities that would render them unable to utilize the salvaged limb. Also if vascular reconstruction is unlikely to succeed or be durable, the best outcome will be provided by primary amputation. This has been shown in terms of quality of life and cost–benefit (12) (level B). There is no evidence pertaining to the benefit of early amputation at a young age, compared with continuing tissue salvage procedures. The final decision to amputate and the level of amputation are decisions that should involve the patient, surgeon, diabetologist, and physiotherapist.

Table 2 Factors Determining Level of Amputation

Factor	Significance
Extent of infection	Component cause in 59% (9)
Vascular status	Component cause in 46% (9)
Quality of tissue	30% associated with hyperkeratosis (13)
Immune status	Poor healing with lymphopenia <1500 cells/mm (3,13)
Nutritional status	Poor healing with albumin <3.5 g/dL (13)

SELECTION OF LEVEL

The decision of level of amputation is multifactorial (Table 2). The ideal level will be one of guaranteed healing, allowing functional rehabilitation and being appropriate for prosthesis.

Techniques to identify safe level for healing include transcutaneous oximetry (14,15), photoplethysmography (16), laser Doppler velocimetry (17,18), and thermography (19). All techniques have evidence confirming correlation between specific values and stump healing. Yet a review of all modalities concluded that they lacked specificity and sensitivity to be recommended in clinical practice (20) (level B). More recent noninvasive methods of evaluating perfusion include hyperspectral technology (OxyVu-1®, HyperMed, Burlington, MA) and skin perfusion pressures (Sensilase®, Vasamed, USA). The OxyVu-1 has been shown to predict foot diabetic ulcer healing with a positive predictive value of 93%, although it has no evidence in amputation wound healing (21) (level C). The Sensilase system combines assessment of micro- and macrocirculatory blood flow assessment by measurement of skin perfusion pressure and pulse volume recording and is presented as a quick noninvasive technique for prediction of wound healing. It has reported equivalence with toe-pressure assessment (22) but is not routinely used to assess healing.

Clinical evaluation including intraoperative decisions reinforced by skin changes and erythema (23), aided by segmental Doppler pressures, at the thigh, ankle, or toe, should allow the surgeon to ascertain the best level for primary healing. It remains true that preoperative methods of determining amputation level are more beneficial in predicting failure than in predicting success (24) (level B).

A simple old study by O'Dwyer et al. demonstrated that below-knee amputations (BKAs) performed when the femoral pulse is absent are unlikely to heal. In that study only 20% of BKAs performed without a palpable femoral pulse healed primarily. This easily measured fact should be born in mind when planning amputation level. Equally they showed that in the presence of a palpable popliteal pulse, more than 90% of BKAs will heal (25) (level B).

Provided the perioperative course is well controlled, there is no evidence that diabetes inhibits wound healing of amputation stumps (20) (level B).

Amputation of single or multiple toes without revascularization is generally not recommended, except in diabetic patients with palpable foot pulses and dry gangrene. In this situation, the tissue has usually demarcated and surgical amputation may merely expedite tissue autoamputation (26).

The capacity for rehabilitation is paramount in selection of level for amputation. Ambulation is an important postoperative goal after major lower limb amputation for patients and physicians alike. Several well-documented studies have shown that energy expenditure with prosthetic ambulation is markedly increased in more proximal amputations (27,28) (level B). Calculating energy expenditure is complex accounting for age, aerobic fitness, and modification in cadence and stride length. Waters et al. concluded that percentage relative energy costs for above knee, below knee, and Syme's amputations were 62, 43, and 42, respectively, in vascular amputees compared with a control group of unimpaired pedestrians unaware of being observed in whom the relative energy cost was 38% (27). In essence, the energy expenditure to ambulate following above-knee amputation (AKA) is two-third greater than normal, and there is a negligible change in energy expense for below knee amputees. The energy a patient expends when walking is inversely proportional to the length of the limb and the number of preserved joints (29). There are as yet no validated studies to predict return to independent mobility with a prosthetic limb.

However, the likelihood of bipedal gait is increased if the knee joint is preserved; Larsson et al. reported that 88% of patients with above ankle amputations as a result of diabetes walked less than 1 km a day at 1 year after transtibial amputation (30). This objective end point may be unrealistic for the majority of amputees, primarily from a physiological standpoint. Rehabilitation following amputation can be arduous, involving a training program to improve strength and balance. It is probably not surprising then that many frail patients faced with the choice of physically demanding activity or a markedly less strenuous primary wheelchair existence eventually choose the latter (31).

The relationship of the amputee and their prosthesis is complex; motivation, comfort, cosmetic appearance, functionality, reliability, ease of use, and degree of energy expenditure during use all combine to the likelihood of independent mobility (32). These factors must be considered when allocating a level of amputation.

Digital Amputation

The best case scenario for diabetes-related ischemia or localized sepsis is single-digit involvement associated with adequate foot vascularity. In this case, simple digit amputation can be performed. This allows for eradication of sepsis while maintaining the structure of a functional foot for the patient. However, in the intermediate to long term, it has been shown that patients with sepsis localized to the forefoot requiring hospitalization and digit amputation have a high incidence of persistent and recurrent sepsis, between 39% and 88% of wounds heal primarily, leading to a modest rate of limb loss, despite adequate forefoot perfusion (33) (level C). Ipsilateral reamputation rates for patients with diabetes following isolated digital amputation have been shown to be as high as 52% at 5 years (34). Yet this is retrospective observational data that may reflect poor diabetic management or surgical decision making. If there is doubt about the perfusion of the foot and there is a realistic option of revascularization, this should be performed to ensure wound healing. In the presence of poor perfusion, it is better to leave toes with partial dry gangrene alone and autoamputation may occur.

Technique

Amputation is performed through the base of the proximal phalanx, as much healthy skin as possible should be preserved. The wound should be left open

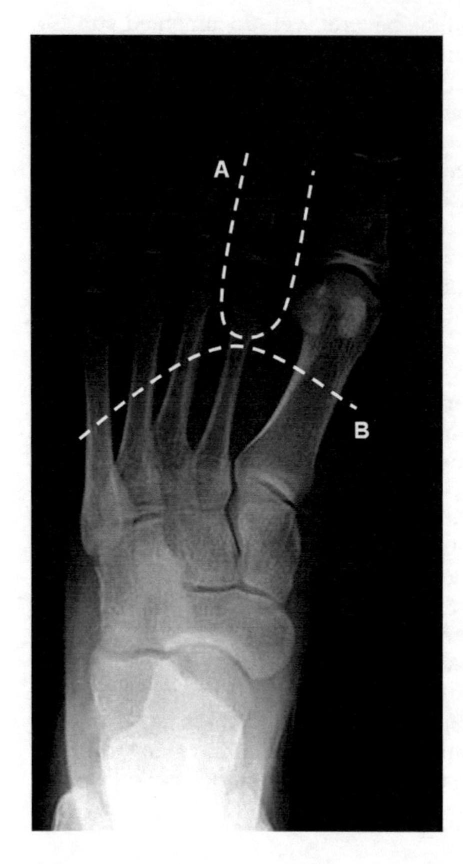

Figure 1 X-ray—AP x-ray of left forefoot. Annotation (level A) second ray amputation and annotation (level B) transmetatarsal amputation.

to heal by secondary intention; even in the presence of adequate skin coverage, closure is not recommended due to the inevitable swelling in the postoperative period. The patient should be encouraged to mobilize promptly after surgery. In the presence of infection extending above the proximal phalanx, a "ray amputation" is indicated (Fig. 1).

Ray Amputation

This is often necessary in patients with diabetes and tracking foot sepsis. The relevant toes are excised and the wedge of infection/necrosis is debrided back, including the metatarsal head to healthy tissue. The wound is left open to heal by secondary intention, or healing may be expedited by application of negative pressure dressing (35–37) (level A). Hallux and first ray amputations are associated with significantly increased risk of recurrent ulceration and more proximal amputation over time (38) (level B). Medial and lateral longitudinal amputations in diabetic patients are highly successful (90% healing) in patients who exhibit adequate circulation (39). To preserve optimal foot function, the first ray should remain intact, the length of the first metatarsal should be preserved as this medial column is important in forward propulsion. Removing two or more central rays is good neither functionally nor cosmetically (40); this dysfunctional forefoot may be better served with a transmetatarsal amputation (TMA).

Bone regrowth following diabetes-related partial foot amputation has the potential to develop new foci of pressure and eventually lead to new ulceration (38). This particularly applies to ray amputations following partial transection of the metatarsal, especially if the resection of the metatarsal had been made distal to the surgical neck of the bone. The redistribution of weight and altered biomechanics of the foot, in combination with new bone growth, can predispose to new ulcer formation, the concept of "transfer ulceration."

Technique

The healthy toes lateral and medial to the infected area should be retracted. This will demonstrate the wedge of tissue to excise. All infected or necrotic tissue should be removed including the metatarsal head (Fig. 2). No bone or tendon should be visible in the wound, as this will delay healing. Hemostasis should be obtained and the wound dressed initially with nonadhesive antiseptic gauze. This can later be changed for a negative pressure dressing, provided there is adequate vascularity.

The dead space following central ray amputation may take time to heal and leave the patient vulnerable to recurrent sepsis. A plantar dermo-fat pad flap has demonstrated efficacy in filling this dead space in patients with diabetes. This plastic surgical technique of mobilizing a rhomboid flap has reported 92% primary healing in a selective patient population (41) (level C).

Simple excision of the metatarsal head, with preservation of the digit, has reported success in primary healing of neuropathic plantar ulceration. In the presence of a plantar wound, the metatarsal head is approached and resected from a dorsal approach under local anaesthetic. This approach has been shown

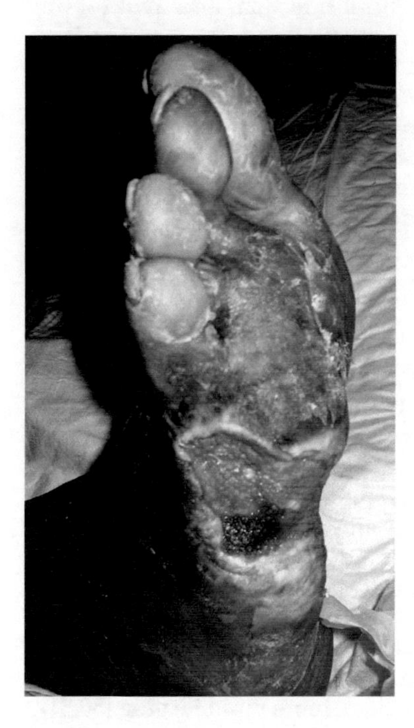

Figure 2 Digit amputation—racquet incision for amputation of fifth digit.

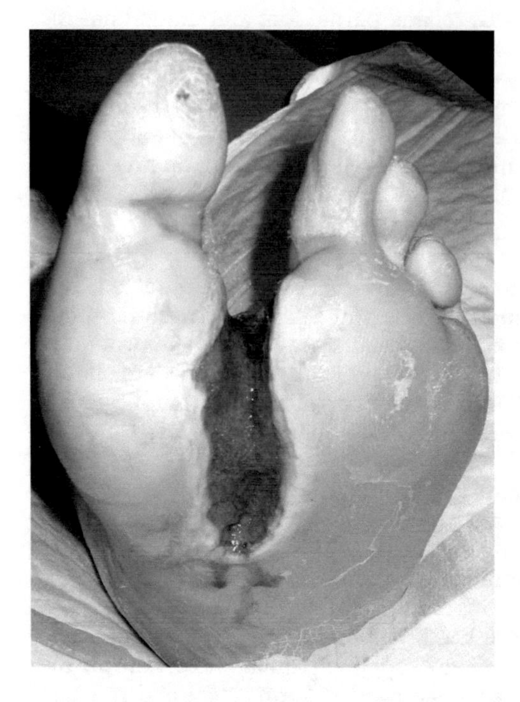

Figure 3 Ray amputation—second ray amputation with granulating wound.

to permit primary healing in 88% of cases, control infection, and avoid more major amputations (42) (level B).

Functionally, preservation of the medial toes is more advantageous than saving the lateral toes. It remains questionable as to whether ray amputation of two or more adjacent toes should be performed. In patients with diabetes, performing amputations that generate gross asymmetry of the forefoot, there is a high rate of tissue breakdown and re-amputation. In these cases, balance, function, and foot integrity will be better provided by a formal primary TMA (43) (level D) (Fig. 3).

Transmetatarsal Amputation

Transmetatarsal amputations (TMAs) for ischemic and infected lower extremities are a viable option for limb salvage and function. It was pioneered by McKittrick for the treatment of forefoot gangrene in patients with diabetes mellitus (44). Its utility is greater for sepsis as opposed to ischemia (45), and while excellent rates of limb salvage have been shown when TMA is combined with revascularization (46,47), the need for primary TMA has been identified as a risk factor predictive of subsequent limb loss (48). Preservation of the hind and mid-foot decreases the overall energy required during function relative to a more proximal amputation. Success is dependent on the arterial supply from the plantar artery. This technique offers best success when the indication is infection as opposed to ischemia (49); in this setting, it is often best to leave the tissue flaps open with delayed closure, again vacuum-assisted closure systems may facilitate more rapid healing (50,51).

Technique

A dorsal skin incision is made in the mid-metatarsal level with a long plantar flap and bone transaction through the metatarsal bases. Transverse sectioning and bevelling of the metatarsals proximal to the surgical neck in the functional metatarsal parabola optimizes the weight-bearing surfaces. Bevel the metatarsals plantarly, with the first and fifth beveled at the medial and lateral aspects, respectively (52). Within the parabola, the second metatarsal is the longest, followed by the first, the third, the fourth, and the fifth. An oblique metatarsal break and graded step down pattern allow propulsion and preserve the gait pattern (53). The plantar flap is then mobilized, so it can be rotated dorsally to cover the bone ends. Often in the presence of significant tissue edema, this cannot be done without tension. Here, a technique of delayed primary closure or healing by secondary intention is used.

Syme's Amputation

First described by James Syme in 1843, this ankle disarticulation is useful if the forefoot cannot be salvaged. The primary benefits include minimization of disability and maintenance of function (54). The preservation of the normal proprioceptive heel pad makes postoperative mobility safer. A Syme's amputation is contraindicated if the tissue of the heel pad is of poor quality or in the presence of an edematous limb compromising healing while its success is dependent on an adequate blood supply via the posterior tibial artery (55). Wagner classified patients as suitable for this level of amputation if they met the following criteria: (*i*) potential to walk with a prosthesis, (*ii*) clinically viable heel pad, (*iii*) no infection at the heel pad, and (*iv*) an adequate vascular inflow demonstrated by minimum ankle-brachial pressure index (ABPI) of 0.5 (56).

The metabolic and energy cost of walking after Syme's ankle disarticulation with a prosthesis is not appreciably greater than that of age matched controls without an amputation (57). It is rarely performed in arterial insufficiency with many surgeons, in the presence of extensive disease precluding a TMA, opting for a BKA (58) (level C).

Failure to heal and compromised future rehabilitation secondary to stump hypermobility have supported vascular surgeons' resistance to this level of amputation; yet a study by Pinzur reported successful healing with Syme's amputation in 81% of cases with ABPI > 0.5 (57) and rehabilitation to walking has been reported in more than 90% of cases of healed stumps (58) (level B).

Technique (57)

A fish-mouth incision is utilized with the apices at the anterior midpoints of the medial and lateral malleoli. The tendons and nerves are cut short under tension and retract. The ankle is disarticulated and the malleoli are removed flush with the articular surface of the distal part of the tibia. The articulate surface of the distal tibia is preserved for weight bearing while the raw osseous surface encourages the heel pad to scar securely to the bones. Oblique drill holes in the anterior tibia allow the heel pad to be further secured in place with nonabsorbable sutures. Low suction drains are sited and the skin is closed with interrupted nylon sutures. Padded dressings are placed over the stump end for comfort.

Transtibial Amputation (Below-Knee Amputation)

The most common major limb amputation in the developed world is transtibial. Surgeons widely regard it as the most likely major limb amputation to result in an independent mobile patient. However, as mentioned earlier, the functional reserve required to ambulate post-BKA is significant. It is probably inappropriate to perform a BKA on patients with limited preoperative ability, older than 70 years, dementia, end-stage renal disease, or advanced coronary artery disease (59). In this setting, the additional risks of non-healing and pressure ulceration in nonambulators are not warranted (level B). The converse is also valid, younger healthy patients do very well with a BKA, and with a prosthesis, can achieve functional outcomes comparable with what might be expected after successful lower extremity revascularization.

Four main reconstructive flaps have been described for transtibial amputation: the long posterior flap technique popularized by Burgess (60), the skew flap technique developed in Roehampton by Robinson (61), equal sagittal flaps (62), and the medially based flap developed in Dundee (63). In the dysvascular diabetic limb, cutaneous blood supply may be compromised. The skew flap technique is based on the arteries that run with the long and short saphenous veins, which provide the main blood supply to the skin. The anteromedial flap contains perforators from the posterior tibial and saphenous arteries, and the posterolateral flap contains perforators from the anterior tibial, sural, and peroneal arteries (64). Comparisons of skew and long posterior flap techniques have shown increased tissue hypoxia in the long posterior flaps (65), but randomized trials have failed to demonstrate any difference in healing between these operations (66) (level A). The benefit shown in the skew flap group was earlier mobility due to a shorter time to limb fitting, thought to be due to the less bulbous stump created.

The use of a tourniquet for control of intraoperative blood loss at amputation has previously been resisted due to fears of further damaging the arterial supply of the ischemic limb. However, two recent prospective trials, one randomized, reported that it was both safe and beneficial by reducing blood loss and consequently reducing the need for postoperative blood transfusion (67,68) (level A). Wolthuis et al. also reported that utilizing a tourniquet led to a 50% reduction in amputation revision rates (68). Although the benefits of limiting intraoperative blood loss are well established, this reduction in revisions may reflect improved patient and level selection rather than a tourniquet effect. In the presence of a functioning infrainguinal bypass graft, it is still advisable to avoid tourniquet use.

All techniques consider an ideal section of the tibia at 12 cm from the tibial tuberosity, with the fibula divided 1.5 cm proximal to this. The weight-bearing point of the prosthesis is the tibial tuberosity, and the distal bone stump should be beveled anteriorly and rounded off to prevent erosions through the skin.

Technique

Burgess long posterior flap. The skin is premarked to preserve the skin overlying gastrocnemius. A surgical tie is used to measure the circumference of the leg at the point of transection. The tape is divided in one-third and two-third lengths. The one-third piece measures the length of the posterior flap. The two-third piece measures the length of the anterior transverse skin incision. Dog ears at each corner are avoided by cutting a curved triangle of skin from the anterior skin at each apex (the rule of thirds) (69). This incision is made preserving enough skin to cover the wound ends without tension. The soft tissues of the lateral compartment are divided to allow access to and division of the fibula below its neck. The tibia is then divided 1.5 cm distal to the fibula transection, it should have an anterior bevel and a smooth finish. This allows access to the posterior compartment and division of the remaining tissues. The muscles of the deep posterior compartment and soleus are filleted out, with the remaining gastrocnemius and its overlying skin forming the distal end of the stump. The fascia is closed using a continuous absorbable braided suture. The skin is opposed using interrupted sutures or skin clips.

A significant modification to the traditional BKA is that of a "bone-bridge". Following BKA, the motionless relationship of the tibia to the fibula diminishes from a stable design to one allowing a "chop-sticking" movement, especially when in prosthesis. This can be a source of pain, or lead to a poor prosthetic fit. Pioneered by Ertl in 1920, the concept of "bone-bridging" was designed to return young amputees to the work force. An osteoperiosteal graft is harvested from the redundant tibia and used to connect the tibia to the fibula. This procedure can increase the morbidity of BKA and is normally the preserve of young, mobile amputees. Recent evidence suggests that the technique may provide a potential benefit by creating a stable platform with an enhanced surface area for load transfer (70,71) (level B). This is also an option as a secondary procedure in the patient who has significant functional pain from bone mobility.

Postoperative dressings now have more advanced roles than simple maintenance of a sterile environment. Dressing strategies now attempt to incorporate a number of postoperative goals including the prevention of knee flexion contractures, reduction of edema, protection from external trauma, facilitating weight bearing, and shaping for early prosthetic management. Smith et al. have reported the utility of nonremovable rigid dressings following BKA, with accelerated rehabilitation times and reduced edema compared with soft gauze (72). Removable rigid dressings have recent evidence supporting their role following BKA. They may reduce time to first prosthetic casting and reduce limb edema, while allowing continued close observation of wound healing (73,74) (level B).

Through-Knee Amputation

Through-knee amputation (TKA) is an alternative if a transtibial amputation is unlikely to heal. The biomechanical benefits of amputation at this level over above knee are that no muscle imbalance is created. A long lever is preserved to maintain an excellent platform for sitting and lever arm for transfer (75). Historically, TKA was associated with less perioperative morbidity than above- or below-knee amputations, as no bone or muscle bellies need to be transacted and there was limited blood loss. The end result, in nonambulatory patients, is a muscle balance amputation with little potential for hip or knee contracture. Other advantages are in pediatric amputation; the epiphyseal growth plates are not disturbed allowing the stump to grow as the child develops. There was resistance from prosthetists to TKA, as it required a lower knee joint than the native limb to accommodate the prosthetic limb. It remained the preserve of the patient in whom transtibial amputation would not heal and who were deemed incapable of walking. This opinion is now changing; it is now the preferred alternative over AKA for patients with vascular disease who are candidates for prosthetic rehabilitation

(76) (level C). The long lever arm decreases the energy expenditure associated with ambulation, while as the TKA provides an end weight-bearing stump, there is greater comfort, proprioception, and stability when compared with AKA (28). The bulbous stump, initially a challenge for fitting a practical prosthesis, aids modern appliance fitting (77), while biomechanically having asymmetrical knee joints does not appear to limit mobility. Two techniques of knee disarticulation have been described. The first by sagittal skin flaps, with the alternative fashioning a posterior myocutaneous flap akin to the Burgess BKA at a more proximal level. The advantage of the myocutaneous flap is the padding that it provides over the stump end aiding comfort and protecting the skin integrity.

Healing rates of 80% to 81% with TKA have been reported (76,78). Synovial fluid leak does not appear to be a significant impediment to healing. Reamputation to a higher level is usually due to inadequate vascularity.

Technique

Symmetrical sagittal skin flaps are fashioned at the level of the tibial tuberosity. The knee joint is then approach anteriorly through the patella tendon (Fig. 4). The cruciate ligaments are divided at the level of the tibia. This allows access to the posterior aspect of the knee exposing the vessels and nerve (Fig. 5). Once all tissues are divided, the patella tendon is secured to the posterior cruciate ligament, preventing dislocation of the patella. The skin edges are then closed with the wound lying in the intercondylar groove. Utilizing the knee disarticulation with myocutaneous flap, the skin flap is fashioned similarly to the BKA, with the long posterior flap reflecting anteriorly to cover the wound end (Fig. 6).

The Gritti-Stokes amputation at the level of the knee has become rarer, as advances in prosthetic design and articulation have made the through-knee procedure more popular.

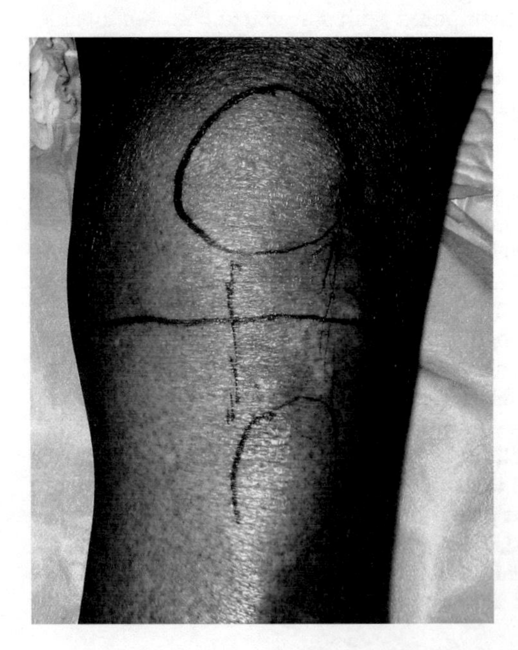

Figure 4 TKA1—Preoperative marking of through-knee amputation (TKA) (patella and tibial tuberosity circled).

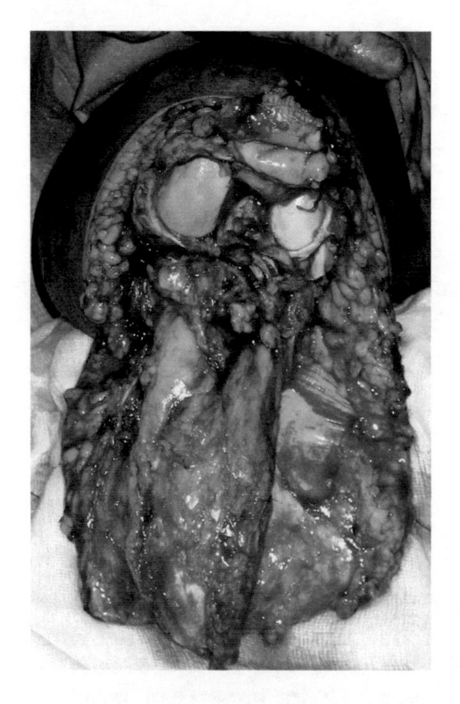

Figure 5 TKA2—Intraoperative image of through-knee amputation (TKA); femoral condyles visible above medial head of gastrocnemius.

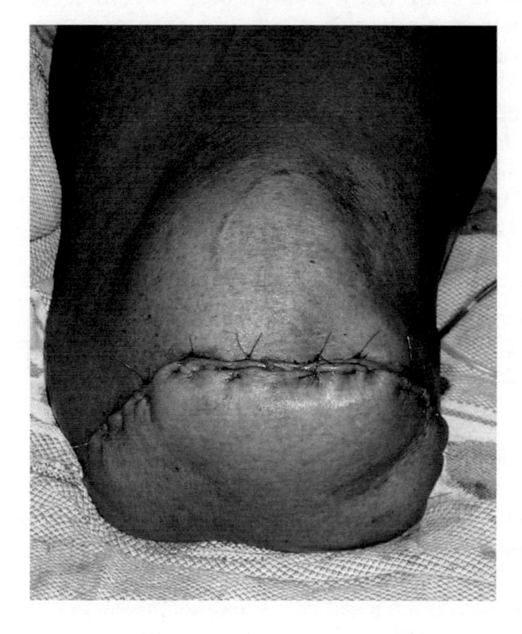

Figure 6 TKA3—Postoperative image of through-knee amputation (TKA) with long posterior flap.

Above-Knee Amputation

Transfemoral amputation is technically straightforward and is likely to heal even in the presence of severe vascular insufficiency. Yet patients rarely return to independent mobility. AKA is traditionally reserved for nonambulatory bedridden patients or if the vascular occlusive disease extends above the knee joint, precluding a more distal amputation. The key problem at this level is muscle imbalance. Disruption of the adductor magnus insertion and the linea aspera allows the residual femur to drift into abduction due to unopposed hip abductors. Technically, it is important that there is adequate myoplastic cover to the cut end of the femur to minimize pain, while allowing balanced action of flexor and extensor muscle groups. A flexor to extensor myoplasty, ignoring the adductors, can lead to an abductor lurch on mobilizing due to the unopposed hip abductors. A method of avoiding this complication is an adductor myodesis, whereby the adductor magnus is secured to the distal femur through drill holes with the leg held in maximal adduction (79).

Technique

Equal anterior and posterior "fish-mouth" skin flaps are fashioned. The soft tissues are divided to allow access to the femur. The medial neurovascular bundle is controlled. The periosteum is elevated and the femur is divided approximately 10 cm from the superior aspect of patella. The wound is closed in layers, with a low-suction drain left in situ for 24 hours. Skin closure is without tension using a continuous subcuticular dissolvable suture. In the presence of fixed hip flexion, or grossly wasted quadriceps and hamstring muscle bulks, a modification using a longer posterior flap may be beneficial. This avoids the often-experienced problem of the femoral shaft eroding through the skin.

In all techniques of amputation, the tendons and nerves are always cut short under tension and allowed to retract into the soft tissue. This improves healing and reduces neuroma formation and subsequent pain. If during amputation bleeding persists from the medullary cavity of the bone, bone wax (a softened beeswax) can be used. This is not a hemostatic agent, it merely tamponades the vascular space in the bone. Bone wax remains in place indefinitely and acts as a foreign body (80). It is known to increase infection rates, interfere with bone healing, and elicit chronic inflammatory reactions (81). Its continued use, in part, reflects the lack of an alternative. A recent animal study has advocated an alternative polymer Ostene® (blend of water-soluble alkylene oxide copolymers; Ceremed, Los Angeles, CA) that when compared with bone wax in an artificial bacterial challenge exhibited reduced rates of postoperative bone infection (82) (level B).

Evidence for Negative Pressure Dressings in Amputation

Amputation wounds can be difficult to heal, particularly if they are left to heal by secondary intention. They can be large, contain residual necrotic material, and be in patients with compromised healing secondary to diabetes or peripheral vascular disease (83). The evolution of vacuum-assisted wound therapy (VAC®, KCI Medical Ltd., UK), where the wound is enclosed in a subatmospheric pressure dressing, has benefited wounds of this kind (Fig. 7). The wound is sealed from the environment and the exudate is drawn away, both advantageous features. Dealing specifically with the diabetic foot, there have been two prospective

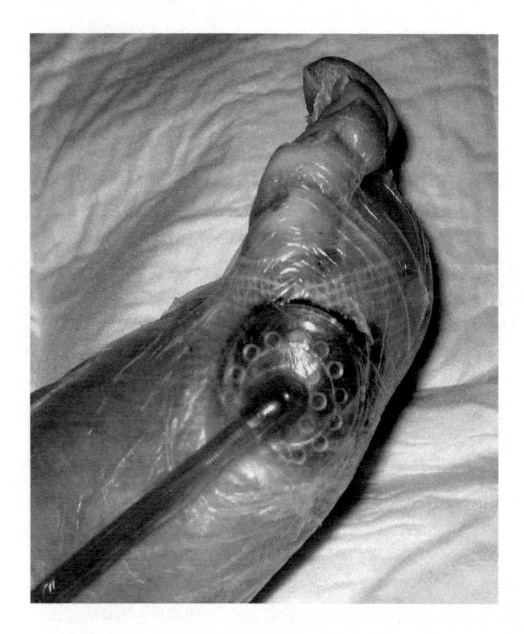

Figure 7 VAC© dressing following lateral foot debridement.

randomized studies. Eginton et al. reported their trial randomizing between VAC and conventional moist dressings in diabetic foot wounds. They concluded that negative pressure may expedite healing of large foot wounds; however, the value of their findings is limited by the fact that only 10 cases were enrolled in the study and only 6 completed the protocol (level B) (36). More recently, a larger ($N = 162$), better powered trial reported by Armstrong and Lavery concluded that VAC therapy was safe for diabetic foot wounds. It was proposed that it may lead to a higher proportion of healed wounds, faster healing, and potentially fewer reamputations than standard care (37) (level A).

COMPLICATIONS

Mortality

There is undoubtedly a selection bias in patients proceeding to major lower limb amputation. Patients are usually diabetic with associated comorbidity. Thirty-day mortality following major amputation is 6% to 18% (84–86), with increasing risk associated with renal impairment, ischemic heart disease, chronic obstructive airways disease, or disseminated malignancy. AKA may be associated with a higher in-hospital mortality compared with below knee (86). A preoperative low serum albumin has also shown to be predictive of 30-day mortality (85). Subramaniam et al. reported a median survival of 20 months following AKA and 52 months following BKA from a large retrospective cohort (level B). They commented that diabetes was not a significant predictor of perioperative mortality, or short-term mortality, but was significant in predicting mortality 10 years following surgery (87) (level B).

The overall cause mortality following lower limb amputation, in the presence of diabetes mellitus, is approximately 60% at 5 years (88,89). These retrospective studies highlighted risk factors for mortality to be duration of diabetes, history of stroke, and elevated serum creatinine.

Delayed Healing and Infection

As previously stated, the most important factor in ensuring a successful amputation is the correct choice of amputation site based on assessment of limb perfusion and functional requirements. Unfortunately, the most common stump-related problem remains wound infection and poor healing, occurring in up to 70% of cases (90). Healing rates vary according to amputation level with AKA stumps healing primarily in 70%, but BKA stumps healing primarily in 30% to 92%, and a reamputation rate up to 30% (91). Important factors in healing and outcome of amputation include the patient's nutritional status, age, active smoking, and coexisting disease, for example, renal failure, diabetes, and anaemia (92) (level B). An interesting retrospective study of 193 operations from Leicester examined clinical and operative factors influencing ambulation after major limb amputation. Univariate analysis confirmed that rate of ambulation was not affected by age, diabetes, or level of amputation, yet importantly fewer patients whose amputations were performed by a junior trainee could walk with a prosthetic limb ($p = 0.03$) (90). (level C). This highlights the specialist nature of amputation surgery, and that targeting optimal functional outcome, the operation should be performed by a specialist and not delegated to a junior surgeon.

Wound infection is a serious complication for the amputee (Fig. 8). Cellulitis may in severe cases lead to septicemia (93). Similarly, severe infection can lead to wound dehiscence requiring further surgical correction (94). Diabetic patients have a five times increased risk of postsurgical wound infections relative to nondiabetics (Fig. 9) (95) (level C). It is vital that postamputation wounds are monitored closely for expedient management of early wound infections. Standard perioperative protocol should include a 5-day course of prophylactic antibiotics aimed at reducing stump infection rates and consequently ensuring prompt discharge (96) (level B). The authors' practice is an intravenous 5-day course of benzyl penicillin 600 mg i.v. q.d.s., or metronidazole 500 mg i.v. t.d.s. for all major lower limb

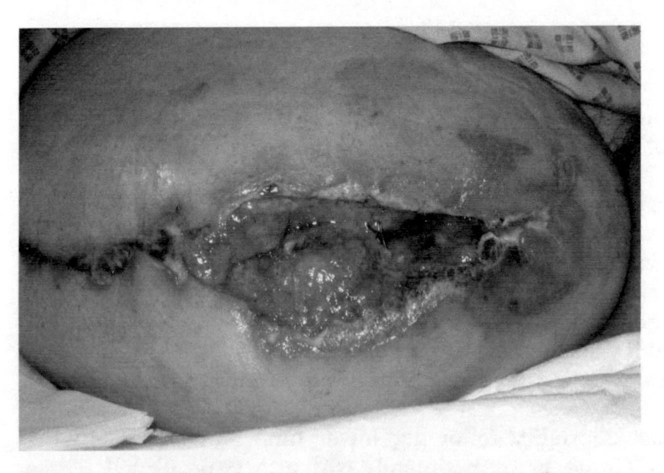

Figure 8 Wound infection following above-knee amputation.

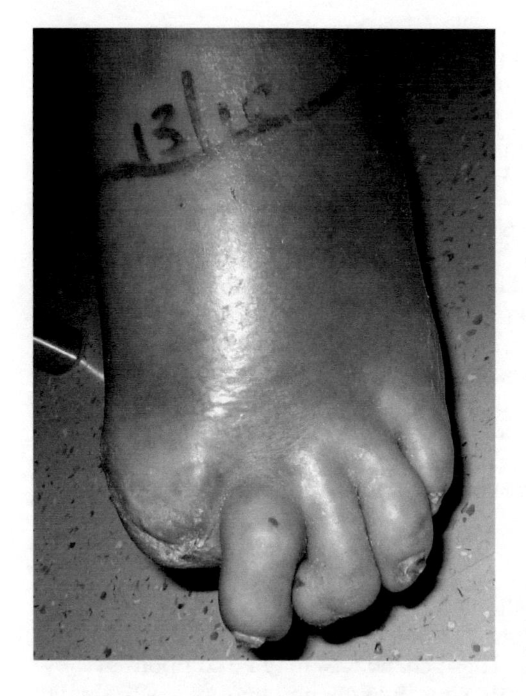

Figure 9 Ischemia—Previously amputated diabetic foot, now critically ischemic

amputations. In the presence of MRSA infection, antibiotic prophylaxis should be in the form of vancomycin or teicoplanin (97).

Postamputation Pain

Stump pain is most common in the immediate postoperative period (98), and its incidence is related to the level of preamputation pain (99). Phantom limb pain (PLP) is a noxious sensory phenomenon of the missing limb and occurs in 60% to 80% of major limb amputations (98). It is typically burning, shooting, throbbing, or boring. The incidence of PLP is increased if the patient has severe pain prior to the amputation; the PLP will often mimic this pain (100).

There is no conclusive evidence regarding techniques to prevent PLP preoperatively. Preemptive analgesia using lumbar epidural block showed initial promise (101), but further randomized studies have all had apparent flaws and provided mixed results (102,103). Overall, the protective effects of epidural anaesthesia are promising. This has been reinforced by a recent randomized trial of preemptive ketamine epidural versus bupivacaine, which showed that persistent pain at 1 year was much less in both groups than in comparable studies (45% incidence of PLP at 1 year), although no difference was identified between the groups (104) (level A).

Although peripheral nerve sheath catheters provide excellent analgesia in the perioperative period, they have no proven benefit in PLP (102) (level B).

Once established, there is no ideal therapy for PLP. There is evidence for parenteral calcitonin (105); a randomized study demonstrated benefit in three-fourth of patients with the majority having no recurrence of PLP, yet the mechanism of modulation of pain perception remains unknown (level A).

The role of oral pharmacotherapy is limited in PLP. Gabapentin has been proven in a double-blind, placebo-controlled, crossover study to be significantly better than placebo for PLP (106) (level A). Pregabalin, like gabapentin, is an amino acid–derivative of gamma-aminobutyric acid. It has been shown to provide equivalent analgesia to gabapentin, but at lower doses, and is therefore likely to have fewer dose-related adverse effects (107). This is related to pregabalin's higher bioavailability (90 vs. 33% to 66%), its rapid absorbance (peak at 1 hour), and linear dose–effect relationship (108). As pregabalin is primarily excreted by the kidneys, the dosage should be reduced in compromised renal function (creatinine clearance < 60 mL/min) (109); other oral pharmacological therapies lack anything other than anecdotal evidence.

Nonpharmacological modalities include TENS machines, acupuncture, and psychological therapies. TENS and acupuncture may work by enhancing sensory inflow to the stump, yet no randomized studies evidence this. Anxiety and depression are common in amputees; these feelings may magnify the pain experience, and efforts to preemptively treat should be part of preoperative counselling and perioperative rehabilitation.

REHABILITATION

Diabetic amputees present the rehabilitation team with the same set of challenges that likely led to the amputation. These include ischemia and/or neuropathy in the amputated or contralateral limb. These challenges may be compounded by a combination of poor muscle strength, coordination, and endurance. Systemic issues of visual impairment, balance problems, cognitive impairment, and lack of motivation to walk again may all hamper rehabilitation (110). There remains during and following rehabilitation a 50% risk of contralateral amputation at 5 years (111). Therefore, the continuing close surveillance of patients with diabetes following amputation is imperative to avoid further tissue loss. This should be identified to all patients, medical staff, and allied health care professionals.

The British Society of Rehabilitation Medicine (BSRM) has published standards and guidelines in amputee and prosthetic rehabilitation (112). They describe how rehabilitation should start at the preamputation phase with emphasis on likely function, prosthesis, and meeting with other amputees. Postoperatively, all patients must be assessed by a multidisciplinary team, advised and counseled regarding the conclusions. The rehabilitation pathway should be dynamic relative to the patients changing needs, and validated outcome measures should be used to document progress. Specific follow-up procedures should be in place, while again during the maintenance phase of established amputees, the service should be responsive to the changing needs of the patient.

Successful postoperative rehabilitation depends strongly on the patients' acceptance and adaptation to limb loss (113). Rehabilitation should start psychologically prior to surgery, but physically starts day 1 postoperatively. Dependent on the patient's general condition and pain control, the physiotherapist will initiate bed mobility, joint movements, transferring, and wheelchair mobility. It is essential that the amputee maintains power and full range of movement in proximal joints and is optimized regarding cardiovascular function. Clinical guidelines in the United Kingdom recommend that patients should be made aware that concurrent pathologies and previous mobility affect realistic goal setting and the outcomes of prosthetic rehabilitation (114). Occupational and physical therapists should ensure an effective and timely rehabilitation program. Integral to this is assessment of the home environment; necessary adaptations; and advice regarding driving, employment, and continued care.

The importance of level of amputation has been shown on rehabilitation to ambulation; there is also evidence to support psychological factors influencing rehabilitation (115). Although depression, due to its variability, cannot be correlated with poor rehabilitation (116), poor learning ability has been shown to limit rehabilitation potential following major limb amputation.

Prosthetics

Early mobilization on two limbs is essential for maximal rehabilitation. It is important, once stump healing is proven, that early walking using aids is initiated. This is beneficial in terms of patient motivation and physical training while minimizing stump edema and pain.

The Vessa® (Vessa Ltd., UK) pneumatic postamputation mobility aid (Ppam aid) is a prosthetic utilized in early postoperative rehabilitation. It comprises an inner air-filled cushion surrounded by an outer metal frame. The cushion pressure is increased proportional to patient tolerance, and allows both initial upright mobility and stump moulding.

Once the stump has healed and the sutures removed, the patient can be referred for fitting for their own prosthesis. Modern prosthetics incorporates thermoplastic materials and laminated plastics as socket materials. Artificial limbs are also constructed in lightweight carbon fibre and alloys. The ICEROSS® (Ossur, Manchester, UK) prosthesis utilized in transtibial amputees may provide a more comfortable interface between stump and socket. This system incorporates a silicon sleeve that fits over the stump, this articulates directly with the prosthesis. There is mixed evidence in the literature regarding the benefits of this system in terms of comfort and performance, with a probable overall slight advantage in terms of comfort (117) (level C).

The final outcome from rehabilitation remains unpredictable, and despite a low rate of postoperative ambulation, most patients remain living in the community (31).

Diabetic foot care should be aimed at limb preservation, but in the presence of significant sepsis or ischemia, amputation may be necessary. All levels of amputation have risks, and preoperative preparation and planning should be optimum to avoid these. If revascularization is required to ensure healing, this should be performed expediently. Amputation should be a single operation that allows prompt wound healing and rehabilitation. Efficient holistic care by the multidisciplinary team ensures that the patient can move on from this stage in their care back to independent living.

Overall length of stay and financial impacts of surgery and rehabilitation are difficult to calculate as they are multifactorial and will be biased. Recent series reported in the United Kingdom described median length of stay as 45 to 50 days (118,119). The NHS costs database published by the United Kingdom by the Department of Health describes the mean average cost of a major lower limb amputation as £5828 (range 4048 to 6953). The average length of stay was 22 days; however, this does not include rehabilitation time and rehabilitation cost (120).

Geographical variation in the rates of many surgical procedures has been described. This is equally the case for amputations in diabetic populations as shown in the U.S. (121) and European studies (122). The reasons behind this variation in procedures and overall care are unclear and not corrected by age, sex, or race adjustment. This may be due to systematic differences in preventative care and treatment decision making. Unfortunately, this type of data does not identify where the best care is provided or confirm what the optimal care pathway is. Uniform evidence-based approaches to care should be adopted worldwide providing consistency for all patients.

CONCLUSIONS

Every effort should be made to prevent the need for amputation in diabetic patients. When it is necessary, the perioperative planning should emphasize the optimal functional outcome for the patient following amputation dependent on their rehabilitation potential. A holistic approach to care governed by input from a multidisciplinary team, combined with skilled surgery from a specialist in the field, should meet this end. Once a patient with diabetes requires an amputation, strict and close follow-up surveillance should be implemented to limit further tissue loss.

REFERENCES

1. Datta D, Atkinson G. Amputation, rehabilitation and prosthetic developments. In: Beard JD, Gaines PA, eds. Vascular and Endovascular Surgery. London, England; Elsevier Ltd., 2006:105–114.
2. Akbari CM, LoGerfo FW. Diabetes and peripheral vascular disease. J Vasc Surg 1999; 30(2):373–384.
3. Asano M, Rushton P, Miller WC, et al. Predictors of quality of life among individuals who have a lower limb amputation. Prosthet Orthot Int 2008; 32(2):231–243.
4. The St Vincent Declaration. In: Diabetes Care and Research in Europe. St Vincent, Italy, 1989.
5. Prompers L, Huijberts M, Apelqvist J, et al. Delivery of care to diabetic patients with foot ulcers in daily practice: Results of the Eurodiale study, a prospective cohort study. Diabet Med 2008; 25:700–707.
6. Houghton AD, Taylor PR, Thurlow S, et al. Success rates for rehabilitation of vascular amputees: implications for preoperative assessment and amputation level. Br J Surg 1992; 79(8):753–755.
7. Bakker K. The international consensus and practical guidelines on the diabetic foot. In: Andrew JM, Boulton HC, Peter R. Cavanagh, eds. The Foot in Diabetes. 3rd ed. Chichester, UK: John Wiley and Sons, Ltd., 2002:323–344.
8. Lavery LA, Armstrong DG, Vela SA, et al. Practical criteria for screening patients at high risk for diabetic foot ulceration. Arch Intern Med 1998; 158:157–162.
9. Pecoraro J, Reiber GE, Burgess EM. Pathways to diabetic limb amputation. Basis for prevention. Diabetes Care 1990; 13:513–521.
10. Sinacore DR. Total contact casting for diabetic neuropathic ulcers. Physical Therapy 1996; 76:296–301.
11. Mueller MJ, Sinacore DR, Hastings MK, et al. Effect of Achilles tendon lengthening on neuropathic plantar ulcers. J Bone Joint Surg 2003; 85-A(8):1436–1445.
12. Johnson B, Evans L, Datta D, et al. Surgery for limb threatening ischaemia. A reappraisal of costs and benefits. Eur J Vasc Endovasc Surg 1995; 9:181–188.
13. Reiber GE, Vileikyte L, Boyko EJ, et al. Causal pathways for incident lower-extremity ulcers in patients with diabetes from two settings. Diabetes Care 1999; 22:157–162.
14. Ratcliffe DA, Clyne CAC, Chant ADB, et al. Prediction of amputation wound healing: The role of transcutaneous pO2 assessment. Br J Surg 1984; 71:219–222.

15. Keyser-Dekker CMG, Moerman E, Leijdekkers VJ, et al. Can transcutaneous oxygen tension measurement determine re-amputation levels? J wound care 2006; 15(1): 27–30.
16. Van Den Broek TAA, Dwars BJ, Rauwerda JA, et al. Photoplethysmographic selection of amputation level in peripheral vascular disease. J Vasc Surg 1988; 8:10–13.
17. Karanfilian RG, Lynch TG, Zinsl VT, et al. The value of laser Doppler velocimetry and transcutaneous oxygen tension determination in predicting healing of ischaemic foot ulcerations and amputations in diabetic and non-diabetic patients. J Vasc Surg 1986; 4:511–516.
18. Adera HM, James K, Castronuovo JJ, et al. Prediction of amputation wound healing with skin perfusion pressure. J Vasc Surg 1995; 21:823–829.
19. Stoner HB, Taylor L, Marcuson RW. The value of skin temperature measurements in forecasting healing of below-knee amputation for end-stage ischaemia of the leg in peripheral vascular disease. Eur J Vasc Surg 1989; 3:355–361.
20. Sarin S, Shami S, Shields DA, et al. Selection of amputation level: A review. Eur J Vasc Surg 1991; 5(6):611–620.
21. Khaodhiar L, Dinh T, Schomacker KT, et al. The use of medical hyperspectral technology to evaluate microcirculatory changes in diabetic foot ulcers and to predict clinical outcomes. Diabetes Care 2007; 30:903–910.
22. Tsai FW, Tulsyan N, Jones DN, et al. Skin perfusion pressure of the foot is a good substitute for toe pressure in the assessment of limb ischaemia. J Vasc Surg 2000; 32:32–36.
23. Barber GG, McPhail NV, Scobie TK, et al. A prospective study of lower limb amputations. Can J Surg 1983; 26:339–341.
24. Burgess EM, Matsen FA. Determining amputation levels in peripheral vascular disease. J Bone Joint Surg 1981; 63:1493–1497.
25. O'Dwyer KJ, Edwards MH. The association between lowest palpable pulse and wound healing in below knee amputations. Ann R Coll Surg Eng 1985; 67:232–234.
26. Jarrett DC. Current concepts in diabetic foot surgery. Podiatry Today 2007; 20(3): 40–46.
27. Waters RL, Perry J, Antonelli D, et al. Energy cost of walking of amputees: The influence of level of amputation. J Bone Joint Surg 1976; 58:42–46.
28. Pinzur MS. Gait analysis in peripheral vascular insufficiency through-knee amputation. J Rehabil Res Dev 1993; 30:388–392.
29. Philbin TM, Berlet GC, Lee TH. Lower-extremity amputations in association with diabetes mellitus. Foot Ankle Clin 2006; 11(4):791–804.
30. Larsson J, Agardh CD, Apelqvist J, et al. Long term prognosis after healed amputations in patients with diabetes. Clin Orthop Rel Res 1998; 350:149–158.
31. Nehler MR, Coll JR, Hiatt WR, et al. Functional outcome in a contemporary series of major lower extremity amputations. J Vasc Surg 2003; 38:7–14.
32. Cumming JCO, Barr S, Howe TE. Prosthetic rehabilitation for older dysvascular people following a unilateral transfemoral amputation. Cochrane Database Syst Rev 2008; 3:1–15.
33. Nehler MR, Whitehill TA, Bowers SP, et al. Intermediate-term outcome of primary digit amputations in patients with diabetes mellitus who have forefoot sepsis requiring hospitalisation and presumed adequate circulatory status. J Vasc Surg 1999; 30: 509–518.
34. Izumi Y, Satterfield K, Lee S, et al. Risk of reamputation in diabetic patients stratified by limb and level of amputation: A 10 year observation. Diabetes Care 2006; 29:566–570.
35. Flack S, Apelqvist J, Keith M, et al. An economic evaluation of VAC therapy compared with wound dressings in the treatment of diabetic foot ulcers. J Wound Care 2008; 17(2):71–78.
36. Eginton MT, Brown KR, Seabrook GR, et al. A prospective randomised evaluation of negative-pressure wound dressings for diabetic foot wounds. Ann Vasc Surg 2003; 17:645–649.

37. Armstrong DG, Lavery LA. Negative pressure wound therapy after partial diabetic foot amputation: A multicentre, randomised controlled trial. Lancet 2005;366: 1704–1710.
38. Armstrong DG, Hadi S, Nguyen HC, et al. Factors associated with bone regrowth following diabetes-related partial amputation of the foot. J Bone Joint Surg 1999; 81–A(11):1561–1565.
39. Wagner FW. Orthopaedic rehabilitation of the dysvascular limb. Orthop Clin North Am 1978; 9:325–350.
40. Bowker JH. Medical and surgical considerations in the care of patients with insensate dysvascular feet. J Prosthet Orthot 1992; 4(1):23–30.
41. Atindas M, Cinar C. Promoting primary healing after ray amputations in the diabetic foot: The plantar dermo-fat pad flap. Plast Reconstr Surg 2005; 116:1029–1034.
42. Wieman TJ, Mercke YK, Cerrito PB, et al. Resection of the metatarsal head for diabetic foot ulcers. Am J Surg 1998; 176:436–441.
43. Atnip RG. Toe and partial foot amputations. In: Operative Techniques in General Surgery. 2005; 7(2):67–73.
44. McKittrick IS, McKittrick JB, Rixley TS. Transmetatarsal amputations for infection or gangrene in patients with diabetes. Ann Surg 1949; 130:826–842.
45. Hoach J, Quiroga C, Bosma J, et al. Outcomes of transmetatarsal amputations in patients with diabetes mellitus. J Foot Ankle Surg 1997; 36:430–434.
46. Geroukalos G, May AR. Transmetatarsal amputation in patients with peripheral vascular disease. Eur J Vasc Surg 1991; 5:655–658.
47. Miller N, Dardick H, Wolodiger F, et al. Transmetatarsal amputation: The role of adjunctive revascularization. J Vasc Surg 1991; 13:705–711.
48. Sheahan MG, Hamdan AD, Veraldi JR, et al. Lower extremity minor amputations: The roles of diabetes mellitus and timing of revascularisation. J Vasc Surg 2005; 42: 476–480.
49. Hosch J, Quiroga C, Bosma J, et al. Outcomes of transmetatarsal amputations in patients with diabetes mellitus. J Foot Ankle Surg 1997; 36(6):430–434.
50. Ballard K, McGregor F. Use of vacuum-assisted closure therapy following foot amputation. Br J Nurs 2001; 10(suppl 15):S6–S12.
51. Andros G, Armstrong DG, Attinger CE, et al. Consensus statement on negative pressure wound therapy (V.A.C. Therapy) for the management of diabetic foot wounds. Ostomy Wound Manage 2006; (suppl):1–32.
52. Funk C, Young G. Subtotal pedal amputations: Biomechanical and intraoperative considerations. J Am Podiatr Med Assoc 2001; 91(1):6–12.
53. Salonga C, Blume P. A guide to transmetatarsal amputations in patients with diabetes. Podiatry Today 2006; 19(7):82–90.
54. Pinzur MS, Morrison C, Sage R, et al. Syme's two-stage amputation in insulin-requiring diabetics with gangrene of the forefoot. Foot Ankle 1991; 11: 394–396.
55. Francis H, Roberts JR, Clagett GP, et al. The Syme amputation: Success in elderly diabetic patients with palpable foot pulses. J Vasc Surg 1990; 12:237–240.
56. Wagner FW. Amputations of the foot and ankle. Current Status. Clin Orthop 1977; 122:62–69.
57. Pinzur MS, Stuck RM, Sage R, et al. Syme ankle disarticulation in patients with diabetes. J Bone Joint Surg 2003; 85-A(9):1667–1672.
58. Weaver FA, Chambers RB, Hood DB. Syme amputation. Perspectives in vascular and endovascular therapy. 1999; 10:89–95.
59. Taylor SM, Kalbaugh C, Blackhurst DW, et al. Preoperative clinical factors predict postoperative functional outcomes after major lower limb amputation: An analysis of 553 consecutive patients. J Vasc Surg 2005; 42:227–235.
60. Burgess EM, Romano RL. The management of lower extremity amputees using immediate post surgical prostheses. Clin Ortho 1968; 57:137–156.
61. Robinson KP, Hoile R, Coddington T. Skew flap myoplastic below-knee amputation: A preliminary report. Br J Surg 1982; 69(9):554–557.

62. Persson BM. Sagittal incision for below-knee amputation in ischaemic gangrene. J Bone Joint Surg 1974; 56B:110–114.
63. Jain AS, Stewart CPU, Turner MS. Transtibial amputation using a medially based flap. J R Coll Surg Edinb 1995; 40:263–265.
64. Humzah MD, Gilbert PM. Fasciocutaneous blood supply in below-knee amputation. J Bone Joint Surg (Br) 1997; 79-B:441–443.
65. Johnson WC, Watkins MT, Hamilton J, et al. Transcutaneous partial oxygen pressure changes following skew flap and Burgess-type below knee amputations. Arch Surg 1997; 132:261–263.
66. Ruckley CV, Stonebridge PA, Prescott RJ. Skew flap versus long posterior flap in below-knee amputations: Multicenter trial. J Vasc Surg 1991; 13(3):423–427.
67. Choksy SA, Lee Chong P, Smith C, et al. A randomised controlled trial of the use of a tourniquet to reduce blood loss during transtibial amputation for peripheral arterial disease. Eur J Vasc Endovasc Surg 2006; 31(6):646–650.
68. Wolthuis AM, Whitehead E, Ridler BM, et al. Use of a pneumatic tourniquet improves outcome following trans-tibial amputation. Eur J Vasc Endovasc Surg 2006; 31(6): 642–645.
69. Sanders RJ, Augspurger R. Skin flap measurement for below-knee amputation. Surg Gynecol Obstet 1977; 145(5):740–742.
70. Pinzur MS, Gottschalk FA, Pinto MA, et al. Controversies in lower-extremity amputation. J Bone Joint Surg Am 2007; 89(5):1118–1127.
71. Pinzur MS, Pinto MA, Saltzman M, et al. Health-related quality of life in patients with transtibial amputation and reconstruction with bone bridging of the distal tibia and fibula. Foot Ankle Int 2006; 27:907–912.
72. Smith DJ, Mcfarland LV, Sangeorzan BJ, et al. Postoperative dressings and management strategies for transtibial amputations: A critical review. J Prosthet Orthot 2004; 16(3s):15–25.
73. Nawijn SE, Van der Linde H, Emmelot CH, et al. Stump management after trans-tibial amputation: A systematic review. Prosthet Orthot Int 2005; 29(1):13–26.
74. Taylor L, Cavenett S, Stephen JM, et al. Removable rigid dressings: A retrospective case-note audit to determine the validity of post-amputation application. Prosthet Orthot Int 2008; 32(2):223–230.
75. Pinzur MS, Bowker JH. Knee disarticulation. Clin Orthop Rel Res 1999; 361:23–28.
76. Morse BC, Cull DL, Kalbaugh C, et al. Through-knee amputation in patients with peripheral arterial disease: A review of 50 cases. J Vasc Surg 2008; 48:638–643.
77. Moran BJ, Buttenshaw P, Mulcahy M, et al. Through-knee amputation in high-risk patients with vascular disease: Indications, complications and rehabilitation. Br J Surg 1990; 77(10):1118–1120.
78. Cull DL, Taylor SM, Hamontree SE, et al. A reappraisal of a modified through-knee amputation in patients with peripheral vascular disease. Am J Surg 2001; 182:44–48.
79. Gottschalk F. Transfemoral amputation: Biomechanics and surgery. Clin Orthop Relat Res 1999; 361:15–22.
80. Randon C, Deroose J. How to perform a below knee amputation (Technical note). Acta Chir Belg 2003; 103:238–240.
81. Schonauer C, Tessitore E, Barbagallo G, et al. The use of local agents: Bone wax, gelatin, collagen, oxidised cellulose. Eur Spine J 2004; 13(suppl 1):S89–S96.
82. Wellisz T, An YH, Wen X, et al. Infection rates and healing using bone wax and a soluble polymer material. Clin Orthop Relat Res 2008; 466:481–486.
83. Armstrong DG, Frykberg RG. Classification of diabetic foot surgery: Toward a rational definition. Diabet Med 2003; 20:329–331.
84. O'Hare AM, Feinglass J, Reiber GE, et al. Postoperative mortality after nontraumatic extremity amputation in patients with renal insufficiency. J Am Soc Nephrol 2004; 15:427–434.
85. Feinglass J, Pearce WH, Martin GJ, et al. Postoperative and late survival outcomes after major amputation: Findings from the Department of Veterans Affairs National Quality Improvement Program. Surgery 2001; 130:21–29.

86. Ploeg AJ, Lardenoye JW, Vrancken Peeters M-P, et al. Contemporary series of morbidity and mortality after lower limb amputation. Eur J Vasc Endovasc Surg 2005; 29:633–637.
87. Subramaniam B, Pomposelli FB, Talmor D, et al. Perioperative and long-term morbidity and mortality after above-knee and below-knee amputations in diabetics and nondiabetics. Anaesth Analg 2005;100(5):1241–1247.
88. Tentolouris N, Al-Sabbagh S, Walker MG, et al. Mortality in diabetic and nondiabetic patients after amputations performed from 1990 to 1995: A 5-year follow-up study. Diabetes Care 2004; 27(7):1598–1604.
89. Faglia E, Favales F, Morabito A. New ulceration, new major amputation, and survival rates in diabetic subjects hospitalised for foot ulceration from 1990 to 1993. Diabetes Care 2001; 24:78–83.
90. White SA, Thompson MM, Zickerman AM, et al. Lower limb amputation and the grade of surgeon. Br J Surg 1997; 84(4):509–511.
91. Dormandy J, Heeck L, Vig S. Major amputations: Clinical patterns and predictors. Semin Vasc Surg 1999; 12(2):154–161.
92. Eneroth M, Persson BM. Risk factors for failed healing in amputation for vascular disease. A prospective, consecutive study of 177 cases. Acta Orthop Scand 1993; 64(3):369–372.
93. Grey JE. Cellulitis associated with wounds. J Wound Care 1998; 7(7):338–339.
94. Baxter H. Management of surgical wounds. Nurs Times 2003; 99(13):66–68.
95. Ray RL. Complications of lower extremity amputations. Topics Emergency Med 2000; 22(3):35–42.
96. Sadat U, Chaudhuri A, Hayes PD, et al. Five day antibiotic prophylaxis for major lower limb amputation reduces wound infection rates and the length of in-hospital stay. Eur J Vasc Surg 2008; 35(1):75–78.
97. Grimble SAJ, Magee TR, Galland RB. Methicillin resistant *Staphylococcus aureus* in patients undergoing major amputation. Eur J Vasc Endovasc Surg 2001; 22: 215–218.
98. Nikolajsen L, Jensen TS. Phantom limb pain. Br J Anaesth 2001; 87(1):107–116.
99. Nikolajsen L, Ilkjaer S, Kroner K, et al. The influence of preamputation pain on post amputation stump and phantom pain. Pain 1997; 72(3):393–405.
100. Katz J, Melzack R. Pain "memories" in phantom limbs: Review and clinical observations. Pain 1990; 43(3): 7–12.
101. Bach S, Noreng MF, Tjellden NU. Phantom limb pain in amputees during the first twelve months following limb amputation, after preoperative lumbar blockade. Pain 1988; 33(3):297–301.
102. Lambert A, Dashfield A, Cosgrove C. Randomised prospective study comparing preoperative epidural and intraoperative perineural analgesia for the prevention of postoperative stump and phantom limb pain following major amputation. Reg Anesth Pain Med 2001; 26(4):316–321.
103. Nikolajsen L, Ilkjaer S, Christensen JH, et al. Pain after amputation. Br J Anaesth 1998; 81(3):486.
104. Wilson JA, Nimmo AF, Fleetwood-Walker SM, et al. A randomised double-blind trial of the effect of pre-emptive epidural ketamine on persistent pain after lower limb amputation. Pain 2008; 135:108–118.
105. Jaeger H, Maier C. Calcitonin in phantom limb pain: A double blind study. Pain 1992; 48(1):21–27.
106. Bone M, Critchley P, Buggy DJ. Gabapentin in post amputation phantom limb pain: A randomised, double blind, placebo controlled, cross-over study. Reg Anesth Pain Med 2002; 27(5):481–486.
107. Lesser H, Sharma U, LaMoreaux L, et al. Pregabalin relieves symptoms of painful diabetic neuropathy: A randomized controlled trial. Neurology 2004; 63(11): 2104–2110.
108. Gajraj NM. Pregabalin: Its pharmacology and use in pain management. Anaesth Analg 2007; 105:1805–1815.

109. Randinitis EJ, Posvar EL, Alvey CW, et al. Pharmacokinetics of Pregabalin in subjects with various degrees of renal function. J Clin Pharmacol 2003; 43:277–283.
110. Call JD. Prosthetic implications of diabetes. Virginia Prosthetics Update 2000; 32:1–2.
111. Reiber GE, Lipsky BA, Gibbons GW. The burden of diabetic foot ulcers. Am J Surg 1998; 176(2A, suppl):5S–10S.
112. BSRM. Standards and guidelines in amputee and prosthetic rehabilitation, 2003. http://www.bsrm.co.uk/Publications/Publications.htm.
113. Gagnon CG, Grise M, Potvin D. Predisposing factors related to prosthetic use by people with transtibial and transfemoral amputation. J Prosthet Orthot 1998; 10:99–109.
114. Broomhead P, Dawes D, Lambert A, et al. Evidence based clinical guidelines for the physiotherapy management of adults with lower limb prostheses: Chartered society of physiotherapy, 2003. http://www.csp.org.uk/uploads/documents/csp_guideline_bacpar.pdf.
115. Larner S, van Ross E, Hale C. Do psychological measures predict the ability of lower limb amputees to learn to use a prosthesis? Clin Rehabil 2002; 17:493–498.
116. Schubert DSP, Burns R, Paras W, et al. Increase in medical length of stay by depression in stroke and amputation patients. Psychother Psychosom 1992; 57:61–66.
117. Dasgupta AK, McCluskie PJA, Patel VS, et al. The performance of the ICEROSS prostheses amongst transtibial amputees with a special reference to the workplace—a preliminary study. Occup Med 1997; 47:228–236.
118. Lim TS, Finlayson A, Thorpe JM. Outcomes of a contemporary amputation series. ANZ J Surg 2006; 76(5):300–305.
119. Turney BW, Kent SJS, Walker RT, et al. Amputation is no longer the end of the road. J R Coll Surg Edinb 2001; 46:271–273.
120. DOH. National Schedule of Reference Costs: DOH, 2006.
121. Wrobel JS, Mayfield JA, Reiber GE. Geographical variation of lower-extremity major amputation in individuals with and without diabetes in the medicare population. Diabetes Care 2001; 24:860–864.
122. Van Houtem WH, Lavery LA. Regional variation in the incidence of diabetes-related amputations in The Netherlands. Diabetes Res Clin Pract 1996; 31:125–132.

13 Preventing foot complications

Lawrence A. Lavery and Agbor Ndip

There are several low-cost prevention strategies to reduce the incidence of foot ulcerations and amputations. The standard approach to prevent ulceration is to provide padded insoles and protective shoes, educate the patients and their family, and provide regular foot inspection by the patients' primary care physician or podiatrist. Several studies support the effectiveness of this type of approach to reduce the incidence of ulceration and amputation (1–3). The benefit of a team approach to prevent foot ulceration and to reduce amputations has been described multiple times in the United States and Europe.

Understanding the etiology of foot wounds is pivotal to appreciate the rationale for prevention and to educate the patient about the severity of disease and self-care strategies. Foot ulcers usually develop in patients with peripheral sensory neuropathy with enough sensory loss that allows them to injure themselves without recognizing or perceiving the injury. It is a level of neuropathy referred to as, neuropathy with loss of protective sensation. Ulcers on the sole of the foot commonly occur at sites of abnormal or prolonged pressure and shear forces. The site of these ulcers can be associated with callus, limited joint mobility, and structural foot deformity such as clawing of the toes, hallux valgus deformity, and ankle equinus. In addition, ulcers may be caused by ill-fitting shoes, penetrating puncture injuries and burns from hot bathwater, sidewalks, or road surfaces. If normal sensation is present, pain usually protects the injured foot from deep tissue damage.

One of the most common components in the causal pathway to limb amputation in persons with diabetes is a neuropathic foot ulcer (4). The etiology of ulcerations in persons with diabetes is commonly associated with the presence of peripheral neuropathy and repetitive trauma due to normal walking activities to areas on the sole of the foot that are subject to moderate or high pressures and shear (5). However, penetrating trauma and ill-fitting shoes are also common mechanisms of injury.

RISK CLASSIFICATION

Classifying patients into groups on the basis of perceived risk status is a practical approach to target and prioritize high risk for prevention services. Every health care system is challenged to assess and prioritize patients to receive specialized prevention services. The naïve assume the diagnosis of diabetes is the threshold to begin prevention of foot ulcerations and amputations rather than diabetes-related comorbidities that have been associated with increased risk of ulceration, infection, and amputation. In most centers, even basic foot risk assessment is not performed even though the criteria and procedures are inexpensive, practical, and easy to execute. A trained technician can perform many of the tests to identify risk factors and begin the risk stratification and referral process. The first challenge in prevention is to identify who to target first.

There are several risk stratification tools that have been used to assess the diabetic foot. Most classification schemes are based on the foot risk classification devised at the Carville Hansen Disease Center. International Working Group on the Diabetic Foot's (IWGDF) risk classification was designed from a consensus panel (6). The most important factors for risk classification include assessment of sensory neuropathy; peripheral vascular disease; severe foot deformity; and history of foot pathology such as ulceration, amputation, Charcot arthropathy, and lower extremity bypass. History is the least expensive and the most reliable factor to identify who is at the greatest risk of developing a foot complication in the next year. Several studies have validated the system to predict foot ulcers and amputations (7,8).

In separate studies Mayfield et al. and Lavery et al. used risk classifications similar to the International Working Group's Diabetic Foot Risk Classification to demonstrate that the frequency of foot complications increases as the risk criteria increases (9,10). Lavery and Peters evaluated a cohort of 1666 patients with diabetes who participated in a diabetes disease management program for more than two years (Table 1). They expanded the IWGDF classification and compared groups with peripheral arterial disease (PAD), neuropathy and neuropathy with foot deformity, PAD, history of foot ulcer, and history of amputation. In the study, there was no difference in ulceration in patients with neuropathy and neuropathy and foot deformity. However, there was a significant increase in incident foot ulceration, reulceration, infection, amputation, and hospitalization in patients with PAD compared to patients with neuropathy and neuropathy and foot deformity. In addition, there were more ulcers in patients with a history of ulcers and amputations compared to patients with PAD or neuropathy, but there was no difference in incident ulcers when groups with a history of ulcers were compared to patients with a history of amputation (7). Overall, there were increasing trends in the frequency of foot ulcers, infections, and amputations with the stratification in a modified version of the IWGDF risk classification.

Targeting the correct risk group is important to provide cost effective preventative care. The risk groups that include patients with peripheral vascular disease and history of ulcers or amputations are the highest risk groups for ulcers. For instance, 20% of the patients account for 70% of diabetic foot ulcers (DFUs) and 90% of foot-related hospitalizations (7). These are the obvious groups to focus intensive prevention therapies. The risk of developing an ulceration is more than 50 times greater in patients with a history of an ulcer or amputation compared to patients with no neuropathy or PAD.

Based on the results of the study, a modification of the foot risk classification was proposed (Table 2) (7). The groups with neuropathy but without PAD were combined, and PAD was stratified into a separate risk group. As proposed in other risk classifications, patients with previous foot ulcers or amputations were included in the highest-risk group. The alternative diabetic foot risk classification reported by Lavery and Peters simplifies the previous systems by stratifying groups on the basis of peripheral neuropathy, peripheral vascular disease, and history of ulceration or amputation. These simple criteria help to predict who will develop ulcers, infections, and amputations (Table 2).

Table 1 Outcomes by Modified International Working Group's Diabetic Foot Risk Classification: Data is Reported in the Percent of Yearly Incidence of Complications and the Odds Ratio of Each Risk Strata Compared to Group 0 (7)

n = 1666	Ulcer	Infection	Amputation
Risk group 1	2.0%	1.2%	0.04%
No neuropathy			
No PAD			
Neuropathy	4.5%	1.8%	0
No PAD			
Odds ratios 0	2.4	1.9	3.3
compared to 1	(1.9–3.1)	(1.1–3.3)	(0.02–631.1)
Risk group 2A	3.0%	2.3%	0.7%
Neuropathy and			
foot deformity			
Odds ratios 0	1.5	2.3	11.1
compared to 2A	(1.3–1.8)	(1.8–2.9)	(1.9–64.1)
Risk group 2B	13.8%	11.0%	3.7%
PAD			
Odds ratios 0	9.3	13.6	61.1
compared to 2B	(8.4–10.4)	(11.6–15.9)	(13.9–268.4)
Risk group 3A	31.7%	14.2%	2.2%
Ulcer history			
Odds ratios 0	51.2	19.3	36.4
compared to 3A	(45.2–57.8)	(16.5–22.6)	(7.2–185.3)
Risk group 3B	32.2%	26.8%	20.7%
Amputation History			
Odds ratios 0	54.4	62.6	576.6
compared to 3B	(44.1–67.1)	(50.0–78.3)	(136.3–2439.0)

THERAPEUTIC SHOES AND INSOLES

Many studies have linked plantar pressures to the sites of ulceration in neuropathic patients (11–14). Duckworth and associates evaluated neuropathic and non-neuropathic diabetic patients, using a computerized optical pedobarograph, and demonstrated that all ulcerated neuropathic patients had a "barefoot" peak pressure greater than 112 N/cm^2 (13). However, other work suggests that "threshold pressures" may be substantially less than that previously reported. In fact, the average peak pressures at the site of ulceration in the two separate studies were 92 N/cm^2 (15) and 82 N/cm^2. In addition, many patients with low or moderate foot pressures developed ulcerations suggesting that shear may be another component in many patients who develop wounds in the presence of relatively moderate vertical forces (16).

Observations about abnormal pressure and shear stresses on the foot have translated into clinical efforts to develop special shoes and insoles to prevent ulcers in high-risk diabetics. Many studies have investigated the effectiveness of insoles to reduce plantar pressures (17–21). Ashry et al. investigated five footwear-insole treatments and found that peak pressures were significantly reduced when an insole was used in an extra-depth shoe. However, there was no difference

Table 2 Diabetic Foot Risk Classifications

Original international working group's diabetic foot risk classification	Modified international working group's diabetic classification	Lavery–Peters diabetic foot risk classification
Risk group 0 No neuropathy, No PAD	**Risk group 0** No neuropathy, No PAD	**Risk group 1** No neuropathy, No PAD
Risk group 1 Peripheral neuropathy No deformity or PAD	**Risk group 1** Peripheral neuropathy No deformity or PAD	**Risk group 2** Neuropathy
Risk group 2 Peripheral neuropathy and deformity or PAD	**Risk group 2A** Peripheral neuropathy and deformity	
	Risk group 2B PAD	**Risk group 3** PAD
Risk group 3 History of ulcer or amputation	**Risk group 3A** History of ulcer **Risk group 3B** History of amputation	**Risk group 4** History of ulcer or amputation

in pressure reduction when modifications to the insoles were made (6). Bus et al. looked at plantar pressure changes with custom insoles in diabetics with neuropathy and foot deformity. Similarly, they found that custom insoles were more effective than flat insoles, but there was considerable variability of this effect among patients. Some patients had no benefit and some patients had an increase in foot pressures rather than a reduction (22).

There is little clinical evidence to help us prescribe specific modifications for shoes and insoles, but there are several studies that consistently demonstrate better clinical outcomes (level A, Table 3). There are a variety of rocker designs and outer sole modifications for shoes, and there are many choices for insole materials and designs. Most of the decisions for protective shoes and insoles are left to technicians who have no working knowledge of the medical literature. Their decisions are based on a hands-on tradition. When patients develop an ulcer, the technicians have no feedback concerning the effectiveness of their work because patients return to medical clinics and not to the shoe and insole maker. It is important to provide feedback to the technician who fabricates special shoes and insoles for high-risk patients.

Providing a shoe and insole to reduce the risk of ulceration entails a prescription for compromise for many patients. The first efforts must be to eliminate the patient's shoe as a source of underlying pathology. Many ulcers are the result of ill-fitting shoes. Finding a shoe fitter that gets the fit correct is essential. The second focus should be to get shoes for inside and outside the home that are cosmetically acceptable and can protect the foot. It does little good for a patient to have shoes they will never use, or refuse prescribed footwear only to go back to a shoe that will cause an ulcer. Often patients with neuropathy and postural instability cannot tolerate rocker soles and thick accommodative insoles. In addition, patients often will go barefoot at home rather than wear any shoes. It is probably unreasonable to ask a patient to wear the same shoes in from the snow and rain when they return home. Yet, often our prescriptions for self-care lack common sense and reason.

There are only two randomized clinical studies that evaluated insoles to prevent ulcers. One study's population had a high proportion of subjects without sensory neuropathy (23). And the other study used only custom molded shoes and insoles (24). Both randomized controlled trials (RCTs) compared a treatment of interest to "self-selected shoes."

Reiber et al. conducted a randomized clinical study and compared custom bilaminar cork and neoprene insoles (n = 121), prefabricated polyurethane insoles (n = 119), and a control group (n = 160) in which patients selected their own shoes (23). Over a two-year evaluation, ulceration was identified in 15% of the custom insole group, 14% of the prefabricated insole group, and 17% of the controls. Unfortunately, most of the study subjects did not have sensory neuropathy and would not have been considered "high risk" by Medicare criteria. In addition, neither insole design would meet the current Medicare standards for therapeutic insoles. Reiber's study was the only negative study of therapeutic shoes and insole for high-risk patients with diabetes. It was also the study with the lowest reulceration rate in the control arm treated with self-selected shoes (17%). The rate of ulceration was lower in the control arm of Reiber's study than many of the therapeutic shoe treatment groups in other studies (Table 3).

Table 3 Clinical Studies of Therapeutic Shoes and Insoles to Prevent Reulceration

Author (year)	Study design and duration	n	Intervention groups	Ulcerations (%)
Reiber (2002)	RCT	121	Custom cork–neoprene	15
	24 months	119	Prefabricated polyurethane insole	14
		160	Self-selected shoes	17
Uccioli[a] (1995)	RCT	33	Custom made shoe and insoles	27.7
	12 months	36	Self-selected shoes	58.3
Busch[a] (2003)	Prospective cohort	60	Rocker sole shoe and standard insole	15
	12 months	32	Self-selected shoes	60
Dargis[a] (1999)	Prospective cohort	56	Therapeutic shoes	30.4
	24 months	89	Self-selected shoes	58.4
Striesow[a] (1998)	Retrospective cohort	30	Therapeutic shoes	26.7
	12 months	27	Self-selected shoes	66.7
Viswanathan (2004)	Prospective cohort	100	Insole with microcellular rubber	4.0
		59	Insole with polyurethane foam	3.4
		32	Custom molded insole with ethylene vinyl acetate and cork	3.1
		50	Insole with leather board insoles	66.0

[a]Ref. 25.

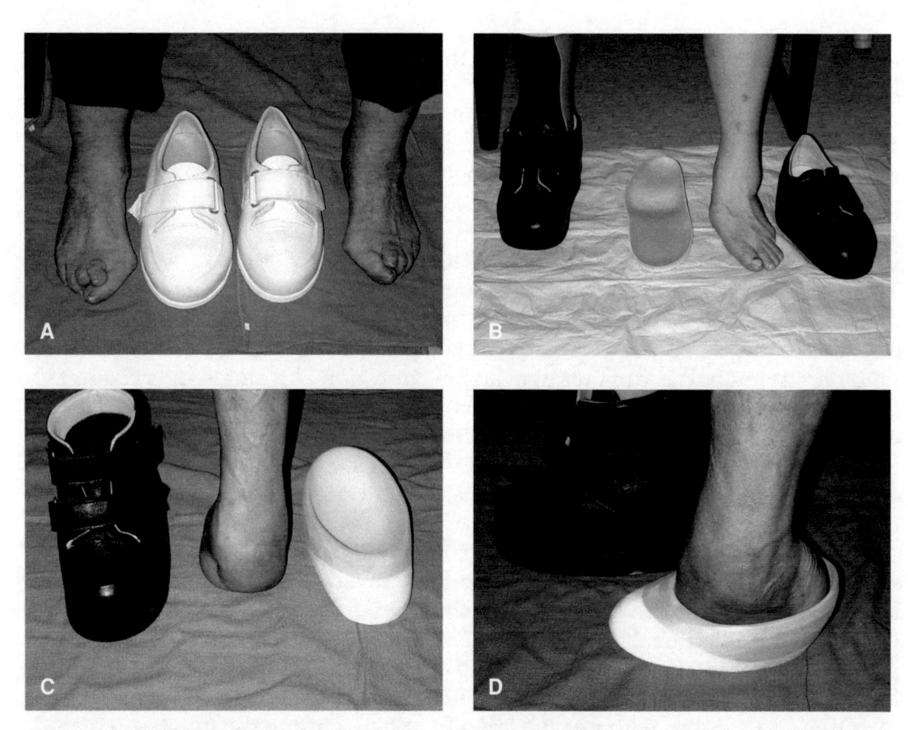

Figure 1 (**A**) Inlay depth shoes with a wide and extra deep toe box to allow room for the severe hallux valgus and hammertoe deformities. (**B**) Custom shoes and insoles to accommodate a foot deformity caused by Charcot Arthropathy. (**C** and **D**) Custom shoe and insole to protect the stump of a Chopart's amputation.

Uccioli and coworkers conducted a multicenter RCT of patients with previous foot ulceration for one year (24). Patients were randomized to custom made shoes and insoles (n = 33) or self-selected shoes (n = 36). Reulceration was significantly lower in the custom shoe treatment group (27.7%) compared with patients who selected their own footwear (58.2%, p = 0.009). Most patients who require therapeutic shoes and insoles do not require a custom made shoe. Usually custom shoes are only necessary when the foot is so deformed that the foot will not fit in a ready-made shoe (Fig. 1).

In addition to the two RCTs, there are several prospective and retrospective cohort studies that describe the benefit of various types of shoes and insoles for high-risk patients with diabetes (Table 3). Most shoe and insole studies evaluated patients who have had previous foot ulceration, because their risk of developing another ulceration in the next 12 months is very high (Table 1). The patients in the control group used "self-selected" shoes. In some studies, this is because they cannot afford therapeutic shoes (25), they refuse recommended shoes (26), or their insurance does not pay for shoes and insoles (27). Most studies were performed at specialty foot centers with a focus on diabetes. Even in these centers, the risk of reinjury was very high (Table 1). In groups that selected their own shoes, the incidence of foot ulceration was 58% to 66% per year. And in patients who received therapeutic shoes and insoles, the incidence of foot ulcerations was as high as 30% a year and as low as 4%.

Therapeutic shoes and insoles are obviously important, but for many high-risk patients they are not enough. To improve clinical outcomes, we need to expand our approach to prevention. Other opportunities may involve enhancing patient education, cooperation, compliance, and self-assessment.

EDUCATION AND SELF-CARE PRACTICES

There is little disagreement that education is important for patients with chronic diseases. This may be especially important in the prevention of foot ulcerations and amputations because self-care and compliance are the key components of limb preservation. It is difficult to evaluate education as a single intervention to prevent foot complications because part of the education process must focus on engaging other subspecialties and prevention strategies. Several studies to evaluate diabetic foot education also incorporate other standard prevention strategies such as education of primary care physicians and recommendations for consultations for high-risk patients for foot care and protective shoes (28,29).

Results of clinical studies report conflicting results. Some studies report significant clinical outcomes with education. Several studies report improved knowledge and self-care behavior, but the change in knowledge is not always linked to improved clinical outcomes. For instance, Malone et al. conducted a prospective randomized clinical study to evaluate the influence of education on lower extremity amputations. Patient were randomized into an education group ($n = 103$) and a group with no education ($n = 100$). During the follow-up period there were significantly few ulceration (education 8, no education 26, $p < 0.005$) and amputation (education 7, no education 21, $p = 0.025$) (30).

Litzelman et al. randomized 395 patients with diabetes to be assigned to either a multifaceted education and prevention program or usual care. The program included patient education with telephone and post card reminders and physician prompts to do foot examination and reinforce education. Patients in the intervention group were less likely to have foot ulcer ($p = 0.05$), more likely to report recommended self-care practices, and more likely to have their feet examined by their physician (intervention group 68%, control 28%) (28) (level A).

In contrast, Lincoln et al. found that education improved knowledge, but there was no difference in foot ulcers or amputations. Lincoln randomized 172 patients with newly healed DFUs to receive usual care or one-to-one education (level A). The incidence of foot ulcers at six months was 30% in the education group and 21% in the control group. At 12 months the incidence of ulceration was the same in both groups (41%) (31).

There are a number of reasons why knowledge may improve but clinical outcomes may not. Often high-risk patients have physical limitations that prevent them from adequately examining their feet (10). Patients have poor vision, limited joint mobility of their hips and knees, and obesity, so they cannot see the bottom or lateral side of their feet. Sometimes well-intentioned clinicians provide mirrors without considering that the patients lack the visual acuity to see with or without a mirror. In a study by Locking-Cusolito et al., 25% of study patients had impaired vision and 45% lacked flexibility to adequately examine their feet (32).

In addition, some of the visual signs we admonish patients to look for may be too subtle to be recognized. In a prospective prevention study, two control groups were given instructions on self-assessment and warning signs of ulceration such as swelling, discoloration, or temperature changes by touching their feet with the back of their hands. When patients identified an abnormality they were to contact the study nurse, so they could be seen in clinic. In 97% of the cases, by the time the patients identified areas of concern, the skin had already ulcerated. Visual changes and self-inspection may not be effective for many patients to prevent foot ulcers (33).

TEMPERATURE SELF-ASSESSMENT

Temperature assessment has been used in clinical practice to diagnose neuropathy and soft tissue injury in patients with neuropathy, and it has been used as a tool for self-assessment and monitoring. The rationale to use temperature as part of a daily foot assessment is that temperatures could provide an objective measurement of tissue injury that can be measured before the subtle signs of tissue injury and inflammation can be visualized. Swelling or color changes associated with trauma are probably too difficult for patients to assess and determine if there is an abnormality or a change over time. Temperature changes could help to locate sites on the foot that are injured and inflamed and at the same time provide a simple measurement a patient can perform by themselves.

There are three randomized clinical studies that compare standard prevention therapies consisting of therapeutic shoes and insoles, regular foot care by a podiatrist, and a standard, foot-specific education to temperature monitoring intervention (level A, Table 4). The temperature treatment group received standard care in addition to being provided a handheld infrared thermometer to record foot temperatures. The patients in all three studies measured temperatures on six sites on each foot and compared the difference to the contralateral foot. If there was a 4°F difference, the patients were to consider this as a preulcerative area. They were instructed to reduce their activity until temperatures returned

Table 4 Temperature Studies to Prevent Reulceration

Author (year)	Study population	Study duration	Study groups	Ulceration (%)	Odds ratio (confidence interval)
Lavery (2004)	Foot ulcer history	6 months n = 85	1. Standard therapy 2. Temperature monitoring	2 20	10.3 (1.2–85.3)
Lavery (2007)	Foot ulcer history	15 months n = 173	1. Standard therapy 2. Structured examination 3. Temperature monitoring	29.30 30.40 8.50	4.4 (1.5–12.8) 4.7 (1.6–13.9)
Armstrong (2007)	Foot ulcer history or neuropathy and deformity	18 months n = 225	1. Standard therapy 2. Temperature monitoring	12.20 4.70	3.0 (1.0–8.5)

to a normal range. In each of the studies, there was a significant reduction in the incidence of foot ulcerations. Patients in the standard therapy groups had a 3- to 10-fold increased risk of developing an ulceration.

FAT PAD AUGMENTATION

Injectable silicone oil has been used for 50 years. Inappropriate applications, the use of silicone that is not medical grade, as well as the controversies surrounding breast implant litigation in the United States have probably limited its acceptance and use, even though PodiSil is approved for marketing in Europe. Balkin reported the use of injectable silicon for the treatment of metatarsalgia, callus, scars, and DFU since 1964 (34,35). He reported data on 1585 patients who were treated for metatarsal and DFUs. He reported information from clinical examinations and surgical and postmortem specimens with no long-term adverse events. There were no granulomas, infection, or inflammation identified (36). Likewise, Zappi et al. examined 35 skin biopsies from soft tissue augmentation procedures and found no adverse reactions (37). A microdroplet technique has been advocated for the injection of silicone to prevent complications (38,39). Benedetto and Lewis describe a technique to inject 0.01 cc or less (39). Injections of small amounts of medical grade silicone (<1 mL per session) have been suggested to carry little risk (40).

Prospective studies have demonstrated that injectable silicone significantly increased tissue thickness on the sole of the foot and reduced peak foot pressures in high-risk diabetes compared with a placebo-injected controls after one and two years (20,41). During the two-year follow-up period, the fat pad thickness and peak pressures were unchanged (level A). There are still no prospective randomized studies that demonstrate a change in clinical outcomes such as ulceration or amputation using this approach, although preliminary results are very promising.

CONCLUSION

Prevention is overlooked and underutilized, even in very high-risk patients who have already experienced an amputation. In the United States, the Therapeutic Shoe Bill has provided shoes and insoles for high-risk persons with diabetes since 1993, and diabetes-specific education is widely available. The cost of prevention is modest and the risk of complications from therapy is negligible. Yet, prevention services are not regularly implemented by clinicians or patients. There is a tremendous opportunity to reduce the incidence of ulcers and the cost of medical care with basic prevention practices.

REFERENCES

1. Ronnemaa T, Hamalainen H, Toikka T, et al. Evaluation of the impact of podiatrist care in the primary prevention of foot problems in diabetic subjects. Diabetes Care 1997; 20:1833–1837.
2. Plank J, Haas W, Rakovac I, et al. Evaluation of the impact of chiropodist care in the secondary prevention of foot ulcerations in diabetic subjects. Diabetes Care 2003; 26:1691–1695.
3. Armstrong DG, Harkless LB. Outcomes of preventative care in a diabetic foot specialty clinic. J Foot Ankle Surg 1998; 37:460–466.

4. Pecoraro RE, Reiber GE, Burgess EM. Pathways to diabetic limb amputation. Basis for prevention. Diabetes Care 1990; 13:513–521.
5. Brand P. The diabetic foot. In: Ellenberg M, Rifkin H, eds. Diabetes Mellitus, Theory and Practice. New York, NY: Medical Examination Publishing, 1983:874–878.
6. Ashry HR, Lavery LA, Murdoch DP, et al. Effectiveness of diabetic insoles to reduce foot pressures. J Foot Ankle Surg 1997; 36:268–271; discussion 328–329.
7. Lavery LA, Peters EJ, Williams JR, et al. Reevaluating the way we classify the diabetic foot: Restructuring the diabetic foot risk classification system of the International Working Group on the Diabetic Foot. Diabetes Care 2008; 31:154–156.
8. Peters EJ, Lavery LA. Effectiveness of the diabetic foot risk classification system of the International Working Group on the Diabetic Foot. Diabetes Care 2001; 24:1442–1447.
9. Mayfield JA, Reiber GE, Nelson RG, et al. A foot risk classification system to predict diabetic amputation in Pima Indians. Diabetes Care 1996; 19:704–709.
10. Lavery LA, Armstrong DG, Vela SA, et al. Practical criteria for screening patients at high risk for diabetic foot ulceration. Arch Intern Med 1998; 158:157–162.
11. Bauman JH, Brand PW. Measurement of pressure between foot and shoe. Lancet 1963; 1:629–632.
12. Boulton AJ, Hardisty CA, Betts RP, et al. Dynamic foot pressure and other studies as diagnostic and management aids in diabetic neuropathy. Diabetes Care 1983; 6:26–33.
13. Duckworth T, Boulton AJ, Betts RP, et al. Plantar pressure measurements and the prevention of ulceration in the diabetic foot. J Bone Joint Surg Br 1985; 67:79–85.
14. Barrett JP, Mooney V. Neuropathy and diabetic pressure lesions. Orthop Clin North Am 1973; 4:43–47.
15. Armstrong DG, Lavery LA, Bushman TR. Peak foot pressures influence the healing time of diabetic foot ulcers treated with total contact casts. J Rehabil Res Dev 1998; 35:1–5.
16. Lavery LA, Lanctot DR, Constantinides G, et al. Wear and biomechanical characteristics of a novel shear-reducing insole with implications for high-risk persons with diabetes. Diabetes Technol Ther 2005; 7:638–646.
17. Boulton AJ. The diabetic foot. Med Clin North Am 1988; 72:1513–1530.
18. Boulton AJ, Franks CI, Betts RP, et al. Reduction of abnormal foot pressures in diabetic neuropathy using a new polymer insole material. Diabetes Care 1984; 7:42–46.
19. Lavery LA, Vela SA, Fleischli JG, et al. Reducing plantar pressure in the neuropathic foot. A comparison of footwear. Diabetes Care 1997; 20:1706–1710.
20. van Schie CH, Whalley A, Armstrong DG, et al. The effect of silicone injections in the diabetic foot on peak plantar pressure and plantar tissue thickness: A 2-year follow-up. Arch Phys Med Rehabil 2002; 83:919–923.
21. Veves A, Masson EA, Fernando DJ, et al. Studies of experimental hosiery in diabetic neuropathic patients with high foot pressures. Diabet Med 1990; 7:324–326.
22. Bus SA, Ulbrecht JS, Cavanagh PR. Pressure relief and load redistribution by custom-made insoles in diabetic patients with neuropathy and foot deformity. Clin Biomech (Bristol, Avon) 2004; 19:629–638.
23. Reiber GE, Smith DG, Wallace C, et al. Effect of therapeutic footwear on foot reulceration in patients with diabetes: A randomized controlled trial. JAMA 2002; 287:2552–2558.
24. Uccioli L, Faglia E, Monticone G, et al. Manufactured shoes in the prevention of diabetic foot ulcers. Diabetes Care 1995; 18:1376–1378.
25. Viswanathan V, Madhavan S, Gnanasundaram S, et al. Effectiveness of different types of footwear insoles for the diabetic neuropathic foot: A follow-up study. Diabetes Care 2004; 27:474–477.
26. Edmonds ME, Blundell MP, Morris ME, et al. Improved survival of the diabetic foot: The role of a specialized foot clinic. Q J Med 1986; 60:763–771.
27. Busch K, Chantelau E. Effectiveness of a new brand of stock 'diabetic' shoes to protect against diabetic foot ulcer relapse. A prospective cohort study. Diabet Med 2003; 20:665–669.
28. Litzelman DK, Slemenda CW, Langefeld CD, et al. Reduction of lower extremity

clinical abnormalities in patients with non-insulin-dependent diabetes mellitus. A randomized, controlled trial. Ann Intern Med 1993; 119:36–41.
29. Donohoe ME, Fletton JA, Hook A, et al. Improving foot care for people with diabetes mellitus–a randomized controlled trial of an integrated care approach. Diabet Med 2000; 17:581–587.
30. Malone JM, Snyder M, Anderson G, et al. Prevention of amputation by diabetic education. Am J Surg 1989; 158:520–523; discussion 523–524.
31. Lincoln NB, Radford KA, Game FL, et al. Education for secondary prevention of foot ulcers in people with diabetes: A randomised controlled trial. Diabetologia 2008; 51:1954–1961.
32. Locking-Cusolito H, Harwood L, Wilson B, et al. Prevalence of risk factors predisposing to foot problems in patients on hemodialysis. Nephrol Nurs J 2005; 32:373–384.
33. Lavery LA, Higgins KR, Lanctot DR, et al. Preventing diabetic foot ulcer recurrence in high-risk patients: Use of temperature monitoring as a self-assessment tool. Diabetes Care 2007; 30:14–20.
34. Balkin SW. Silicone injection for plantar keratoses. Preliminary report. J Am Podiatry Assoc 1966; 56:1–11.
35. Balkin SW. Treatment of painful scars on soles and digits with injections of fluid silicone. J Dermatol Surg Oncol 1977; 3:612–614.
36. Balkin SW. Injectable silicone and the foot: A 41-year clinical and histologic history. Dermatol Surg 2005; 31:1555–1559; discussion 1560.
37. Zappi E, Barnett JG, Zappi M, et al. The long-term host response to liquid silicone injected during soft tissue augmentation procedures: A microscopic appraisal. Dermatol Surg 2007; 33(suppl 2):S186–S192; discussion S92.
38. Naoum C, Dasiou-Plakida D, Pantelidaki K, et al. A histological and immunohistochemical study of medical-grade fluid silicone. Dermatol Surg 1998; 24:867–870.
39. Benedetto AV, Lewis AT. Injecting 1000 centistoke liquid silicone with ease and precision. Dermatol Surg 2003; 29:211–214.
40. Clark DP, Hanke CW, Swanson NA. Dermal implants: Safety of products injected for soft tissue augmentation. J Am Acad Dermatol 1989; 21:992–998.
41. van Schie CH, Whalley A, Vileikyte L, et al. Efficacy of injected liquid silicone in the diabetic foot to reduce risk factors for ulceration: A randomized double-blind placebo-controlled trial. Diabetes Care 2000; 23:634–638.

14 Impact of specialized foot clinics

Kristien Van Acker

INTRODUCTION

Since the Saint Vincent Declaration of 1989, our mission has been to reduce the amputation rate in patients with diabetes by 50% (1). To date we have partially failed in our mission. In 2005, we had a call to action and "the diabetic Foot" was clearly identified as a priority by the International Diabetes Federation (IDF) who, together with the International Working Group of the Diabetic Foot (IWGDF), published a new book: "Time to Act": Diabetes and Foot Care, Put Feet First, Prevent Amputations.

It is well known that the vast majority of amputations can be prevented with well-organized diabetic foot care, and so considerable attention was given to organizational items in this book. Working together, we developed a model of different levels of organization, a model that will form the basis of this chapter. It has been shown that, through appropriate prevention and management of the diabetic foot, it is possible to achieve a reduction in amputations and reduce the suffering of people living with diabetes (2,3). In some countries the approach to foot care is exemplary and provides a model of a Specialized Foot Clinic, frequently called multidisciplinary diabetic foot clinic. These clinics serve to inspire others who are charged with the delivery of diabetic foot care. The core components of a successful foot clinic, can be measured by improved outcome markers such as a reduction in the number of amputations, reduced healing time, better survival, and reduced reulceration rates. In addition, screening procedures, such as regular and thorough examination of the feet of diabetic patients, patient education, organization, research, and guidelines all contribute to a successful diabetic foot clinic. As the magnitude of the problem has grown so too our level of understanding the challenges that confront us. Nevertheless, there are many barriers to the implementation of appropriate care. If we can gain better insights into, and understanding of, these barriers,we will be better able to improve our regional, national, and international organization and in the end succeed in our mission . . . achieve a worldwide reduction of amputations in patients suffering from diabetes. Ralph Abermathy once said: "I don't know what the future may hold, but I know who holds the future." In the Diabetic Foot World, I am personally convinced that the future is in hands of our young enthusiastic clinicians and researchers, who will act as champions in harmony with one another and who together can convince their local and national policymakers to create the funding for improving structures and professionalism by education. Early detection and early intervention are key to improving outcomes in people with diabetic foot problems and to reduce the unacceptable amputation and mortality rates (4,5). The importance of education for patients with diabetes, their family and health care providers, and investment in such strategies cannot be underestimated (6,7).

Only when the local and national policymakers acknowledge the need for such strategies will we witness the introduction of regional strategies and national programs.

WHY SPECIALIZED MULTIDISCIPLINARY FOOT CLINICS?

Eye Opener

From 1999 to 2001, which coincided with our national prevention program in Belgium (1993–2001), we performed regional workshops for primary health care providers, as well as for nurses, pharmacists, and general practitioners (GPs) and other health care professionals. During this period, more than 4000 primary health care providers attended 100 workshops in the North part of the country. From this experience we learned that prior to the introduction of multidisciplinary foot clinics, GPs did not know who to refer the patient with a diabetic foot to. A dermatologist? A diabetologist? An orthopedic Surgeon? A podiatrist or perhaps a vascular surgeon? They simply did not know. Such referral issues constitute a major barrier to delivery of diabetic foot care with predictable variations in outcome. The following case clearly demonstrates the importance of clearly defined referral strategies. It is meant to be a "wake-up" call to all who read it.

Case Example with Different Approach and Outcome Depending on Referral

A 48-year-old male with Diabetes Mellitus since 12 years developed a plantar ulcer, without knowing when and how it started. The DM patient has a good diabetic control with a HBA1C of 6.2% and no other important complications, except a positive microalbuminuria. The treatment consisted of oral antidiabetics, low dose of aspirin, and statines. He consulted his GP who treated this wound with an antiseptic bandage and after two weeks there was no improvement. The patient was referred to a dermatologist who treated the wound with a specialized wound dressing, Aquacell®. After two weeks with no improvement, a two-week course of antibiotics was initiated (Ciproxine® 2 × 500 mg). Again there was no spectacular improvement.

We will now follow two different possible approaches:

* After 5 weeks there was no improvement so the GP referred the patient to a *vascular surgeon:*

The vascular surgeon immediately initiated an assessment of the vascular status. After the clinical examination, it had become clear that the pulses were weak and a dupplex-doppler examination was performed. At the site of the plantar ulcer a significant stenosis was explored at the Arteria Femoralis Superficialis and one at the Arteria Tibialis Anterior.

Together with the nephrologist, an arteriogram was performed during a simultaneous angioplasty involving the placement of a stent. The patient is referred back to the GP for follow-up. Although the wound was smaller, further improvement after two weeks failed to materialize.

* After 5 weeks there was no improvement so the GP referred the patient to *a diabetologist:*

This diabetologist decided to hospitalize the patient and to start a combination of antibiotics (Clindamycine combined with Quinolones). A deep tissue sample was taken and sent to the microbiologist. After three days, the antibiotics were changed to Amoxyclavic acid. At the same time, the patient was sent to the radiologist and a classical radiography and MRI showed an important osteomyelitis. The orthopedic surgeon was asked for an advice and together they decided to perform a minor amputation of the first ray. The patient has to wait one week for this surgery. After 10 days the patient was discharged and went home. After one week, the boarders of the wound were black and necrosis was present. The GP decided to send the patient to a vascular surgeon who elected to treat this patient with an angioplasty and stenting at the same levels discussed earlier. The patient was discharged and returned to his home. It took four weeks before any noticeable improvement was present.

* After 5 weeks there was no improvement so the GP referred the patient to *a multidisciplinary diabetic foot clinic:*

At the specialized foot clinic, the patient was first seen by the diabetologist together with the wound care nurse and the podiatrist. They convinced the patient to stay in the hospital. That same day, the patient was seen by the vascular surgeon, who convinced the staff members and the patient to have a revascularization the next day. The team immediately recognized an osteomyelitis. The nurse had demonstrated bone contact by probing and the osteomyelitis was confirmed by standard radiography. On day 4, a minor amputation of the first ray was performed. One week before the procedure the patient was given oral antibiotics. These were stopped after 24 hours post amputation. After 10 days, the patient was sent home with the specific message not to walk on the wound. One week later the patient was seen at the outpatient foot clinic. The progression was so good that the patient received an adapted bandage shoe.

The GP was asked to see the patient every week. After one month, the patient was seen again and the nurse and podiatrist gave some preventive education and semiorthopedic shoes were prescribed. With the aid of his partner, the patient was asked to monitor his feet every day. Thereafter, regular follow-up with the podiatrist was initiated. The patient was active again two months after discharge.

Discussion: Even without any comment and discussion this case clearly demonstrates that a multidisciplinary team-based approach can bring about significant improvements in outcome, including a faster healing of the ulcer, a better mental and improved social outcome for the patient. It could be argued that this approach will deliver a reduction of the financial burden for society and, given the high "hotel" costs associated with hospitalization, also for the patient. In another chapter, Professor Snoeck discusses the important role the psychosocial impact has on the patient with diabetic foot ulcers in this book.

In addition, we will look more closely at the barriers and the different problems associated with working in a team . . . . The challenge of performing a good multidisciplinary approach is huge!

DEFINITION OF A MULTIDISCIPLINARY TEAM

Over the years there have been several attempts to define exactly what we mean when we refer to a "multidisciplinary team" without coming to a general consensus. Therefore, we completed some research on our own. You will not be surprised to learn that we found an assortment of definitions. "A *group* of people with different kinds of training and experience working together, usually on an ongoing basis. *Professionals* often use the word *'discipline'* to mean a field of study such as medicine, social work, or education" (8).

"A *group* composed of members with varied but complementary experience, qualifications, and skills that contribute to the achievement of the organization's specific *objectives*" (9).

"A *group* of health care and social care professionals who provide different services for patients in a *co-ordinated way*. Members of the team may vary and will depend on the patient's needs and the condition or disease being treated" (10).

"A multidisciplinary team is composed of members from different health care professions with specialized skills and expertise. The members *coordinate and communicate* with each other to provide quality patient care. Coordination and teamwork among clinicians results in greater efficiency and improved clinical outcomes" (11).

We ask you to pay special attention to words such as *group, professionals against disciplines, objectives, co-ordinate, and communicate*. We will discuss these words and their meaning further, because these items play an important role in the success of multidisciplinary teams.

MEMBERSHIP OF THE MULTIDISCIPLINARY FOOT CLINIC TEAMS

The multidisciplinary approach of a diabetic foot clinic is determined by skills and experience necessary for making a good diagnosis, treatment, and prevention. Due to a rather complex physiopathology the diagnosis can be complex. Neuropathy, vasculopathy, and limited joint mobility are the fundamental problems. The trigger for an ulcer is most often a trauma (12). The trigger to an amputation is often an infection of the wound (13). Therefore, it is essential that team members are familiar with this process and understand the capabilities and limitations of the clinic. Not all clinics will have access to and have the necessary skills required to use the modern techniques of diagnosis of neuropathy and vasculopathy. This is especially so when considering access to a vascular lab and advanced imaging techniques such as MRI, angiography and, CT angiography. Moreover, not all service providers may be aware of just how essential new diagnostic tools are in setting up modern reference centers in the Western World. These diagnostic tools include the latest advance in microbiology, MRI and, bone biopsy such as that used for the detection of osteomyelitis. The same is true for the knowledge and skills concerning treatment of diabetic foot ulcers. Therefore, the members of the diabetic foot team will vary depending on the location of the service, the makeup of the team in terms of clinical background, level, and type of education of the health care providers, with a clear delineation of roles and responsibilities of each team member. It is evident for all of us—after reading the previous chapters—that prevention is the key to us achieving our mission. We will only reduce the amputation rates and prevent reulceration if we adopt the necessary preventive measures. However, this will only be possible if team members are given the necessary training in educational skills and, even more importantly, in "therapeutical education practice."

Before discussing the different models of teams involved in diabetic foot care, and the importance of understanding the stepwise process, we first want to review the history of "the diabetic foot" and the experience of previous attempts to introduce teams in the past.

HISTORY OF MULTIDISCIPLINARY DIABETIC FOOT CLINICS

In a recent manuscript, Dr. Henry Connor discusses the reasons why it took so many years before "the diabetic foot" was seen as an important complication and, why it took even a longer period before diabetologists recognized this complication not only in daily practice but also for research reasons (14). Marchal de Calvi first recognized the association between gangrene and diabetes in 1852 and he also suggested a causal relationship between diabetes and peripheral nerve damage in 1864 (15,16). Nonetheless, ischemia and infection were seen as the major causes of diabetic foot disease, resulting in the neglect of the role of neuropathy with the ensuing prolonged period of therapeutic stagnation. For many years, disease of the lower limb in diabetic patients was conceptualized as "diabetic gangrene." Even today, the presence of local thrombosis, with gangrene as a consequence, due to severe infection is still not recognized by some clinicians. It was the surgeon Godlee who was among the first to recognize the distinction was important because the prognosis in case of gangrene associated with neuropathy and infection was potentially much better than in those due to vascular disease (17). For many years, "diabetic gangrene" was equal to major amputation and frequently followed by hyperglycemic coma and death. All of which resulted in diabetic foot being considered to be equal to a "fatal process."

The discovery of insulin reduced the risk of surgical intervention; diabetic foot replaced hyperglycemic coma as the major cause of diabetic mortality. Together with the introduction of aseptic surgery, and later by the discovery of penicillin, the survival of diabetic patients with gangrene improved. The risk of infection and gangrene in the stump was diminished and survival improved (18,19). The teaching of diabetic foot care was considered so important that by 1928 the clinic at the Deaconess Hospital in Boston had assigned one graduate nurse and two pupil nurses to that duty (20), considered by many to be the first multidisciplinary approach to diabetic foot care.

The conclusion of Dr. Henry Connor and lessons we have learned from history remain true to this day: "So long as clinicians continued to think of diabetic foot lesions predominantly in negative terms like gangrene and amputation, it was—*and it is*—almost inevitable that they would—*will*—do so in an area of therapeutic nihilism . . . . It took us some time till the 1980s when the more neutral terms such as neuropathic ulcer, "diabetic foot disease," were used and when the minds of diabetologists and surgeons opened to the possibility of therapeutic advance . . . ." History is young in this field and we must recognize that recent advances, especially interventional revascularization with angioplasty and stents, play a more important role in a complex patient with Diabetes Mellitus combined with serious comorbidity (21).

Between 1987 and 1993 a large number of new interventional devices have been introduced. Some, like lasers, are less effective than hoped for while others have been approved and are in use worldwide. These devices include rotational arterectomy devices (Rotablator), intravascular ultrasound (IVUS), and stents. In the period 1994 to 1997, stents become commonplace and eliminated many complications. In 2001, almost two million angioplasties (percutaneous transluminal angioplasty [PTA] and percutaneous coronary transluminal angioplasty [PTCA]) were performed worldwide, with an estimated increase of 8% annually and in 2003 the first drug-eluting stent, the CYPHER® sirolimus-eluting stent was approved by the FDA, marking a major advance in the battle to reduce restenosis to single digits. The introduction of these new techniques and devices is accompanied by the addition of new "crew members" . . . and this will be the case in the future (22,23)! More and more we also see a distinction in foot care programs in developing countries and in developed countries; in the former more attention must still be given to neuropathy and prevention and in the latter the accent and success of treatment lies more in revascularization. We believe that the longer life expectancy of the diabetic patients together with available resources will play a role in this evolution of the so-called Western World.

It has become clear that the successful introduction of new technologies with associated parity, or superior outcomes, is matched by an increase in level of interest in the topic. Modern markers of interest such as Pub Med and Google^{TM} can demonstrate this increase in interest by the number of enquiries or "hits" they record.

For example, a search on Pub Med for articles published during 2007 on the *diabetic foot* identified 274 articles, in contrast with the 14 published during the year 1980 (24) (from 2008 till June 2009:1116 articles) (25). "Googling" on the item "diabetic *foot*" gives a result of 2,280,000 items in July 2009.

HOW TO ORGANIZE A DIABETIC FOOT CLINIC?

In the 1980s, the growth in diabetic foot clinics, with no consistency in terms of the makeup and numbers of the team members, the situation was further complicated by the different specialists from different disciplines involved in leading the teams. Models were adapted to different local, regional, and national circumstances.

At our international meetings, newcomers frequently ask for advice on how to start a diabetic foot clinic. As a result, the IWGDF convened a roundtable meeting to discuss the principles of organizing a diabetic foot clinic. We published these data in the Time to Act in the year of the "Diabetic Foot," 2005 (26). Subsequently, this concept was incorporated into the new consensus document of 2007 (27). The idea of the working group was to make a distinction between three models: The minimal model or basic model, the intermediate model, and the centers of excellence also called tertiary referral centers. All worldwide-known diabetic foot clinics, the so-called centers of excellence, were created one step at a time, beginning with the basic model. In practice, the gradual process toward excellence is initiated by a dedicated individual, "local champion," working in a very small team. More often than not, this person drives the project for many years and he or she assumes much of the responsibility from the start.

By accepting the concept of this "3-level model," we are aware that referral patterns between these levels of care in this global organization must be clearly defined. This will only be possible if the organization in the country has a well-established center of excellence. This was not the case in the 1980s but today, looking at the network of the IWGDF, many countries are offering intermediate to tertiary referral centers. In the following part, we cite some local examples in order to clarify some principles (*see* * *further in text*). In Belgium, we had the opportunity to start in 1989 at the university of Antwerp with a first multidisciplinary foot clinic. It was the only existing foot clinic at that time. This number has grown to 22 diabetic foot clinics recognized by the government (2005). Today we have a well-defined referral pattern and a quality control system with benchmarking in a country of 10 million inhabitants and about 125 recognized diabetic clinics.

Table 1 The Minimal Model

Staff	Doctor Podiatrist and/or nurse
Aim	Prevention and basic curative care
Patients	Own population
Setting	General practitioner's office, health centre, or small regional hospital
Facilitating elements	Close collaboration with a referral center
Equipment	Scalpel handles, scalpel blades, nail nippers, nail files, 10 g monofilaments, 128 Hz tunning fork, dressings (simple gauze), bandges, antiseptic instrument-cleaning equipment

We have officially recognized education institutes for podiatry, but still no official recognition of the profession of podiatry (28).

Tables 1, 2, and 3 show who are the staff members, what is the aim of the team, which population the team cares for, the setting of the team, facilitating elements, and the necessary equipment. The steps and all these items can be used as guidelines suitable for adapting to local circumstances and settings.

MINIMAL MODEL/BASIC MODEL

Because of limited resources the goal of this foot clinic is modest: the central goal is to prevent ulcers and to prevent further deterioration of small ulcers. The core business of this small team will be: foot examination of their own diabetic patients, screening for feet at risk, basic treatment of foot problems (e.g., Wagner 1 and 2), and preventive care with regular education of patients, family members, and own team members. The team (a doctor and a nurse/podiatrist) should refer the patient with complicated problems to, for example, an intermediate or center of reference. For this reason it is preferable that the team members establish good contacts with other centers, sharing ideas and exchanging information with each other.

Table 2 The Intermediate Model

Staff	Diabetologist or general physician Surgeon Podiatrist and/or nurse Orthotist
Aim	Prevention and curative care for all types of patients and more advanced assessment and diagnosis
Patients	From the regional catchment area of the hospital with possibly some referrals from outside the region
Setting	Hospital
Facilitating elements	Motivated coordinator to inspire team Exchange of experiences with other centers Staff meetings to discuss diabetic foot patients Active collaboration with other departments within the hospital Active collaboration with extra mural facilities (general practitioners, nursing homes, etc.)
Equipment	10 g monofilaments, 128 Hz tuning fork, blostheslometer, Doppler, operating theatre, full sets of podiatry instruments including tissue nippers, probes, x-ray, lab facilities for microbiology, blood testing, etc.

Table 3 The Centre of Excellence

Staff	Diabetologist Surgeon (orthopedic, and/or vascular, and/or general, and/or plastic) Podiatrists Physiotherapist Microbiologist Dermatologist Psychiatrist Nurses Educators Casting technician Orthotist Administrative, reception, and secretarial staff
Aim	Prevention and specialized curative care for complex cases To teach other centers To develop innovative care strategies
Patients	National, regional, or even international referral center
Setting	Usually a large teaching or university hospital
Facilitating elements	Organize regional, national, or international meetings Allow providers to visit to improve knowledge and practical skills Active collaboration with other reference centers Active participation in the development of guidelines
Equipment	As for intermediate centre plus: Transcutaneous oxymetry, angiography, angioplasty, arterial bypass, fully equipped operating theatre, duplex scan, intensive care unit, beds, CT scans, ultrasound, laser Doppler, pedobarogram, patient and operator's chairs, computerized records, fully equipped teaching facilities, fully equipped orthotics service, grinder, etc., telephones, computerized record systems

INTERMEDIATE MODEL

In this model, we agreed that the team must have more professions involved: the coordinator will attract motivated experts in the field: A diabetologist (or internal medicine doctor with a special interest in diabetology), a surgeon (depending on the interest and availability: general, vascular, orthopedic or even a plastic surgeon), a nurse and/or podiatrist, and orthotist or shoemaker. In addition to the basic services provided by the basic model, the intermediate level center will be expected to treat all types of ulcer and infection. Exchange of experiences with other diabetic foot centers is important. Regular staff meeting to discuss patient cases together with improvements in the organization of the center is also leading to improvements in quality which, in turn, results in improved team building. All of which leads to success. The same is true for the discussion of patient cases during ward rounds. Furthermore, improvement in the communication within the team and with the patient ensures that the whole team is sharing the decision-making process associated with the selection of the appropriate therapy for each patient. At this level the relationship with hospital administrators, staff members from other departments within the hospital (e.g., microbiology, radiology, pharmacy) should be carefully fostered by the coordinator. Not only intramuros relationships but also the extramuros links (e.g., GPs, nursing homes, and rehabilitation facilities) are important. The "intermediate" team should also provide support to community health care practitioners, who are working with people with diabetic foot problems, especially with the local podiatrists and the home nurses.

* The criteria used in the recognition by government of diabetic foot centers in Belgium are based on this model. The team must consist of a diabetologist, a surgeon, a nurse with knowledge of diabetes and preferably with a knowledge of wound care, a podiatrist, and an orthotist/shoemaker. They have to work together for the minimum of a half-day (4 hours a week) in an adapted location in the hospital, where there is a recognized diabetes center. There must be an availability of 24 hours of diabetic foot care. Before recognition they must show some experience in the field: having 52 new cases of diabetic foot ulcers with a minimum degree of Wagner 2. This is foreseen in the criteria to encourage that the recognized teams form networks for referral with other centers. The willingness to fulfill a register for quality control and benchmarking is asked from the government.

CENTRE OF EXCELLENCE/TERTIARY REFERRAL CENTRE

These teams should provide optimal diagnosis and treatment and integrate knew knowledge and skills into their daily practice. They must serve as center of excellence in two directions: treating patients with difficult diabetic foot ulcers (e.g., cases with difficult revascularization problems or with neuro-osteoarthropathy/Charcot), referred to them and also they should play a major role by providing a working example for other health care professionals and help generate improved diabetic foot services throughout their country and perhaps even throughout the world. The team is drawn from multiple, highly specialized disciplines, including diabetology, vascular and orthopedic surgery, physiotherapy, microbiology, radiology, dermatology, psychiatry, nursing, diabetes educators, podiatry, casting specialists, orthotist/shoemaker, administration .... The challenge of the coordinator is great: inspire colleagues to further levels of excellence, creating a good team atmosphere, and develop further good relations with the hospital administration to optimize the resources.

The overall goal is to minimize amputation rates and for this there is a responsibility to set up an organization that can prevent ulcers and amputations not only in a local setting. This team will play a major role in regional, pan-regional, national, and even in international diabetic foot care and related programs.

Moving from a local to a more international level will require staff at this center to be experts in teaching and being excellent in the following items: organizing local meetings and creating prevention and treatment programs in collaboration with other specialized centers, attending and presenting at international meetings, receiving visitors from other centers and from other countries, offering training opportunities, create good cooperation with national diabetes patient organization and forming partnerships with corporate interests to ensure a firm base for funding services, designing and testing innovative care strategies, and conducting clinical trials.

* In Belgium a few of the recognized centers, most of the time academic centers, are in this position. Together with key opinion leaders, team leaders

---

*In the Belgian model today we accept that all recognized diabetic centers have to take these tasks.

form a discussion group with the reimbursement system, the government, and the patient association, the latter having a special foot community. They will be responsible for the two yearly quality reports and the yearly formation of the teams of all the diabetic foot centers in Belgium.

Enthusiasm and belief in the importance of diabetic foot care are key elements of all successful foot teams.

As Karel Bakker, the president of the IWGDF mentioned: "The challenge of building, sustaining, and organizing a center of excellence for the diabetic foot is huge, but the rewards in terms of reduction of amputations and improved quality of life for people with diabetes and job satisfaction for the team are very high. Newcomers will receive a warm welcome from established centers of the IWGDF, who will be keen to offer advice and encouragement" (26).

THE ROLE OF THE COORDINATOR

From the models presented, it has become clear that the role of the coordinator will depend on the level of the organization. As stated the team leader is the person that drives the project and assumes much of the responsibilities from the start. Typically, the project leader is able to motivate health care professionals and inspire people with diabetes; set up facilities and organizational structures; establish attainable goals; recruit, train, and retrain team members; establish contacts with administrative, governmental, and health care bodies to ensure support for, and the survival of, the foot clinic, and raise the funding required for salaries, materials, training, and equipment.

In one word: keep order in the chaos!

SKILLS NECESSARY TO WORK IN A MULTIDISCIPLINARY TEAM

In the definition of multidisciplinary teams we draw special attention to words as *group, professionals against disciplines, objectives, coordinate, and communicate.* We will discuss these items further in depth because they play a major role in the success of these teams. We will start with an approach of the so-called business world and we use the "*businessdictionary.com.*"

Group: Collection of individuals who have regular contact and frequent interaction, mutual influence, common feeling of camaraderie, and who work together to achieve a common set of goals and objectives.

Objective: Mission, purpose, or standard that can be reasonably achieved within the expected timeframe and with the available resources. In general, an objective is broader in scope than a goal and may comprise of several different goals. Objectives are the most basic planning tools underlying all planning and strategy activities. They serve as the basis for policy and performance appraisals, and act as the glue that binds the entire organization together. For the performance appraisal, the team leader, together with the individual team members, evaluates the members, documents the results, and provides feedback to the individual.

We can learn a lot from the expert Paul Gordon who wrote several articles and books about multidisciplinary teams. From his work we can learn a lot about the differences and nuances: *professionals against disciplines* (29).

The very nature of multidisciplinary teams (MTs) means: bring in together different expertise, different value systems, and different organizational hierarchies. The team leader has the task of maximizing the strengths of the individuals so as the make the team stronger than the individuals. To understand the necessary skills for this MTs, it is necessary to question the different *disciplines*. The generic versus specialist debate has been going on for years and will continue for years to come. Paul Gordon wrote: "In our evolution as human being we have learnt that specialization enables us to know more about things. This greater depth of knowledge gives us greater control over that part of our world. At the same time, other people have specialist knowledge about other things. If we come together we will have greater breadth of knowledge." If a person with psychosocial skills work together with some one who has the medical technical skills they can treat the patient better. Also in health care we have arranged this knowledge into distinct disciplines. "However, it is not simply knowledge which is divided by the boundaries of profession and disciplines. Status, reward, and power are also divided. So, doctors get paid better than nurses and in some environments, have more status and power. Gender too plays a crucial role in the way professions operate internally and the way they interact with each other. This lead to define the mission statements of the professional bodies (e.g., podiatry, chiropody, and nursing); the professional bodies act as gatekeepers to the *professions*, thus controlling the right to practice and protect the public from charlatans. Working in MT can change our feeling of boundaries around our role and responsibilities. Because professions have an element of exclusivity about them, this exclusivity is unhelpful in the provision of high quality of care provided in MT. For this reason it is preferable to speak in terms of *multidisciplinary teams instead of multiprofessional teams*, where members of staff, like auxiliaries, receptionists, porters and all the others have also a central role. Most of the time they even have the highest level of contact with the patients."

The importance of the patient and their families to the success of the diabetic foot team must not be overlooked (30). A fact that might be neglected in a multiprofessional team, but less likely in a multidisciplinary team. In our modern health care systems where the impact of new technology is huge, biotechnology offers amazing prospects, telemedicine can bring world expertise together, and Internet access is open for many of our patients. This all leads to expansion of the expectations of the patient, fuelled by the introduction of initiatives like the Patient's Charter in the United Kingdom by the National Health Service, which have reinforced the message about individual choices. However, the introduction of new technologies and the development of international consensus and guidelines that define strategies for diagnosis and appropriate treatment have not been matched by the inflexibility of budgetary management and the ensuing willingness to commit sufficient resources to health care. Restrictions on these resources are the daily reality of not only the national health care system but also for the local hospital managers. All of which the diabetic team must face on a daily basis.

In considering these different terminologies we are agreed that the most important skills to develop are:

- To be keep an open mind when considering the role of other specialists
- To accept their knowledge
- Not to forget the central position of the patient and their relatives

- *Communication* between the team members and the patients and their relatives will be of great importance as well with the team leader accepting the responsibility for the *coordination* of communication. "Business dictionaries" reveal some interesting definitions (31).

Communication: Two-way process of reaching mutual understanding, in which participants not only exchange (encode–decode) information but also create and share meaning. *Coordination:* Synchronization and integration of activities, responsibilities, and command and control structures to ensure that the resources are used most efficiently in pursuit of the specified objectives. Along with organizing, monitoring, and controlling, coordinating is one of the key functions of management.

In 2007, Rebecca L. Jessup from Australia was one of the first to adopt the concept of interdisciplinary teams and their skills and behavior (32).

"We are continuously challenged to find better, evidence-based ways of doing things that will not only improve patient care (our number one priority), but will reduce costs and increase staff satisfaction and retention rates. The move away from *multidisciplinary teams* toward *interdisciplinary teams* is a change that may help us to meet these challenges. Therefore it is essential that we have a common understanding of the differences between the terms, and thus the operational differences between the teams."

Multidisciplinary team: utilize the skills and experience of individuals from different disciplines, with each discipline approaching the patient from their own perspective. Most often, this approach involves separate individual consultations. These may occur in a "one-stop-shop" fashion with all consultations occurring as part of a single appointment on a single day. It is common for this teams to meet regularly, in the absence of the patient, to "case conference" findings and discuss future directions for the patient's care. MTs provide more knowledge and experience than disciplines operating in isolation.

Interdisciplinary team: integrate separate discipline approaches into a single consultation. That is, the patient-history taking team, together with the patient, conducts assessment, diagnosis, intervention, and short- and long-term management goals at one time. The patient is intimately involved in any discussions regarding their condition or prognosis and the plans about their care. A common understanding and holistic view of all aspects of the patient's care ensues, with the patient empowered to form part of the decision-making process, including the setting of long- and short-term goals. Individuals from different disciplines, as well as the patient themselves, are encouraged to question each other and explore alternate avenues, stepping out of discipline silos to work toward the best outcome for the patient.

In his book "Managing multidisciplinary teams in the NHS," Paul Gorman, in 1989, described a widely accepted model of multidisciplinary working (29).

We will try to put a synthesis of some golden rules together and only hope that it will help us in the future to take this more into account in our daily work. Perhaps we have to introduce team building interventions on a regularly basis as for example, the so-called Interprofessional collaboration (IPC)—practice-based interventions (*see further* *).

In the literature of the diabetic foot no articles in this field were found. As "believers" many of us started with MTs and many of us discussed in our international " support" contacts our daily team problems we have to deal with. Unlike colleagues from industry, most of us have never had training in skills such as team building. Many experts recognized the numerous barriers to the implementation of good care, and by a combination of good luck and knowledge they were able to solve many of the problems they faced. However, many of the problems were not solved. All of which suggests that we might learn some golden rules taken from management course and the literature (33–37).

Practical "Golden Rules" for Team Building

- Activity or project management has four characteristics: (*i*) definite duration, (*ii*) logic relationship with other activities in the project, (*iii*) resource consumption (information, energy, know how, time financial resources), and (*iv*) associated cost.
- Define roles and boundaries: Everyone needs clarity on their own role and to be clear about what other team members do.
- Be aware of power dynamics: Are certain members competing for control? Do some have more status than others?
- Taking decisions: How, who, and when is important. Team members must learn to value each other's contributions, look at how the group communicates.
- Be aware " different professionals have different views."
- Do not underestimate the value of listening to service users (patients).
- Team building within your organization is a dynamic process. New and exciting concepts continually develop to increase your success in corporate team building and business team building.
- The challenge is to stay current and aware of your team's strengths and weaknesses.
- The number one success factor within a team is a strong leader who is cognizant of member needs and abilities. For that reason: Improve the leader's ability to foster teamwork. Skilled team leaders are able to build teams with a common purpose and a sense of camaraderie, so together they work as one.
- Train team members to find team-building solutions.
- Avoid barriers to success with team-building workshops.

Most Frequent Barriers to Team Success

- Often small details are the biggest barriers to team success, so pay attention to possible or current problems within your team. Some of the biggest barriers include unclear goals, unhealthy communication, playing it "safe," individual goals, and poor leadership.

In a modern world where evidence-based medicine plays a crucial role we need to ask ourselves if these theories are proven in a scientific way and ask, for example: Is there evidence to support the premise that teams are one of the most effective organizational forms for bringing together the wisdom and skills of the various disciplines with a better medical outcome?

EVIDENCE OF BETTER OUTCOME RELATED TO MULTIDISCIPLINARY CARE?

In General

In their review article "Interprofessional Collaboration: Effects of Practice-Based Interventions on Professional Practice and Health Care Outcomes," Zwarenstein et al. suggested that: "The extent to which different health care professionals work well together can affect the quality of the health care that they provide. If there are problems in how health care professionals communicate and interact with each other, then problems in patient care can occur. Interprofessional collaboration (IPC) can lead to positive changes in health care" (38).

IPC–practice-based interventions are strategies put into place in health care settings so as to improve work interactions and processes between two or more types of health care professionals. The following are examples: interprofessional rounds, interprofessional meetings, and externally facilitated interprofessional audit.

In his review, he found five randomized controlled trial (RCT) studies that evaluated the effects of practice-based IPC interventions. Three of these studies found that these interventions led to improvements in patient care, such as drug use, length of hospital stay, and total hospital charges. One study showed no impact, and one study showed mixed outcomes.

The authors concluded that more rigorous, cluster randomized studies with an explicit focus on IPC and its measurement, are needed to provide better evidence of the impact of practice-based IPC interventions on professional practice and health care outcomes. These studies should include qualitative methods to provide insight into how the interventions affect collaboration and how improved collaboration contributes to changes in outcome.

IN THE CASE OF GENERAL DIABETES CARE

Research has shown that for patient with Type 2 diabetes, a multidisciplinary approach can actually lead to the improvement of glycemic control and improved quality of life (39). A 2004 National Institute for Clinical Excellence (NICE) guideline for Type 1 diabetes in adults (2004) says that a range of professional skills are needed for the best service delivery model (40). An MT is specifically recommended and it is suggested that the team have professionals in education, nutrition, and medical and mental health care.

IN THE CASE OF DIABETIC FOOT CARE

On the fifth International Symposium on the Diabetic Foot in The Netherlands, Prof. Peter R. Cavanagh from Cleveland, USA was receiving the prestigious Diabetic Foot Award and was presenting his view on the future for the diabetic foot world in this lecture. He explained how, after contacting many experts, he divided their predictions into three areas: innovators, policy makers, and implementers (24). Special attention was given to implementation: "several experts suggested that better organization and health care delivery would improve diabetic foot care". He himself reported in 2008 that diabetes-related lower extremity amputations in the North England reduced over a 5-year period of time during which improvements in the organization of diabetes care were implemented (41).

Today we all believe that a multidisciplinary approach is mandatory in order to have a better outcome for the diabetic foot with a reduction of amputation. But what is the evidence of this believe?

As earlier mentioned, perhaps the first multidisciplinary diabetic foot clinic is as old as the one in the Joslin Clinic. By 1928, the clinic at the Deaconess Hospital in Boston had assigned one graduate nurse and two pupil nurses to the duty of diabetic foot care (42). In the same hospital, the mortality for major amputations fell from 11.6% in the years 1923 to 1943 to 6.6% in 1944 to 1949 (43). Was this related to this team and educational skills of this new team? By reading the literature of Joslin the introduction of penicillin played the major role. So new therapies and new team approach were going hand in hand . . . . Looking for evidence of a better outcome related only to the team approach will be difficult. These days it is hard to find good randomized control studies concerning noninvasive revascularization techniques. Together with changes in team approach the evolution of new techniques is extremely fast . . . .

In more recent literature, it has become clear that the first article of importance to the item of multidisciplinary is the one of Mike Edmonds who started in 1981 with a MT, published in 1986 (44).

"A specialized foot clinic has brought together the skills of chiropodist, shoe-fitter, nurse, physician and surgeon to manage the distinctive lesions of the neuropathic and ischemic diabetic foot. Over three years it has achieved a high rate of ulcer healing and reduced the number of major amputations. Essential aspects of management are specially constructed shoes, intensive chiropody and precise antibiotic treatment. Healing was achieved in 204 out of 238 (86 per cent) neuropathic ulcers and 107 out of 148 (72 per cent) ischemic ulcers. Relapse rate in special shoes was 26 per cent compared with 83 per cent who preferred to wear their own shoes. In the two years before the establishment of the clinic, there were 11 and 12 major amputations yearly. This rate has been reduced to seven, seven and five amputations yearly."

From a review of the literature on the term "multidisciplinary" we learn that many authors are mixing up different parts of the "process of care" and also the aim of care existing in primary prevention, curative care, and secondary prevention. The multidisciplinary approach starts from when the patient involvement is fully integrated into this specific area of care in the national health care system. In Figure 1 we want to stress the different parts of the "process of care of the diabetic foot" to clarify the principle key players in the process and their influence of outcome. Healing time of ulcers, reduction of number of minor or major amputations, reduction of costs and reduction of new ulcers are frequently used as outcome parameters to measure the impact of a process of care as for example the MTs as intervention. It will be clear that all parts will play a role in outcome and that especially delay of referral is one of the most important interfering parameter in the process influencing these outcome results. We will also discuss further how important it is to use the correct outcome parameters.

PATIENT AS KEY PLAYER

At this level prevention of foot ulcers and amputation the patient is central to the success of the strategy. Together with the Primary Health Care System, the education of the patient and his relatives plays a major role in prevention, a fact

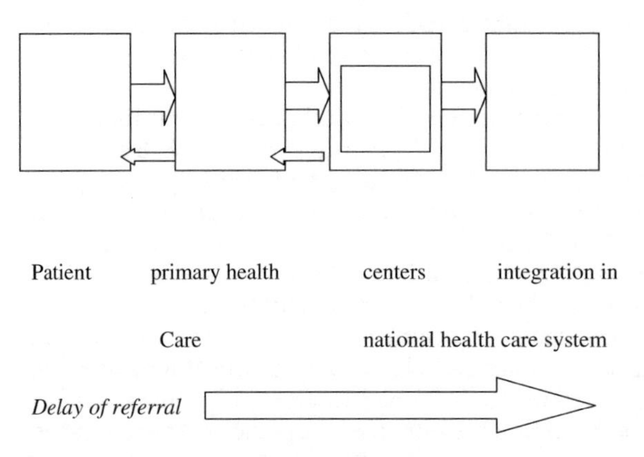

Figure 1 Process of care of the diabetic foot.

clearly defined in the literature. The self-responsibility is crucial and central in a model of chronic disease management (45).

In 1985, sixty-five patients with diabetes were studied in order to describe the contributions of the patient, the physician, and the health care system to the performance of a preventive foot examination. The data suggest that all play an important role in the success of a foot-screening program and the most significant determinants of physician foot examination were patient recall of foot-related education received at the clinic and also the inter-physician variability (46).

Singh, Armstrong, and Lipsky published in 2005 an extent clinical review while retrieving literature for pertinent information, paying particular attention to prospective cohort studies and randomized clinical trials on "Preventing Foot Ulcers in Patients with Diabetes" (1980–2004 review period). They concluded: Screening all patients with diabetes to identify those at risk for foot ulceration is supported by substantial evidence. Following prophylactic intervention might be useful: patient education, prescription footwear, intensive podiatric care, and evaluation for surgical intervention (25).

Because no major differences have been found in risk factors for diabetic foot ulceration throughout Europe, widespread adoption of educational and preventive strategies may be equally successful in different European countries and should result in a reduction of ulceration (47).

Education seems to improve people's foot care knowledge and behavior, but the research is not strong. Valk et al. concluded in their study, where only nine prospective randomized controlled trails (Rat's) were included: RCTs evaluating education for people with diabetes, aimed at preventing diabetic foot ulceration, are mostly of poor methodological quality. Weak evidence suggests that patient education may reduce foot ulceration and amputations, especially in high-risk patients. Foot care knowledge and behavior of patients seem positively influenced by patient education in the short term (48).

GPS AND HOME NURSES, *PRIMARY HEALTH CARE*, AS KEY PLAYER

Primary Care clinicians should inquire about factors known to be associated with foot ulcers, namely, previous foot ulceration (49), prior lower extremity amputation (49), long duration of having diabetes (50), poor glycemic control (HBA1c > 9%) (50), and impaired vision (49). Clinicians should also examine the feet for structural abnormalities, reduced joint mobility, dry or fissured skin, tinea, or mycosis (51,52), and also inspect footwear to ensure proper fit. In an Italian study conducted in 2005, Type 2 diabetic patients were asked if they had been offered adequate foot care by their health care system. Overall, 125 diabetic outpatient clinics and 103 GPs recruited 3564 patients. GPs tended to perform foot examination less frequent than diabetologists. Foot self-examination was not performed by 33% of the patients. Even in the presence of major risk factors, Type 2 diabetic patients were not offered adequate foot care and it was observed that patient knowledge and practices were strongly related to physicians' attitude (53).

From the South Central District Health of Washington we can learn about how the implementation of a rural model led to an increase of annual foot examinations. Being the region known for the lowest percentage of foot examinations in the State, they developed a comprehensive program with limited resources and increased this examination by 13.8%, above the state average. Key program components include: development of a curriculum on CD-ROM called 2 Minute Diabetes Foot Examination, training area physicians and nurses in the curriculum, incorporating the curriculum into the nursing program at the local college, offering free foot-screening clinics to targeted populations, and conducting public education and outreach (54).

For that reason we will discuss further the importance of integration of responsibilities of the key players in a national program.

In our opinion such implementation programs can be best installed by recognized and specialized centers.

SPECIALIZED CENTRES AS KEY PLAYER

Only a few studies have assessed the role of a foot specialist as the main intervention in *preventing* diabetic foot ulcers (55–57) and other studies have used multidisciplinary (e.g., podiatrists, internists, surgeons, nurses, dieticians, social workers) care teams. In one of the studies, patients were randomized during a period of three years in a group receiving twice a year podiatric care and the other group received no podiatric treatment. There was surprisingly no difference in the incidence of foot ulcers, but the podiatric care group had fewer deep ulcers, infected ulcers, and hospital admission days (57).

In one of the multidisciplinary care team studies, after three years, the incidence of lower extremity amputation was only 1.1 per 1000 persons per year. In this study, special attention was paid to the high-risk persons and those who missed more than 50% of their appointments with the team: This subgroup were 54 times more likely to develop an ulcer and 20 times more likely to require an amputation than those who kept most appointments (58,59). In my personal opinion, we must conduct research into our organization so as to gain a better understanding of the main factors that influence patients keeping their appointments at the diabetic foot clinic (e.g., transport, costs, availability of our services).

Over the last 20 years many studies were designed so as to illustrate the superior "outcome" of a multidisciplinary approach. The most frequent used design of the first studies reported was a retrospective study one. Most of the time reduction of amputation was used as the important outcome parameter. Karel

Bakker and his team published his data from the Heemstede hospital. It was a retrospective study in which 4323 diabetic checkups were completed during the period from 1987 to 1991. Hospital admission for diabetic foot problems decreased from 48 to 29 days with 30 admissions being prevented. The number of amputations decreased by 43%. The reduction in costs was significant (60).

The group of Gerry Ryman illustrated a significant reduction in total and *major amputation* rates in a defined U.K. population measured over an 11-year period (1995–2005) following improvements in foot care services including multidisciplinary teamwork. Expressed as incidence per 10,000 people with diabetes total amputations fell 70%, from 53.2% to 16.0%, and major amputations fell 82%, from 36.4% to 6.7%. This was also the result of a continuous prospective audit (61).

The fourfold regional variation in incidence of major amputation reported some years later by Van Houtem and Canavan both in the Netherlands and in the United Kingdom (62,63) suggests that patients are not always as informed and influential as they should be.

The needs and wishes of the patient and their relatives in influencing management choices are critical, and informed decisions by the patient should be an essential part of the process. This is one of the cornerstones of modern management in "chronic disease management," as mentioned by the World Health Organization.

In his review in the Lancet of 2003, William Jeffcoate discussed in detail all the items related to outcome parameters (64). Some specialists have reported a reduction in major amputations rates (65–69). In some cases, however, the initial rate was rather high (66,67). Other studies record no change in incidence of amputation (70–72), or even an increase (73,74). However, Jeffcoate stated that the amputation rate may not be a good marker of the quality of clinical care and better endpoints are required. Moreover, amputation is a marker not just of disease but also of disease management. The decision to operate in a health care system is determined by many factors, which vary between centers and patients and local culture and habits. "A high amputation rate might result from high disease prevalence, late presentation, and inadequate resources, but could also reflect a particular approach by local surgeons. In many cases, major amputation is not a mutilating admission of failure but the most appropriate way of ensuring an early return to a relatively independent existence. Conversely, a low rate of amputation might reflect better care, but might also conceal the effects of an inappropriately conservative approach—namely, protracted incapacity, suffering, and death with ulcers unhealed."

"Effectiveness can be judged in terms of outcomes relating to the ulcer, the limb, and the patient, and all three should be considered together." The most appropriate end point is complete healing without amputation, but this is often not achieved (75,76). However, despite good management, healing rates in large multicenter trials were 24% at 12 weeks and 31% at 20 weeks (77).

Survival, functional outcomes, and quality of life should be assessed. For this reason we selected some studies looking at other outcomes and with a prospective design.

Andrew Boulton and others stressed our attention to the *recurrence of diabetic foot ulcers*, which is another important quality marker for the multidisciplinary approach. This prospective study has demonstrated the effectiveness of a multidisciplinary approach to diabetic foot care together with the provision of specialty footwear in the long-term management of high-risk patients with a history of neuropathic foot ulcers in Lithuania. A total of 145 patients were included in this two-year prospective study and significantly fewer recurrent ulcers were seen in the intervention group (multidisciplinary follow-up with regular podiatry and reeducation every three months and provision of specialty footwear) than in the standard treatment group (30.4% vs. 58.4%, $P < 0.001$) (78).

A holistic approach of a patient with diabetic foot ulcer is also an important quality marker of this kind of multidisciplinary approach. Theoretically it will ameliorate the survival of these patients. Matthew Young and coworkers published data on improved survival of diabetic foot ulcer patients from 1995 to 2008. The purpose of this study was to demonstrate whether a strategy of aggressive cardiovascular risk management reduced the mortality associated with diabetic foot ulceration. The research design is a typical example of the role of audit cycles. Overall five-year mortality was reduced from 48% before this intervention to 26.8% in the group who received this aggressive cardiovascular risk management. Interestingly, the reduction was seen in both neuroischemic patients (relative reduction of 38%) and neuropathic patients (relative reduction of 47%, both $P < 0.001$) (79). Concerning survival we can find that the United States has a better survival rate than Europe, which could reflect faster access to specialized care, or a greater readiness to do amputations in young and otherwise fit people.

Mortality seems also to be influenced by the state of depression of these patients. Mike Edmonds and his coworkers evaluated a cohort of 253 patients with their first foot ulcer over a period of 18 months and studied whether depression was associated with mortality. They found that one-third of them suffered from clinical (minor and major) depression and this was associated with an approximately threefold hazard risk for mortality compared with no depression [3.23 (95% CI, 1.39–7.51)] (80).

Using the psychological adjustment to illness scale and hospital anxiety and depression scale, Carrington et al. showed worse adjustment to illness and significantly more depression in patients with active ulcers than in diabetic controls (77). In addition to these generic measures, one disease-specific scale has recently been developed and validated and its use considered for future clinical studies (81).

DELAY IN REFERRAL

Elsewhere in this chapter we explained the important central role specialized centers play in a well-defined referral pattern and which are crucial in the success of this approach. There is some research in this field. William Jeffcoate et al. undertook a prospective study of the presentation of all 669 ulcers seen in their multidisciplinary foot clinic in Nottingham from 1993 till 1996, with particular reference to any delay in referral. 61.3% of all lesions was first detected by the patient or a relative. The median time, which elapsed between ulcer onset and first professional review, was 4(0–247) days, and the median time between this review and first referral to the specialist clinic was 15 days (0–608). Overall, professional factors contributed to the development or deterioration of 106 lesions, or 15.8% of the total. Deterioration in a wound is more likely if assessment is delayed. The patient might be unaware of the ulcer or might avoid seeking advice for fear of being a nuisance or in the hope that the ulcer will heal on its own. However, delays are more likely to be caused by lack of speedy access to an informed opinion and by poor communication between specialist departments (82). Jan Apelqvist presented his data showing that by introducing a regional program, where podiatry was playing a central role there was a reduction of a median delay from 188 days to 25 days. The researchers believe that due to this approach they observed a reduction of 79% of the amputations rate.

A SPECIAL ROLE FOR THE PODIATRIST, A FOOT SPECIALIST—WHO IS THE TEAM COORDINATOR?

In some discussion groups the question will be put forward: Who will be the coordinator of the team? Unfortunately, there is very little in the way of literature to help us answer this question. However, there is some research that will help us in the future. For example, if we think medical doctors have the most important influence, a Dutch study published in 2004 suggests that this is not necessarily so. The researchers studied adherence to recently developed diabetes guidelines at Dutch hospital outpatient clinics in order to distinguish determinants for variations in care in hospital, internist, and patient levels. Adherence to all process measures and most of the intermediate outcome indicators was highest in the patients seen by a diabetes specialist nurse.

In a review from 2000, Andrew Boulton stated that it is possible to increase the numbers of foot clinics with the provision of podiatry services by more than 100% (83). However, many countries still lack proper podiatry and specialist nursing provision. Where podiatry is present it is not always the case that this survey is well integrated. The association of British Clinical Diabetologists tried to examine the provision of, and variations in, podiatry and other services for diabetes foot care in the United Kingdom. They demonstrated that the strategy of a coordinated "team" approach to foot care with integration of podiatry still takes place in less than 50% of centers. They conclude that both providers and purchasers of diabetes services may not pay sufficient attention to this area (84).

In case there is a discussion that doctors will be in charge for coordination, Slovakia was publishing an interesting paper. They compared a group of patients treated by "a classical surgical management" and a group of patients treated by intensive surgical therapy, with a maximum possible use of revascularization procedures. Because the patients entered their hospital in a rather advanced stage probably caused by neglect, there was no better outcome in the patient group treated with the maximum use of surgical procedures to prevent amputation. They concluded that the patient with these foot diseases must be treated by someone who can intervene at an earlier stage of the disease in order to better treat infections and the comorbidity. They stated: "It would be most appropriate to delegate this 'frontman' task to diabetologists" (85).

INTEGRATION IN NATIONAL HEALTH CARE AND INTERNATIONAL NETWORKS

We also learned from our model the importance of reference centers. They play a major role in policy and organization in their countries. For example, a Danish publication in 2001 demonstrated that by integrating multidisciplinary centers into an accepted national expert function of wound healing will result in an optimal way to improve the clinical outcome of prophylaxis and treatment of all types of problem wounds. During the first three years of the fully functioning wound healing center a total of 23,802 patient consultations were performed in the outpatient clinic, and 1014 patients were hospitalized. They divided the organization of their center in the following well-described action plan points: aim, clinical activity, scientific and educational activity, and integration. The organization plan is based on two important issues: organization and classification of a new structure for education of staff to get acceptance as an authorized wound healer. Contacts with the national societies of each medical specialty working with wound problems have been established. Integration of such a center of excellence in the National Health Care system is of great importance and it will improve the global care, education of health care personnel, as well as research. The authors believe that their model, with minor adjustments, may be applicable for both industrialized and developing countries (86).

Personally, I believe that in the future it will be good to integrate the diabetic foot centers in a more holistic approach of wound care centers. This opinion is based on the fact that for several types of wounds we need the same relevant diagnostics and therapeutic measures.

Integration in international networks can help national development. These relations with international colleges can be very fruitful.

In 1999, the International Working Group on the Diabetic Foot (IWGDF), a consultative section of the IDF since 2000, published the first *International Consensus on the Diabetic Foot and Practical Guidelines on the Management and the Prevention of the Diabetic Foot*. This was fully updated in 2007. The updated consensus reports on footwear and offloading, wound management, and osteomyelitis are based on sound scientific evidence. In order to implement the International Consensus, IWGDF recruited local "champions" representing 92 countries around the world. These local champions have become highly regarded experts in diabetic foot complications, who with their experience, knowledge, and passion have shown that better care is possible and amputation rates can be reduced. They are also responsible for a successful implementation process of the consensus guidelines in their countries.

The IWGDF conceived "The Step-by-Step project" with a common objective to improve diabetes foot care in the developing world. The project received generous funding from the World Diabetes Foundation and academic support from the IDF and the IWGDF. The first two success stories are from Tanzania and India with financial and mental support from the Diabetic Foot Society of India, and the Muhimbili University College of Health Sciences Dar es Salaam in Tanzania (87,88). Today other projects are also underway, for example, in Egypt and The Caribbean Islands, the last one supported by Rotary clubs.

The strength of the Step-by-Step program is founded on a two-year setup: a basic and an advanced course to be attended by the same delegates. Participation on the first course was conditional on attending the second course. The attendees were each supplied with a free, full set of the appropriate equipment. Combined with the education and teaching materials and the acquired knowledge, the participants were well placed to immediately introduce improvements to the local foot care management service. The use of case report presentations generated a lively and interactive exchange of ideas and experiences that made the delegates more alert to the common pitfalls. A key learning for the delegates was the realization that it is possible to bring improvements to the management of diabetic foot by the use of rather simple and affordable care, such as education of both colleagues and patients. Another strength of the project is the interaction of both doctors and nurses or paramedics in the teams together with an international faculty. The project will be followed by a survey on the cascade of effects of improved foot care in the areas from which the participants have been chosen. The educational grants enabled the invited delegates to participate on the project free of charge.

QUALITY CONTROL

Delivery of good diabetic foot care is also dependent on the need for feedback, self-reflection if we are to witness improvements in the performance of the teams which in turn lead to improvements in the delivery and outcome of medical care. Mike Edmonds wrote: "The need is to keep comprehensive records of the patients, keep close follow up with them and conduct audits of the clinic cases for evaluation with critical analysis" (89).

To evaluate the input, or the intervention (e.g., multidisciplinary diabetic foot clinic) and the process itself we have to register the outcome parameters for our evaluation. There are many examples of such processes. One of the modern techniques used is benchmarking.

"Best practice benchmarking" or "process benchmarking," is a process used in management and particularly in strategic management, in which organizations evaluate various aspects of their processes in relation to best practice, usually within a peer group defined for the purposes of comparison. This then allows organizations to develop plans on how to make improvements or adopt best practice, usually with the aim of increasing some aspect of performance. Benchmarking may be a one-off event, but is often treated as a continuous process in which organizations continually seek to challenge their practices.

The 50% reduction of amputation was one of the benchmarks of improvement, incorporated into the St Vincent Declaration in Europe as one of the proposed targets of improved health care in diabetes.

One of the first important studies to compare differences by centre is the EURODIALE. The EURODIALE study is a prospective cohort study of 1232 consecutive individuals presenting with a new diabetic foot ulcer in 14 centers across Europe in 10 different countries. In Figure 1, you can see the parameters taken into account for input, process, and outcome parameters. The use of management strategies was determined by: referral, use of offloading, vascular imaging, and revascularization. In this study, we learned that treatment of many patients is not in line with current guidelines and there are large differences between countries and centers. Current guidelines seem to be too general and health care organizational barriers and personal beliefs result in underuse of recommended therapies. In my personal opinion offloading and revascularization can be taken as quality markers for our clinics. But closer examination of the results reveals that even in the European centers, the so-called centers of excellence, there is a underuse for these two techniques. At study entry, 77% of the patients had no or inadequate offloading. During follow-up, casting was used in 35% (0–68% variation between countries!) of the plantar fore-or midfoot ulcers. Vascular imaging was performed in 56% (14–86%) of patients with severe limb ischemia; revascularization was (only) performed in 43% (90–92).

In another audit: "Use of pressure offloading devices in diabetic foot ulcers: Do we practice what we preach?" from the group of David Armstrong. A survey was sent to all foot clinics in Columbia in 2005. Of the 895 respondents, shoe modifications (41.2%, $P < 0.03$) were the most common form of pressure mitigation, whereas total contact casts (the gold standard) were used by only 1.7% of the centers (93).

As mentioned earlier, we worked on an audit cycle system by benchmarking in our country. Some opinion leaders together with Scientific Institute of Public Health, Epidemiology in Brussels developed an "Initiative for Quality of Care Promotion and Epidemiology in Belgian Diabetic Foot Clinics", so-called IQED centers. This prospective cohort study is designed to describe, evaluate, and improve the Quality of Care in the Belgian diabetic foot clinics (DFC) by collecting data and providing benchmarking. Data of 542 patients were collected, with wounds from Wagner 2, and with acute Charcot lesions. The majority of the lesions were infected (82.8%). Half of the lesions were Wagner grade 2 (25.4%), 24.7% grade 3, 24.7% grade 4, and 0.6% were grade 5. Offloading was used in 75% of the ulcer patients. A total contact cast was only used in 2.4%. 42.8% of the patients with peripheral arterial disease underwent revascularization and 59.4% was hospitalized. From one DFC to another, the treatment differed. The proportion of offloading for plantar ulcers varied from 100% to 42%; the proportion of revascularization for ischemic ulcers from 47% to 9%. The population studied had severe foot problems. We compared them to the results of EURODIALE. As you can see in Figure 2 there were more peripheral arterial disease (PAD) + patients with vascular disease (80% vs. 49%). The possible explanation is that thanks to the referral system only the most difficult cases selected in these centers. There was a large variation in the treatments used in the different DFC. Benchmarking allowed comparisons of the results. As has been demonstrated in Figure 3, centers with a 42% of offloading result can see that they clearly have to improve their organization regarding this topic. Utilizing the outcome results of this IQED evaluation each year we identify one topic where improvement is necessary. For example, a whole day workshop during which the teams focused on how to improve offloading techniques. Next year the topic will be revascularization. Levels of improvement will be monitored by a survey every two years.

We can evaluate the quality of service provided by our local organization by adopting the "must do's" check list approach of Reiber's. With their study, based on two-day site visits at 10 veterans affairs medical centers using standardized interviews, they tried to determine which of the micro system success characteristics were associated with decreased major lower limb amputations rate. They defined six "must do's" for foot care [the sum of these items described 59% of the variance ($P = 0.006$)]: (*i*) addressing all foot care needs, (*ii*) appropriate referrals, (*iii*) ease in recruiting staff, (*iv*) confidence in staff, (*v*) available stand alone specialized diabetic foot care services, and (*vi*) providers attending diabetic foot care education in the past three years (94).

CONCLUSION

As a believer, who never falls in love with her hypothesis, I strongly believe that all of us interested in the "Diabetic Foot" together with our colleagues from the "first hour," who put the diabetic foot on the international agenda, have contributed to a marked improvement in diabetic foot care in the last 20 years. It is impossible

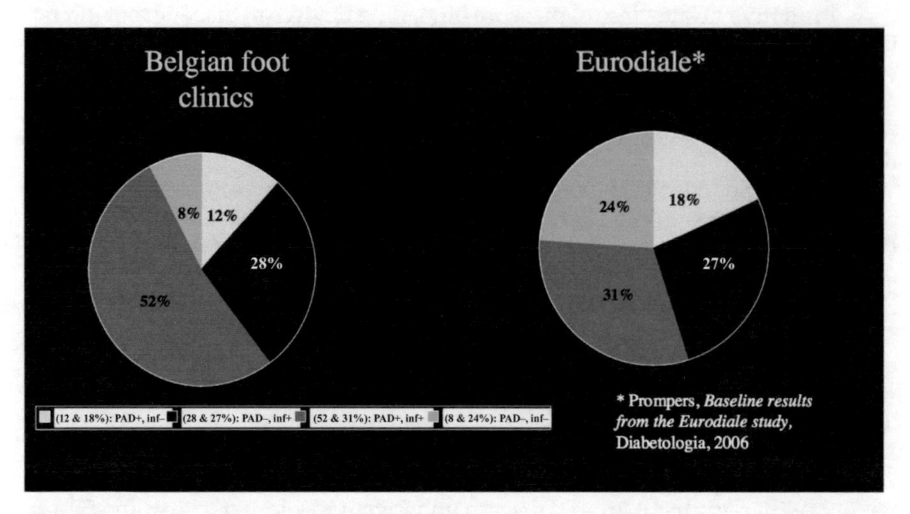

Figure 2 Baseline results from the EURODIALE study. *Abbreviations:* PAD, peripheral arterial disease; inf, infection.

to acknowledge everyone in person but two colleagues deserve special mention. Andrew Boulton and Karel Bakker are two of the most important key role players who brought together an "international multidisciplinary team."

As long as we put the patent central in our team and daily approach, we will improve. This mission is also covered by many definitions of chronic disease management: "chronic disease management in the clinical setting as an organized, proactive, multicomponent, patient-centered approach to health care

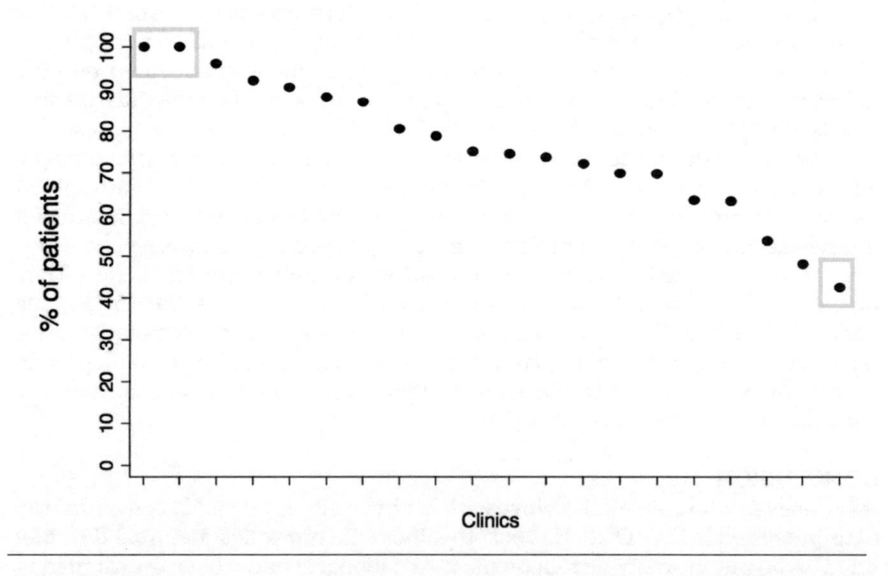

Figure 3 Chart depicting percentage of patients with ulcers treated with offloading per foot clinic in Belgium.

delivery that involves all members of a defined population who have a specific disease entity (or a subpopulation with specific risk factors)."

Looking to the future, it has become clear that we have to work together in consensus groups if we are to further improve our understanding of the evidence and in doing so improve our own knowledge levels. In the near future not only will revascularization be a topic but also the need for more scientific insights into the mechanisms of multidisciplinarity and interdisciplinarity of our teams dealing with diabetic foot care.

Implementation is a "golden word" in the success stories. We hope that the model of standard–intermediate and tertiary referral centers can help us in the near future. Today, the early experience gained from the Step-by-Step programs is producing the initial results achieved in developing countries. Looking to the future, one of the most crucial points will be the need to clearly define our personal, team, and society barriers.

> 'It (modernisation) is about looking at the workforce in a different way, as teams of people rather than as different professional tribes. For too long we have planned and trained staff in a uni-professional/uni-disciplinary way without a clear and comprehensive look at the future.'
>
> —(Hargadon & Staniforth, 2000, 1.3, Ref. 95)

REFERENCES

1. World Health Organization (Europe) and International Diabetes Federation (Europe). Diabetes care and research in Europe: The Saint Vincent declaration. Diabet Med 1990; 7:360.
2. Lavery L, Wunderlich R, Tredwell J. Disease management for the diabetic foot: Effectiveness of a diabetic foot prevention program to reduce amputations and hospitalizations. Diabetes Res Clin Pract 2005; 70(1):31–37.
3. Ragnarson TG, Apelqvist J. Health-related quality of life in patients with diabetes mellitus and foot ulcers. J Diabetes Complicat 2000; 14:235–241.
4. Mason J, O'Keeffe C, Hutchinson A, et al. A systematic review of foot ulcer in patients with type 2 diabetes mellitus, II: Treatment. Diabet Med 1999; 16:889–909.
5. Bruckner M, Mangan M, Godin S, et al. Project LEAP of New Jersey: Lower extremity amputation prevention in persons with type 2 diabetes. Am J Manag Care 1999; 5:609–616.
6. Barth R, Campbell LV, Allen S, et al. Intensive education improves knowledge, compliance, and foot problems in type 2 diabetes. Diabet Med 1991; 8:111–117.
7. McCabe CJ, Stevenson RC, Dolan AM. Evaluation of a diabetic foot screening and protection programme. Diabet Med 1998; 15:80–84.
8. Definition by: http://www.DWP.GOV.UK department for work and pensions. Accessed June 15, 2010.
9. Definition by: Oxford dictionary.
10. Definition by: http://www.bestforhealth.nhs.uk/page.asp. Accessed June 15, 2010.
11. Horak BJ, Pauig J, Keidan B, et al. Patient safety: A case study in team building and interdisciplinary collaboration. J Healthc Qual 2004; 26(2):6–12.
12. Boulton AJ, Kirsner RS, Vileikyte L. Clinical practice. Neuropathic diabetic foot ulcers. N Engl J Med 2004; 351(1):48–55.
13. Lipsky BA, Berendt AR. Principles and practice of antibiotic therapy of diabetic foot infections. Diabetes Metab Res Rev 2000; 16(suppl):42–46.
14. Connor H. Some historical aspects of diabetic foot disease. Diabetes Metab Res Rev 2008; 24(suppl 1):S7–S13.

15. Marchal de Calvi A. Des rapports de la gangrene et de la glycosurie. Gazette des Hôpitaux Civils et militaries 1852; 25:178.
16. Marchal de Calvi A. Récherches sur les Accidents diabétiques, et essai d'une théorie générale du diabète. Paris: Asselin, 1864.
17. Godlee RJ. On amputation for diabetic gangrene. Med Chir Trans 1893; 76:37–55.
18. Treves F. A System of Surgery. Vol 1. London: Cassell and Co. Ltd, 1895:268–269.
19. Keen WW, White JW. A Textbook of Surgery for Practitioners and Students. Vol 1. London: WB Saunders and Co., 1903:67.
20. Joslin EP. The treatment of Diabetes Mellitus. 2nd ed. Philadelphia: Lea and Febiger, 1917: 423–427; 4th ed. 1928: 785–802.
21. Faglia E, Mantero M, Caminiti M, et al. Extensive use of peripheral angioplasty, particular infrapopliteal, in the treatment of ischaemic diabetic foot ulcers: Clinical results of a multicentric study of 221 consecutive diabetic subjects. J Intern Med 2002; 252:225–232.
22. Jacqueminet S, Hartemann-Heurtier A, Izzillo R, et al. Percutaneous transluminal angioplasty in severe diabetic foot ischemia: Outcomes and prognostic factors. Diabetes Metab 2005; 31:370–375.
23. Brophy DP. In: Veves A, Giurini JM, Logerfo FW, eds. Angioplasty and Other Non-invasive Surgical Procedures. The Diabetic Foot: Medical and Surgical Management. Humana Press Inc, 2002:512.
24. Boulton AJM. The diabetic foot: Grand overview, epidemiology and pathogenesis. Diabetes Metab Res Rev 2008; 24(suppl 1):S3–S6.
25. Singh N, Armstrong DG, Lipsky BA. Preventing foot ulcers in patients with diabetes. JAMA 2005; 293:217–228.
26. Time to Act. Put feet first, prevent amputations: Diabetes and foot care. Joint publication of the International Diabetes Federation and the International Working Group on the Diabetic Foot, 2005.
27. International Consensus on the Diabetic Foot & Practical Guidelines and Management and Prevention of the Diabetic Foot. International Working Group on the Diabetic Foot, 2007.
28. Van Acker K, Vandeleene B, Vermassen F, et al. Prise en charge du pied diabétique dans un centre spécialisé. Albe de Coker. 2008.
29. Gorman P. Managing Multidisciplinary Teams in the NHS. Oxfordshire: Marston Lindsay Ross International Ltd, 1989.
30. Malone JM, Snyder M, Anderson G, et al. Prevention of amputation by diabetic education. Am J Surg 1989; 158:520–524.
31. Definitions by http://www.businessdictionary.com. Accessed June 15, 2010.
32. Jessup RL. Interdisciplinary versus multidisciplinary care teams: Do we understand the difference? Aust Health Rev 2007; 31(3):330–331.
33. Logan K. Diabetes—The role of the multidisciplinary team in patient self management. Standards of medical care in diabetes—2008. Diabetes Care 2008; 3(suppl):S12–S54.
34. Multidisciplinary Care. A model for achieving best practice cancer care. A Victorian Government Initiative. www.health.Vic.gov.au/cancer. Accessed June 15, 2010.
35. Fay D, Borrill C, Amir Z, et al. Getting the most out of multidisciplinary teams: A multi-sample study of team innovation in health care. J Occup Organ Psychol 2006; 79(4):553–567.
36. Gorman P. Excellent information is needed for excellent care, but so is good communication. West J Med 2000; 172:319–320.
37. Jenkins VA, Fallowfield LJ, Poole K. Are members of multidisciplinary teams in breast cancer aware of each other's informational roles? Qual Health Care 2001; 10:70–75.
38. Zwarenstein M, Goldman J, Reeves S. Interprofessional collaboration: Effects of practice-based interventions on professional practice and healthcare outcomes. Cochrane Database Syst Rev 2009; (3):CD000072.
39. McGill M, Felton A. New global recommendations: A multidisciplinary approach to improving outcomes in diabetes. Prim Care Diabetes 2007; 1(1):49–55.

40. http://www.nice.org.uk/CG015. Accessed June 15, 2010.
41. Cavanagh RJ, Unwin NC, Connolly VM, et al. Diabetes and non-diabetes related lower extremity amputation incidence before and after the introduction of better organized diabetes foot care. Diabetes Care 2008; 31(3):450–463.
42. McKittrick LS, Root HF. Diabetic Surgery. Philadelphia: Lea and Febiger, 1928:92–104. Chapter V.
43. McKittrick LS. Recent advances in the care of the surgical complications of diabetes mellitus. N Eng J Med 1946; 235:929–932.
44. Edmonds M. Improved survival of the diabetic foot: The role of a specialized foot clinic. Q J Med 1986; 232:763–771.
45. Holman H, Lorig K. Patients as partners in managing chronic disease. B Med J 2000; 320(7234):526–527.
46. Bailey TS, Yu HM, Tayfield EJ. Patterns of foot examination in a diabetes clinic. AM J Med 1985; 78(3):371–374.
47. Veves A, Uccioli L, Manes C, et al. Comparison of risk factors for foot problems in diabetic patients attending teaching hospital outpatient clinics in four different European states. Diabet Med 1994; 11(7):709–713.
48. Valk GD, Kriegsman DM, Assendelft WJ. Patient education for preventing diabetic foot ulceration. Cochrane Database Syst Rev 2001; 4:CD001488.
49. Boyko EJ, Ahroni JH, Stensel V, et al. A prospective study of risk factors for diabetic foot ulcer: The Seattle Diabetic Foot Study. Diabetes Care 1999; 22:1036–1042.
50. Lavery LA, Armstrong DG, Vela SA, et al. Practical criteria for screening patients at high risk for diabetic foot ulceration. Arch Intern Med 1998; 158:157–162.
51. Altman MI, Altman KS. The podiatric assessment of the diabetic lower extremity: Special considerations. Wounds 2000; 12(6 suppl B):64B–71B.
52. Boike AM, Hall JO. A practical guide for examining and treating the diabetic foot. Cleve Clin J Med 2002; 69:342–348.
53. De Berardis G, Pellegrini F, Franciosi M, et al. QuEd Study Group-Quality of Care and outcomes in Type 2 Diabetes. Are Type 2 diabetic patients offered adequate foot care? The role of physician and patient characteristics. J Diabetes Complications 2005; 19(6):319–327.
54. Beem SE, Machala M, Holman C, et al. Aiming at "de feet"and diabetes: A rural model to increase annual foot examinations. Am J Public health 2004; 94(10):1664–1666.
55. Plank J, Haas W, Rokovac I, et al. Evaluation of the impact of chiropodist care in the secondary prevention of foot ulcerations in diabetic subjects. Diabetes Care 2003; 26:1691–1695.
56. Ronnemaa T, Hamalainin H, Toikka T, et al. Evaluation of the impact of podiatrist care in the primary prevention of foot problems in diabetic subjects. Diabetes Care 1997; 20:1833–1837.
57. Van Putten M, Schaper NC. The preventive value of podiatry for the diabetic foot at risk for ulceration. Paper presented at: International Consensus on the Diabetic Foot; May 22–24, 2003; Noordwijkerhout, The Netherlands.
58. Armstrong DG, Lavery LA, Harkless LB. Validation of a diabetic wound classification system: The contribution of depth, infection, and ischemia to risk of amputation. Diabetes Care 1998; 21:855–859.
59. Arsmtrong DG, Harkless LB. Outcomes of preventive care in a diabetic foot specialty clinic. J Foot Ankle Surg 1998; 37:460–466.
60. Bakker K, Dooren J. A specialized outpatient foot clinic for diabetic patients decreases the number of amputations and is cost saving. Ned Tijdschr Geneeskd 1994; 138:565–569.
61. Singhan K, Fiona N, Neil Baker, et al. Reduction in diabetic amputations over 11 years in a defined U.K. population. Diabetes Care 2008; 31:99–101.
62. Van Houtum WH, Lavery LA. Regional variation in the incidence of diabetes-related amputation in The Netherlands. Diabetes Res Clin Pract 1996; 31:125–132.
63. Canavan R, Connolly V, Airey CM, et al. A population based study of lower extremity amputations among four UK centres. Diabet Med 2002; 19(suppl 2):A23.

64. Jeffcoate WJ, Harding KG. Diabetic foot ulcers. Review. Lancet 2003; 361:1545–1551.
65. Faglia E, Favales F, Morabito A. New ulceration, new major amputation, and survival rats in diabetic subjects hospitalised for foot ulceration from 1990 to 1993: A 6.5 year follow-up. Diabetes Care 2001; 24;78–83.
66. Holstein P, Ellitsgaard N, Olsen BB, et al. Decreasing incidence of major amputations in people with diabetes. Diabetologia 2000; 43:844–847.
67. Larsson J, Apelqvist J, Agardh CD, et al. Decreasing incidence of lower limb amputations in diabetic patients: A consequence of a multidisciplinary foot care team approach? Diabet Med 1995; 12:770–776.
68. Calle-Pascual AL, Garcia-Torre N, Moraga I, et al. Epidemiology of nontraumatic lower-extremity amputations in Area 7, Madrid, between 1989 and 1999. Diabetes Care 2001; 24:1686–1689.
69. Faglia E, Favales F, Aldeghi A, et al. Change in major amputation rate in a center dedicated to diabetic foot care during the 1980s: Prognostic determinants for major amputation. J Diabet Complications 1998; 12;96–102.
70. Trautner C, Haastert B, Spraul M, et al. Unchanged incidence of lower-limb amputation in a German City 1990–1998. Diabetes Care 2001; 24;855–859.
71. Mayfield JA, Reiber GE, Maynard C, et al. Trends in lower limb amputation in the Veterans Health Administration, 1989–1998. J Rehabil Res Dev 2000; 37:23–30.
72. Stiegler H, Standl E, Frank S, et al. Failure of reducing lower extremity amputations in diabetic patients: Results of two subsequent population based surveys 1990 and 1995 in Germany. Vasa 1998; 27:10–14.
73. Feinglass J, Brown JL, LoSasso A, et al. Rates of lower-extremity amputation and arterial reconstruction in the United States, 1979 to 1996. Am J Public Health 1999; 89(8):1222–1227.
74. Anon. Hospital discharge rates for nontraumatic lower extremity amputation by diabetes status—United States, 1997. MMWR Morb Mortal Wkly Rep 2001; 50:954–958.
75. Piaggesi A, Schipani E, Campi F, et al. Conservative surgical approach versus non-surgical management for diabetic neuropathic foot ulcers: A randomised trial. Diabet Med 1998; 15:412–417.
76. O'Meara S, Cullum, N, Majid M, et al. Systematic reviews of wound care management: (3) antimicrobial agents for chronic wounds; (4) diabetic foot ulceration. Health Technol Assess 2000; 4:21.
77. Margolis DJ, Kantor J, Berlin JA. Healing of diabetic neuropathic foot ulcers receiving standard treatment: A meta-analysis. Diabetes Care 1999; 22;692–695.
78. Dargis V, Pantelejeva O, Jonushaite A, et al. Benefits of a multidisciplinary approach in the management of recurrent diabetic foot ulceration in Lithuania: A prospective study. Diabetes Care 1999; 22:1428–1431.
79. Young MJ, Mc Cardle E, Randall LE, et al. Improved survival of diabetic foot ulcer patients 1995–2008. Possible impact of aggressive cardiovascular risk management. Diabetes Care 2008; 31:2143–2147.
80. Ismail K, Winkley K, Stahl D, et al. A cohort study of people with diabetes and their first foot ulcer: The role of depression on mortality. Diabetes Care 2007; 30:1473–1479.
81. Abetz L, Sutton M, Brady L, et al. The diabetic foot ulcer scale (DFS): A quality of life instrument for use in clinical trials. Pract Diabetes Int 2002; 19:167–175.
82. Macfarlane RM, Jeffcoate WJ. Factors contributing to the presentation of diabetic foot ulcers. Diabet Med 1997; 14:867–870.
83. Boulton AJ. The Diabetic foot: A global view. Diabetes Metab Res Rev 2000; 16(suppl 1):S2–S5.
84. Association of British Clinical Diabetologists (ABCD). Survey of specialist diabetes care services in the UK, 2000.3. Podiatry services and related foot care issues. Diabet Med 2002; 19(Suppl 4):32–38.
85. Petrasovic M, Carsky S, Holoman M. Care of the diabetic foot. Bratisl Lek Listy 1997; 98:572–576.
86. Gottrup F, Holstein P, Jorgensen B, et al. A new concept of a multidisciplinary wound healing center and a national expert function of wound healing. Arch Surg 2001; 136: 756–772.

87. Bakker K, Abbas ZG, Pendsey S. Step by Step, improving diabetic foot care in the developing world. A pilot study for India, Bangladesh, Sri Lanka and Tanzania. Pract Diabetes Int 2006; 23(8):1–6.
88. Pendsey S, Abbas ZG. The step-by-step program for reducing diabetic foot problems: A model for the developing world. Curr Diab Rep 2007; 7:425–428.
89. Edmonds ME. The Diabetic Foot, 2003. Diabetes Metab Res Rev 2004; 20(Suppl 1):S9–S12.
90. Prompers L, Huijberts M, Apelqvist J, et al. High prevalence of ischaemia, infection and serious comorbidity in patients with diabetic foot disease in Europe. Baseline results from the Eurodiale study. Diabetologia 2007; 50(1):18–25.
91. Prompers L, Huijberts M, Apelqvist J, et al. Optimal organization of health care in diabetic foot disease: Introduction to the Eurodiale study. Int J Low Extrem Wounds 2007; 6(1):11–17.
92. Prompers L, Huijberts M, Apelqvist J, et al. Delivery of care to diabetic patients with foot ulcers in daily practice: Results of the Eurodiale Study, a prospective cohort study. Diabet Med 2008; 25(6):700–707.
93. WU SC, Jensen JL, Weber AK, et al. Use of pressure offloading devices in diabetic foot ulcers: Do we practice what we preach?. Diabetes Care 2008; 31:2118–2119.
94. Wrobel JS, Robbins JM, Charns MP, et al. Diabetes-related foot care at 10 veteran affairs medical centers: Must do's associated with successful microsystems. Jt Comm J Qual Patient Saf 2006; 32:206–213.
95. Hargadon, J, Staniforth, M. A health Service of all the Talents: Developing the NHS Workforce. London: Department of Health, 2000.

Index